AF251553

THE BIOLOGY OF SKELETAL METASTASES

Cancer Treatment and Research
Steven T. Rosen, M.D., *Series Editor*

Klastersky, J. (ed): *Infectious Complications of Cancer.* 1995. ISBN 0-7923-3598-8.

Kurzrock, R., Talpaz, M. (eds): *Cytokines: Interleukins and Their Receptors.* 1995. ISBN 0-7923-3636-4.

Sugarbaker, P. (ed): *Peritoneal Carcinomatosis: Drugs and Diseases.* 1995. ISBN 0-7923-3726-3.

Sugarbaker, P. (ed): *Peritoneal Carcinomatosis: Principles of Management.* 1995. ISBN 0-7923-3727-1.

Dickson, R.B., Lippman, M.E. (eds.): *Mammary Tumor Cell Cycle, Differentiation and Metastasis.* 1995. ISBN 0-7923-3905-3.

Freireich, E.J, Kantarjian, H. (eds): *Molecular Genetics and Therapy of Leukemia.* 1995. ISBN 0-7923-3912-6.

Cabanillas, F., Rodriguez, M.A. (eds): *Advances in Lymphoma Research.* 1996. ISBN 0-7923-3929-0.

Miller, A.B. (ed.): *Advances in Cancer Screening.* 1996. ISBN 0-7923-4019-1.

Hait , W.N. (ed.): *Drug Resistance.* 1996. ISBN 0-7923-4022-1.

Pienta, K.J. (ed.): *Diagnosis and Treatment of Genitourinary Malignancies.* 1996. ISBN 0-7923-4164-3.

Arnold, A.J. (ed.): *Endocrine Neoplasms.* 1997. ISBN 0-7923-4354-9.

Pollock, R.E. (ed.): *Surgical Oncology.* 1997. ISBN 0-7923-9900-5.

Verweij, J., Pinedo, H.M., Suit, H.D. (eds): *Soft Tissue Sarcomas: Present Achievements and Future Prospects.* 1997. ISBN 0-7923-9913-7.

Walterhouse, D.O., Cohn, S. L. (eds.): *Diagnostic and Therapeutic Advances in Pediatric Oncology.* 1997. ISBN 0-7923-9978-1.

Mittal, B.B., Purdy, J.A., Ang, K.K. (eds): *Radiation Therapy.* 1998. ISBN 0-7923-9981-1.

Foon, K.A., Muss, H.B. (eds): *Biological and Hormonal Therapies of Cancer.* 1998. ISBN 0-7923-9997-8.

Ozols, R.F. (ed.): *Gynecologic Oncology.* 1998. ISBN 0-7923-8070-3.

Noskin, G. A. (ed.): *Management of Infectious Complications in Cancer Patients.* 1998. ISBN 0-7923-8150-5

Bennett, C. L. (ed): *Cancer Policy.* 1998. ISBN 0-7923-8203-X

Benson, A. B. (ed): *Gastrointestinal Oncology.* 1998. ISBN 0-7923-8205-6

Tallman, M.S. ,Gordon, L.I. (eds): *Diagnostic and Therapeutic Advances in Hematologic Malignancies.* 1998. ISBN 0-7923-8206-4

von Gunten, C.F. (ed): *Palliative Care and Rehabilitation of Cancer Patients.* 1999. ISBN 0-7923-8525-X

Burt, R.K., Brush, M.M. (eds): *Advances in Allogeneic Hematopoietic Stem Cell Transplantation.* 1999. ISBN 0-7923-7714-1

Angelos, P. (ed): *Ethical Issues in Cancer Patient Care* 2000. ISBN 0-7923-7726-5

Gradishar, W.J., Wood, W.C. (eds): *Advances in Breast Cancer Management.* 2000. ISBN 0-7923-7890-3

Sparano, Joseph A. (ed): *HIV & HTLV-I Associated Malignancies.* 2001. ISBN 0-7923-7220-4.

Ettinger, David S. (ed): *Thoracic Oncology.* 2001. ISBN 0-7923-7248-4.

Bergan, Raymond C. (ed): *Cancer Chemoprevention.* 2001. ISBN 0-7923-7259-X.

Raza, A., Mundle, S.D. (eds): *Myelodysplastic Syndromes & Secondary Acute Myelogenous Leukemia* 2001. ISBN 0-7923-7396.

Talamonti, Mark S. (ed): *Liver Directed Therapy for Primary and Metastatic Liver Tumors.* 2001. ISBN 0-7923-7523-8.

Stack, M.S., Fishman, D.A. (eds): *Ovarian Cancer.* 2001. ISBN 0-7923-7530-0.

Bashey, A., Ball, E.D. (eds): *Non-Myeloablative Allogeneic Transplantation.* 2002. ISBN 0-7923-7646-3

Leong, Stanley P.L. (ed): *Atlas of Selective Sentinel Lymphadenectomy for Melanoma, Breast Cancer and Colon Cancer.* 2002. ISBN 1-4020-7013-6

Andersson , B., Murray D. (eds): *Clinically Relevant Resistance in Cancer Chemotherapy.* 2002. ISBN 1-4020-7200-7.

Beam, C. (ed): *Biostatistical Applications in Cancer Research.* 2002. ISBN 1-4020-7226-0.

Brockstein, B., Masters, G. (eds): *Head and Neck Cancer.* 2003. ISBN 1-4020-7336-4.

Frank, D.A. (ed): *Signal Transduction in Cancer.* 2003. ISBN 1-4020-7340-2.

Figlin, Robert A. (ed): *Kidney Cancer.* 2003. ISBN 1-4020-7457-3.

Kirsch, Matthias; Black, Peter McL. (ed.): *Angiogenesis in Brain Tumors.* 2003. ISBN 1-4020-7704-1

Keller, E.T., Chung, L.W.K. (eds): *The Biology of Skeletal Metastases.* 2004. ISBN 1-4020-7749-1

THE BIOLOGY OF SKELETAL METASTASES

Edited by

Evan T. Keller, DVM, PhD, University of Michigan

Associate Professor of Urology, Comparative Medicine and Pathology

Co-Director, Connective Tissue Oncology Program

University of Michigan Comprehensive Cancer Center

University of Michigan School of Medicine

University of Michigan

Ann Arbor, Michigan, USA

Co-Edited by

Leland W. K. Chung, PhD,

Professor of Urology, Hematology/Oncology, Biochemistry

and the Winship Cancer Institute

Director, Molecular Urology and Therapeutics Program

Emory University School of Medicine

Emory University

Atlanta, Georgia, U.S.A.

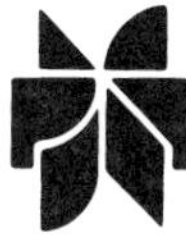

Kluwer Academic Publishers
Boston/Dordrecht/London

Distributors for North, Central and South America:
Kluwer Academic Publishers
101 Philip Drive
Assinippi Park
Norwell, Massachusetts 02061 USA
Telephone (781) 871-6600
Fax (781) 681-9045
E-Mail: kluwer@wkap.com

Distributors for all other countries:
Kluwer Academic Publishers Group
Post Office Box 322
3300 AH Dordrecht, THE NETHERLANDS
Telephone 31 786 576 000
Fax 31 786 576 254
E-Mail: services@wkap.nl

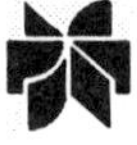 Electronic Services <http://www.wkap.nl>

Library of Congress Cataloging-in-Publication Data

A C.I.P. Catalogue record for this book is available
from the Library of Congress.

Title: The Biology of Skeletal Metastases
Editor: Evan T. Keller and Leland W.K. Chung
ISBN: 1-4020-7749-1

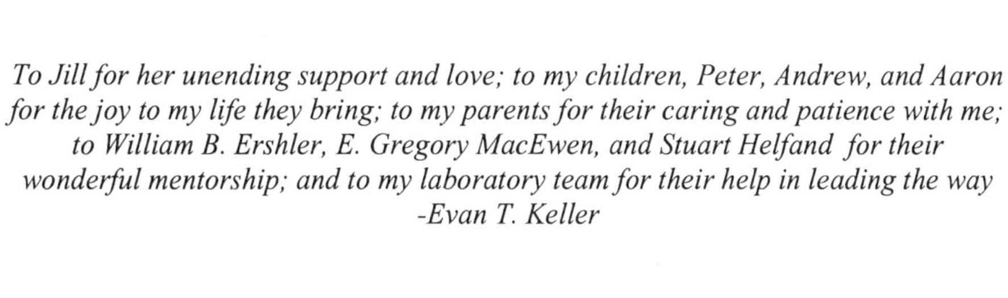

To Jill for her unending support and love; to my children, Peter, Andrew, and Aaron for the joy to my life they bring; to my parents for their caring and patience with me; to William B. Ershler, E. Gregory MacEwen, and Stuart Helfand for their wonderful mentorship; and to my laboratory team for their help in leading the way
-Evan T. Keller

To my wife Haiyen, my teacher, Don Coffey and my students who inspired, taught and supported me over the years"
-Leland W. K. Chung

Contents

Contributing Authors

Angela Alexander, Bachelors Student, Department of Biological Sciences, University of Delaware, Newark, DE 19716, U.S.A.

R. Daniel Bonfil Ph.D., Associate Professor, Departments of Urology and Pathology, Wayne State University School of Medicine and The Barbara Ann Karmanos Cancer Institute, Detroit, MI 48202, U.S.A.

Julie Brown, Ph.D. Leader, Bone Metastasis Group, Oncology Research Centre, UNSW Department of Clinical Medicine, Prince of Wales Hopsital, Randwick, NSW 2031, Australia

Michael Cher, M.D. Associate Professor, Departments of Urology and Pathology, Wayne State University School of Medicine and The Barbara Ann Karmanos Cancer Institute, Detroit, MI 48202, U.S.A.

Sun Jin Choi, Ph.D., Assistant Professor, Division of Hematology and Oncology, Department of Medicine, University of Pittsburgh, E1152 BST, 200 Lothrop St., Pittsburgh, PA 15261, U.S.A.

Leland W. K. Chung, Ph.D., Professor, Departments of Urology, Hematology/Oncology and Biochemistry and the Winship Cancer Institute; Director, Molecular Urology and Therapeutics Program, Emory University School of Medicine, Atlanta, GA 30322, U.S.A.

Carlton Cooper, Ph.D., Assistant Professor, Department of Biological Sciences, Wolf Hall, University of Delaware, Newark, DE 19716, U.S.A

Eva Corey, Ph.D., Research Associate Professor, Department of Urology, University of Washington Medical Center, Seattle, WA 98195, U.S.A.

Stephanie Corn, D.V.M., Postdoctoral Research Fellow, Department of Veterinary Biosciences, College of Veterinary Medicine, The Ohio State University, Columbus, OH 43210, U.S.A.

Mary Farach-Carson, Ph.D., Professor, Department of Biological Sciences, University of Delaware 19716, U.S.A.

Rafael Fridman, Ph.D., Professor, Department of Pathology, Wayne State University School of Medicine and The Barbara Ann Karmanos Cancer Institute, Detroit, MI 48202, U.S.A.

Theresa A. Guise, M.D., Gerald D. Aurbach Professor of Endocrinology and Professor of Medicine, Department of Internal Medicine, Division of Endocrinology and Metabolism, University of Virginia, Charlottesville, VA 22904, U.S.A.

Nobuyuki Hashimoto, M.D., Ph.D., Assistant Professor, Department of Orthopedics, Osaka University Gradauate School of Medicine. Osaka, 565-0871, Japan.

Celestia Higano, M.D., Associate Professor, Department of Medicine-Division of Oncology, University of Washington Medical Center, Seattle, WA 98195, U.S.A.

Toru Hiraga, Ph.D., D.D.S., Assistant Professor, Department of Molecular and Cellular Biochemistry, Osaka University Graduate School of Dentistry, 1-8 Yamadaoka, Suita, Osaka 565-0871, Japan

Chia-Ling Hsieh, Ph.D., Assistant Professor, Department of Urology and the Winship Cancer Institute, Emory University School of Medicine, Atlanta, GA 30322, U.S.A.

Eric Kaufman, B.A., Medical Student, Pritzker School of Medicine, The University of Chicago, Chicago, IL 60637, U.S.A.

Evan T. Keller, D.V.M., Ph.D., Associate Professor, Departments of Urology, ULAM and Pathology, School of Medicine, University of Michigan, 1150 W. Medical Center Drive, Ann Arbor, MI 48109

Jeffrey Kiefer, Ph.D., Postdoctoral Fellow, Cancer Drug Development Laboratory, Translational Genomics Research Institute, Gaithersburg, MD 20878, U.S.A.

Hiroyuki Kubo, MD. PhD, Assistant Professor, Department of Urology, Graduate School of Medical and Dental Sciences, Kagoshima University, Kagoshima 890-8520, Japan.

Sue-Hwa Lin, Ph.D. Ashbel Smith Professor, Department of Genitourinary Medical Oncology and Molecular Pathology, The University of Texas, M.D. Anderson Cancer Center, Houston, TX 77030, U.S.A.

Laurie K. McCauley, Ph.D., D.D.S., Chair and Professor, Department of Periodontics/Prevention/Teriatrics, School of Dentistry, University of Michigan and Department of Pathology, University of Michigan Medical School, Ann Arbor, MI 48109, U.S.A.

Khalid Mohammad, M.D., Ph.D., Assistant Professor, Department of Internal Medicine, Division of Endocrinology and Metabolism, University of Virginia, Charlottesville, VA 22904, U.S.A.

Suresh Mohla, Ph.D. Chief, Tumor Biology and Metastasis Branch Division of Cancer Biology, National Cancer Institute, National Institutes of Health, Bethesda, MD 20892, U.S.A.

Brian Nicholson, M.D., Instructor, Department of Urology, University of Virginia Health Science Center, Charlottesville, VA 22904, U.S.A.

Pamela Osenkowski, Graduate Student, Department of Pathology, Wayne State University School of Medicine and The Barbara Ann Karmanos Cancer Institute, Detroit, MI 48202, U.S.A.

Susan Ott, M.D., Assocaite Professor, Department of Medicine-Division of Metabolism, University of Washington Medical Center, Seattle, WA 98195, U.S.A.

Kenneth Pienta, M.D., Professor, Departments of Internal Medicine and Surgery, University of Michigan, Ann Arbor, MI 48109, U.S.A.

Carrie Rinker-Schaeffer, **Ph.D.**, Associate Professor, Section of Urology, Department of Surgery, and Section of Hematology/Oncology, Department of Medicine, The University of Chicago, The Genitourinary Oncology Research Program, The University of Chicago Comprehensive Cancer Research Center The University of Chicago, Chicago, IL 60637, U.S.A.

Victoria Robinson, B.A., Graduate Student, Cancer Biology, The University of Chicago, Chicago, IL 60637, U.S.A.

G. David Roodman, M.D., Ph.D., Bone Biology Center of the University of Pittsburgh Medical Center, University of Pittsburgh, E1152 BST, 200 Lothrop St., Pittsburgh, PA 15261, U.S.A.

Thomas Rosol, **D.V.M., Ph.D.**, Professor of Veterinary Pathobiology, Adjunct Professor of Urology, Department of Veterinary Biosciences, College of Veterinary Medicine, The Ohio State University, Columbus, OH, 43210, U.S.A.

Martine P. Roudier, M.D., Ph.D., Senior Research Fellow, Department of Urology, University of Washington Medical Center, Seattle, WA 98195, U.S.A.

Abraham Schneider, Ph.D., Research Fellow Department of Periodontics/Prevention/Teriatrics, School of Dentistry, University of Michigan and Department of Pathology, University of Michigan Medical School, Ann Arbor, MI 48109, U.S.A.

Robert Sikes, Ph.D., Assistant Professor, Department of Biological Sciences, Wolf Hall, University of Delaware, Newark, DE 19716, U.S.A

Mitchell Sokoloff, M.D., Assistant Professor, Section of Urology, Department of Surgery, The University of Chicago, Chicago, IL 60637, U.S.A.

Yan-Xi Sun, M.D., Research Fellow, Periodontics/Prevention/Geriatrics, School of Dentistry, University of Michigan, Ann Arbor, MI, 48109, U.S.A.

Russell Taichman, D.M.D., D.M.Sc., Professor, Periodontics/Prevention/Geriatrics, School of Dentistry, University of Michigan, Ann Arbor, MI 48109, U.S.A.

Sarah Tannehill-Gregg, D.V.M., Senior Research Associate, Department of Veterinary Biosciences, College of Veterinary Medicine, The Ohio State University, Columbus, OH 43210, U.S.A.

Lawrence True, M.D., Associate Professor, Department of Pathology, University of Washington Medical Center, Seattle, WA 98195, U.S.A.

Shi-Ming Tu M.D., Associate Professor, Department of Genitourinary Medical Oncology and Molecular Pathology, The University of Texas, M.D. Anderson Cancer Center, Houston, TX 77030, U.S.A.

Robert Vessella, Ph.D. Professor and Director of Genitourinary Cancer Research Laboratory, Department of Urology, Box 356510, University of Washington Medical Center, Seattle, WA, 98195 and the Puget Sound VA Medical Center, Seattle, WA, 98108, U.S.A.

Toshiyuki Yoneda, Ph.D. D.D.S., Professor and Chairman, Department of Biochemistry, Osaka University Graduate School of Dentistry, Osaka, Japan and Heyser Professor, Endocrine Research, Department of Medicine, University of Texas Health Science Center, 7703 Floyd Curl Dr., San Antonio, TX 78229, U.S.A.

Jian Zhang, M.D., Ph.D., Research Investigator, Unit for Laboratory Animal Medicine and Department of Pathology, University of Michigan, 1150 W. Medical Center Drive, Ann Arbor, MI 48109, U.S.A.

Foreword

I am privileged to write this introduction for the Book: "The Biology of Skeletal Metastases" edited by Drs. Evan Keller and Leland Chung.

Skeletal metastases are frequent sites of colonization of tumor cells in a large number of human cancers, and they contribute heavily towards morbidity and mortality. Skeletal metastases are observed in a majority of solid tumors such as breast and prostate cancer, melanoma, renal cell carcinoma and lung cancer, as well as in hematopoietic malignancies including multiple myeloma, and lymphomas. The debilitating symptoms of bone metastasis include bone pain, spinal cord compression, pathological fractures, partial paralysis, hypercalcemia and eventual death. According to the American Cancer Society, approximately 553,000 cancer deaths are expected to occur in the United States in 2003 with at least two thirds of these with bone metastases (1). In certain human cancers the incidence of bone metastasis is extremely high –these include prostate and breast cancer and multiple myeloma. Recognizing this, the United States Congress in the FY2001 National cancer Institute Budget, encouraged the NCI "to conduct research to develop a better understanding of the unique role the bone microenvironment plays in metastasis of cancer to bone, in particular breast cancer, prostate cancer and myeloma, including the development of animal models of bone metastasis and identification of novel therapeutic targets and modalities to prevent and treat bone metastasis". Subsequent NCI budgets, in FY 2002 and FY 2003 have similar language to encourage research in this area.

The NCI organized a "think tank" style workshop on this topic and assembled a multidisciplinary team of bone biologists, clinical investigators and cancer biologists to assess (a) the current state-of-the-science on the available experimental models to study bone metastasis, (b) what is currently known about molecular mechanism of tumor-bone stroma interaction, and (c) some of the critical unresolved issues in tumor metastasis to the bone. Speakers and participants agreed that identification of unique features of bone that encourage homing of tumor cells, delineating the role played by growth factors and cytokines in this process, elucidating the bidirectional interactions between tumor and bone stroma and exploiting the resulting information for diagnostics or therapeutics were areas of high priority (2).

The area of tumor –host interactions continues to be an area of high priority for the NCI. Several initiatives to provide funds to NCI grantees to pursue this area of science have been awarded, and a recent initiative, "Molecular Interactions between Tumor Cells and Bone" supported by three NIH institutes has been funded.

The Book, Biology of Skeletal Metastases provides comprehensive reviews written by well known experts. The Book starts with three informative and insightful reviews on bone metastasis, covering the basic biology, clinical aspects, and animal models. This is followed by several excellent chapters focused on understanding the role of extracellular matrix, cell adhesion molecules, proteases, growth factors and cytokines, immune aspects and bidirectional interactions between tumor-bone stroma in bone metastasis. Finally, highly informative chapters focus on therapeutic aspects related to tissue-specific promoter based targeting, and the effects on bisphosphonates on bone versus visceral metastasis.

Overall, this exciting book provides a comprehensive approach to the current understanding and management of skeletal metastases which contribute so significantly towards overall cancer morbidity and mortality.

Suresh Mohla, Ph.D.
Tumor Biology and Metastasis Branch
Division of Cancer Biology
National Cancer Institute, NIH
Bethesda, MD 20892

References

1. Kakonen, S. M. (2003) Mechanisms of osteolytic none metastasis in breast carcinoma. Cancer, 97, 834-839.

2. Reddi, A.H., Roodman, D., Freeman, C. and Mohla, S. (2003) Mechanisms of tumor metastasis to the bone: challenges and opportunities. J Bone & Miner. Res. 18, 190-194.

Preface

Metastasis is the penultimate signature of most aggressive cancers and is often associated with the cause of death of patients. The pathophysiology of metastasis to any organ is complex and involves many inter-connected steps. Clearly, as predicted by Paget's "seed" and "soil" hypothesis over 100 years ago, the interaction between tumor, the seed, and metastatic site, the soil, is a critical factor in the development, establishment, and progression of metastases. This "cross-talk" between tumor and target organ is readily demonstrated at the site of bone metastases. However, understanding why certain tumors target bone and how they influence bone remodeling, and the mechanisms by which the bone microenvironment influences the ability of tumor cells to colonize in bone have been challenging due to the difficulties of working with cancer bone metastases in general. Bone is unique in comparison to soft tissue sites because it differentiates into mineralized solid bone matrices and physiologically it is constantly being remodeled with the release of large pools of soluble growth factors and insoluble extracellular matrices. Thus, the major focus of this book is on the theme that understanding the biology of bone metastases requires knowledge of both bone biology and tumor pathophysiology.

Our goal in producing this book is to provide an overview on the important aspects of the biology of bone metastases. To that end, we have brought together investigators with expertise in tumor biology and bone biology. The cross-disciplinary approach to bone metastases provides a comprehensive view of both how tumor influences the bone environment and how the bone environment influences metastases.

Dr. Rinker-Schaeffer et al. describe the basic biology of metastasis where metastatic cascade and the factors within the bone microenvironment are emphasized. They describe both the contribution by metastatic suppressor genes and tumor microenvironment in cancer metastases. Drs. Tu and Lin review the clinical aspects of bone metastasis in prostate cancer by providing the readers with some very pertinent information on topics such as clinical features of prostate cancer bone metastasis, radiographic evaluation of bone metastasis and currently available therapies for prostate cancer bone metastasis. Dr. Rosol et al. comprehensively review animal models of cancer bone metastases including models for mammary cancer, prostate cancer, lung cancer, malignant melanoma, renal cell carcinoma, and multiple myeloma. Some of the in vivo imaging approaches of cancer bone metastases in animal models are also described. Drs. Roodman and Choi reviewed in depth one of the osteoclast activating factors, macrophage inflammatory protein-1α (MIP-1α), in myeloma bone disease. They provided the rationale, the identification, putative functions and prognostic values of MIF-1α in myeloma patients. Dr. Kiefer et al. present their cDNA microarray data on human prostate cancer cells plating on type 1 collagen. Based on their analysis of a large series of genes that were changed upon contact with type 1 collagen, they concluded that type 1 collagen may influence the proliferative capability of prostate cancer cells to colonize in bone. The roles of parathyroid hormone-related protein (PTHrP), a highly bone active cytokine, is reviewed by Drs. McCauley and Schneider. The structure and signaling of PTHrP and the role of PTHrP in breast cancer and prostate cancer and therapeutic intervention of PTHrP as a paracrine signaling molecule are particularly emphasized. Dr. Brown et al review in detail OPG, RANKL, and RANK in cancer metastasis with specific focus on the expression and regulation of these factors. They provided useful information on steroid hormones, growth factors, and cytokines that could regulate key regulators of bone resorption and the opportunity of therapeutic targeting of OPG/RANKL/RANK axis. Matrix metalloproteinases (MMPs) and bone metastasis is reviewed by Dr. Bonfil et al. They provide an overview of the roles of matrix MMPs on extracellular matrix turnover and how this may affect tumor stroma interaction and subsequent bone metastasis. They also discuss a protease activating imaging system to determine MMP activity and the opportunity of offering novel clinical imaging. Drs. Guise and Mohammad comprehensively review endothelins in cancer bone metastases. They provide an in depth review of endothelin structure and function and the special role of endothelins in cancer induced osteoblastic reaction and the development of an endothelin receptor antagonist ABT-627 for the treatment of osteoblastic metastases in prostate cancer. Dr. Yoneda et al. review bisphosphonate actions on bone and visceral metastases. They provide the basic action of bisphosphonates and their potential clinical usage in the prevention of bone loss as a result of cancer bone metastases and the rationale of bisphosphonate usage in combination with other anticancer agents on the treatment of cancer in the osteosclerotic bone metastasis and other cancer related metastasis to non-bone sites. Dr. Hsieh et al. review gene therapy for prostate cancer bone metastasis with specific focus on summarizing the viral and non-viral vectors, useful therapeutics genes, and strategies. The potentials of targeting angiogenic pathway, host immune system and the cell surface receptors are emphasized. They also summarize all current ongoing clinical trials using gene therapy for the treatment of both localized and disseminated prostate cancer. The topic of cancer cell homing to bone and the role of chemotaxis and cell adhesion is reviewed by Dr. Cooper et al. They focus on the importance of cancer cell chemotaxis, neutralizing CXCR4/CXCL12 interaction and the interaction of prostate cancer cells with bone-specific extracellular matrix. They suggest an opportunity for the use of anti-chemotaxis and anti-adhesive therapies for the effective treatment of cancer bone metastases. Dr. Roudier et al. provide a comprehensive overview on the histopathological and immunohistochemical aspects of prostate cancer bone metastasis relevant to clinical progression of prostate cancer. They focus specifically on the current status of osteoblastic response both from the clinic and the basic science studies with supplemental information by up-to-date animal model data. The heterogeneity of prostate cancer bone metastasis and the importance of evaluating clinical specimens coupled with appropriate animal models are emphasized and highlighted.

Due to the vastness of the subject and limited space of this book, we could not include all worthy subject areas and apologize to our colleagues in advance for obvious important omissions. We wish to thank our contributors for their time and effort in putting together their chapters and also give thanks to Ms. Laura Walsh and Ms. Maureen Tobin at Kluwer Publishers who helped us with this endeavor. We would also like to thank Ms. Terry Fracala for her dedication and perserverance for typesetting this book.

Evan T. Keller DVM, PhD
Leland W. K. Chung, PhD   September 15th, 2003

Acknowledgments

We would like to thank the many patients afflicted with skeletal metastases whom had the vision, fortitude and selflessness to help cancer investigators learn about the biology of skeletal metastases to help future generations.

Chapter 1

THE BASIC BIOLOGY OF METASTASIS

Victoria L. Robinson[1], Eric C. Kauffman[1], Mitchell H. Sokoloff[1] and Carrie W. Rinker-Schaeffer[1,2]

[1]*Section of Urology, Department of Surgery, The University of Chicago,* [2]*Section of Hematology/Oncology, Department of Medicine, The University of Chicago, The Genitourinary Oncology Research Program, The University of Chicago Comprehensive Cancer Research Center*

METASTASIS: THE CLINICAL CHALLENGE

It is the ability to metastasize that makes cancer a fatal disease. Of the 555,500 cancer-related deaths expected this year in the United States, the vast majority are due to the development of metastatic disease rather than the primary tumor (Jemal et al., 2002). Although treatment is available for patients with metastatic cancer, options are limited and responses can be quite variable. Furthermore, complete remissions tend to be limited in both scope and duration.

As a result, there has been increasing focus on early detection in order to provide curative therapy while a tumor is still confined to the primary organ. However, while clinically localized cancer may be curable, standard parameters of assessing localization (i.e., size, grade and stage) cannot rule out the possibility that cancer cells have already disseminated to distant sites at the time of diagnosis. As a result, a significant number of patients treated for localized disease will ultimately develop metastases. Advances in molecular staging techniques have enhanced our ability to detect disseminated cancer cells, and it is apparent that dissemination may occur earlier and more frequently than once believed (Christiano et al., 2000; Kauffman et al., 2003). Nevertheless, not all patients with tumor cells at the secondary site ultimately develop overt metastatic lesions, even in the absence of therapy (Cher et al., 1999; Ellis et al., 1998; Melchior et al., 1997; Sokoloff et al., 1996). This observation has lent new support to the long-standing idea that like cells at early steps in the metastatic cascade, disseminated cells are subject to significant growth control mechanisms at the secondary (metastatic) site. Identification of such growth control mechanisms may improve our ability to predict the clinical course of an individual patient's disease and to identify targets for antimetastatic therapies.

The physiologic steps that allow a cancer cell to form a metastatic lesion are well defined and the collective process is known to be quite inefficient (Weiss, 1990). Initially, escape from the primary tumor was considered to be the rate-limiting step for metastasis formation, however recent studies suggest that post-extravasation steps may play a significant role in metastatic inefficiency (Luzzi et al., 1998). In addition, little is known regarding the genes and molecular pathways that govern each step. Roles for numerous genes in either the promotion or suppression of metastasis have been proposed based on 1) functions demonstrated *in vitro* that correlate with metastatic potential *in vivo* (e.g., gene X promotes invasion *in vitro*, therefore it promotes metastasis), or 2) *in vivo* expression patterns that correlate with the presence of metastases or clinicopathological parameters predicting metastasis (Shevde and Welch, 2003). However, in order to demonstrate that a gene has a causal role in metastasis, the gene must be shown to directly alter metastatic potential *in vivo*. In this regard, the identification and characterization of metastasis suppressor genes, which are defined by their ability to directly suppress metastasis *in vivo*, may provide valuable insight into the mechanisms that regulate metastasis (Steeg, 2003; Yoshida et al., 2000; Shevde and Welch, 2003).

In this chapter, we will provide and overview of the metastatic process, and provide a detailed discussion of growth control of disseminated cancer cells at the secondary site as an important determinant of metastatic efficiency, and the clinical significance and applicability of these findings will also be discussed. Although the development of prostate cancer bone metastases is the emphasis of this chapter, we anticipate that the fundamental mechanisms regulating metastatic growth will be conserved among a variety of cancers. In addition, molecules with established roles in metastasis are discussed.

THE METASTATIC CASCADE

In order to become a metastasis, a cell must complete a series of steps known as the metastatic cascade (Figure 1) (Poste and Fidler, 1980). The diversity of these steps requires that <u>multiple cellular changes take place.</u> During the progression of cancer from normal tissue to a tumor with metastatic ability, cells can undergo multiple genetic and epigenetic alterations which give rise to altered cellular functions. Histologically, this change is marked by a progressively less- differentiated phenotype in which the normal structures of the tissue are lost and often cells have invaded the underlying basement membrane (local invasion). Intravasation is the process of cells invading into lymphatic or blood vessels. In order to survive within the circulation, tumor cells must be anchorage independent, evade immune recognition, and be able to survive a variety and physical and biochemical stresses. Upon reaching a target organ, cancer cells may adhere to and proliferate within the vessel, eventually rupturing it as it continues to grow into a secondary tumor. Alternatively, cancer cells can extravasate, or actively migrate though endothelium into the target tissue. In either case, the cell must be able to survive and proliferate at the secondary site, a process known as metastatic colonization. Metastatic colonization can be further subdivided into tumor cell survival and proliferation followed by development of a blood supply through vessel recruitment, angiogenesis, channel formation, or perhaps vasculogenesis.

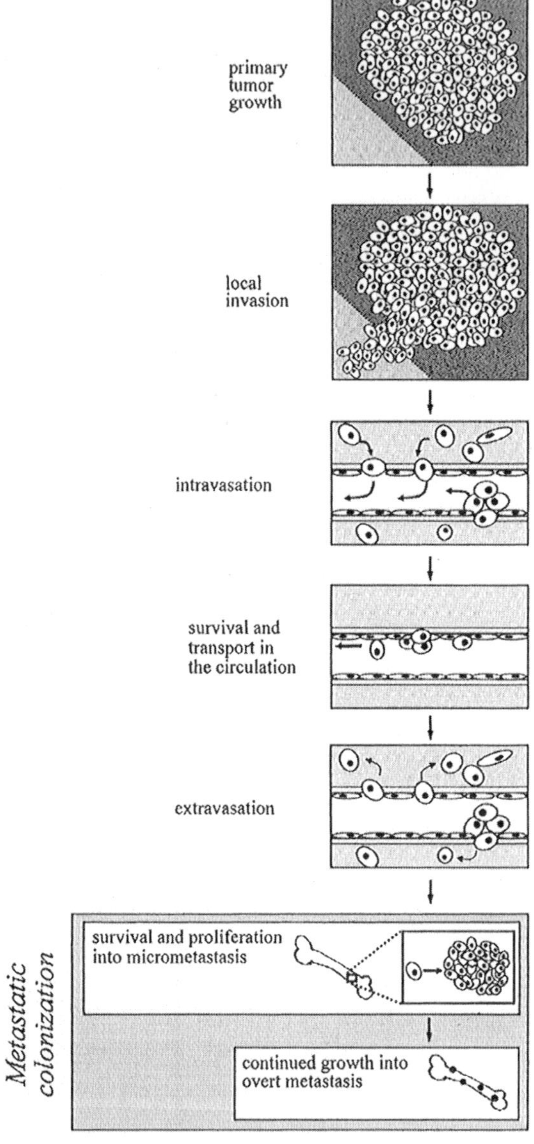

Figure 1. Metastatic cascade. For cancer cell to form metastasis it must complete series of steps, including 1) growth within primary tumor, 2) invasion of local tissue, 3) intravasation into the bloodstream or lymphatics, 4) survival in bloodstream or lymphatics as single cell or as part of embolus, 5) arrest in microvasculature at secondary site with subsequent extravasation into tissue parenchyma (extravasation may not be required), and 6) survival and proliferation into micrometastasis, followed by continued growth into overt metastatic lesion. Angiogenesis may be required during metastatic colonization only after lesion has achieved critical size. Metastasis suppressor genes are defined by ability to prevent metastasis without affecting primary tumor growth. (Continued on next page)

(Fig. 1 legend continued). Therefore, these genes could inhibit steps 2 to 6 but not 1. At least 2 know metastasis suppressor genes can inhibit early metastatic colonization, that is step 6. From: Kauffman: J Urol. Volume 169(3). March 2003, 1122-1133. Reproduced with permission from Lippincott Williams & Wilkins.

The inability of a cancer cell to complete any one step in the metastatic cascade will result in its failure to form a clinically significant metastasis. Each step in the cascade thus represents a potential target for anti-metastasis therapies. The most promising targets, however, are those steps that are most highly regulated— that is, the rate-limiting steps. Because a cancer cell can more efficiently complete the less regulated steps, the clinical window for identifying and therapeutically targeting such steps is likely to be brief and unpredictable (Chambers et al., 2000). In contrast, cancer cells will spend more time arrested in the rate-limiting steps, thus providing a more practical clinical target (Chambers et al., 2000). Furthermore, it is also during the rate limiting steps that the greatest fraction of cancer cells are likely to die, and the characterization of the molecular mechanisms responsible for this effect may lead to novel therapeutic strategies for preventing clinical metastasis.

ARRIVAL AT THE SECONDARY SITE- AN EARLY CLINICAL EVENT

The inherent inefficiency of metastasis suggests that one or more steps in the metastatic cascade are rate limiting (Weiss, 1990). Traditionally, those steps occurring prior to arrival at the secondary site (local invasion, intravasation and survival in the circulation) have been considered key rate-limiting steps. This paradigm has been challenged over recent years by the clinical finding that cancer cells frequently disseminate to the secondary site while the primary tumor is still clinically localized. This observation holds true for prostate cancer as well as most other solid tumor cancers (Hermanek, 1999; Funke and Schraut, 1998). Using immunohistochemistry, disseminated cancer cells can be identified at the secondary site as solitary cells or small clusters termed "micrometastases" early in the clinical course of the disease (Hermanek, 1999). The presence of these cells has become more readily demonstrated with PCR-based methods that allow detection of a single epithelial cell among 10^6 non-epithelial cells (Bockmann et al., 2001). Although a criticism of PCR-detection has been its potential for false positives, specificity approaches 100% in prostate cancer patients when PSA mRNA is used as the cell marker (Sokoloff et al., 1996; Su et al., 2000). Studies employing PCR detection of PSA report the presence of disseminated prostate cells in bone marrow aspirates for ~20-70% of patients with clinically or pathologically localized prostate cancer (Cher et al., 1999; Melchior et al., 1997; Deguchi et al., 1997; Wood et al., 1994; Corey et al., 1997; Wood et al., 1998) and comparable incidences are observed for many other clinically localized malignancies (Funke and Schraut, 1998).

Riethmuller et al have recently discussed two additional clinical observations which support further the notion that cancer cell dissemination to the secondary site is an early event in clinical disease (Riethmuller and Klein, 2001). The first line of support comes from "unknown primary carcinoma" (UPC), cancers detected by their metastases rather than a primary lesion and which represent 5% of all malignancies. In many UPC cases, the primary lesion is later identified (e.g., at autopsy) and is noted to be small and well differentiated, despite the presence of metastases. In genitourinary oncology this scenario is well described in germ-cell tumor patients presenting with retroperitoneal masses. The second line of evidence supporting early dissemination of cancer cells is provided by the transmission of metastatic cancer from organ donors who have been diagnosed as being tumor-free or as having localized lesions. Transmitted cancer is thought to result from the presence of disseminated tumor cells present in the donor organ prior to organ harvest. In a particularly striking case, a transplant recipient developed osteoblastic metastases involving the ribs and spine after receiving a heart from a donor with regional prostatic disease, suggesting that prostate cancer cells were arrested in the heart at the time of transplant (Riethmuller and Klein, 2001).

Taken together, these observations suggest that dissemination to the secondary site may be an early and frequent clinical event. The implication is that the steps in the metastatic cascade preceding arrival at the secondary site may be completed with much more efficiency than traditionally believed.

GROWTH AT THE SECONDARY SITE- A KEY REGULATORY STEP IN METASTASIS

Both clinical findings and experimental models suggest that significant control of metastasis may occur after cancer cell arrival at the secondary site, during metastatic colonization. Clinically, this conclusion is drawn from two observations. First, it is clear that some patients with disseminated cancer cells at the secondary site will not go on to develop metastases. This is not only observed in prostate cancer patients (Cher et al., 1999; Melchior et al., 1997), but is also evidenced by the fact that other cancers- namely colonic, gastric, and esophageal- commonly disseminate to bone, but infrequently develop into metastases there (Jauch et al., 1996; Lindemann et al., 1992; Thorban et al., 1996). Second, for those cases in which metastases do develop, there is a significant delay- sometimes years- between the initial detection of the disseminated cells and the clinical presentation of overt lesions (Christiano et al., 2000). Together, these clinical findings support the existence of significant growth-control mechanisms at the secondary site.

Experimental support for growth control at the secondary site has come from animal metastasis models. Two types of *in vivo* metastasis assays, "experimental" and "spontaneous", are commonly used. These methods are described in *"Laboratory Techniques In Biochemistry and Molecular Biology*; Cancer Metastasis: Experimental Approaches." (Rusciano et al., 2000). Traditionally, these models have been limited by the ability to observe only the endpoint of the assays (i.e., presence or absence of lesions) and not the individual steps as they happen *in vivo*. Regulatory mechanisms in metastasis have therefore been based largely on inference rather than direct observation. However, this has changed in recent years with the advent of new technologies, including *in vivo* videomicroscopy (IVVM) and fluorescent cell tagging, which allow for detailed *in vivo* monitoring. By coupling these techniques with a method for quantifying cancer cell survival at specific steps of the metastatic cascade, Chambers and colleagues have shown that the vast majority (at least 70-90%) of cancer cells injected intravenously manage not only to survive in the circulation but to arrest in the microvasculature and extravasate (Naumov et al., 2001); (Chambers et al., 2002). Completion of these steps is rapid and efficient, so that as early as 24 hours post-injection, all cells have exited the circulation and are present entirely in the target organ parenchyma. Subsequent growth, however, is remarkably less efficient, and less than 0.1% of cancer cells reaching the target organ parenchyma go on to form metastases. Interestingly, most micrometastases appear to die off rapidly, while most solitary cells remain growth-arrested, with some still present in the target tissue even after 21 days (Luzzi et al., 1998). Thus, the inefficiency of metastatic colonization exists during microscopic growth, prior to the need for blood supply and therefore independent of angiogenesis. These observations have been confirmed, although not independently, in multiple studies using different cancer cell lines and with different animal models and target organs (Luzzi et al., 1998; Morris et al., 1994; Varghese et al., 2002). An independent study using IVVM reports the extravasation step to be inefficient (Al-Mehdi et al., 2000).

Additional support for growth control at the secondary site comes from animal model studies that correlate a lower metastatic potential specifically with a lesser ability to grow at the secondary site (Kuo et al., 1995; Aslakson et al., 1991). For example, when engrafted into mice, metastatic and non-metastatic human colon cancers demonstrate equal ability to invade local tissue and intravasate; however, only the metastatic cancers are able to grow at the secondary site, as demonstrated by both spontaneous metastasis assays and direct injection or engraftment at the target organ (Kuo et al., 1995). Such findings further support the idea that reaching the secondary site is not by itself sufficient for metastasis.

Seed and Soil- importance of microenvironment in regulating growth at the secondary site

Bone is one of the most common sites of metastases, in part due to the fact that many of the most common solid tumors frequently metastasize to bone, including cancers of the breast, lung and prostate. Clinically, bone metastasis is often characterized by severe bone pain, pathological fractures, and nerve compression syndromes (Mundy, 1997). Clearly, understanding the biology of bone metastasis is an important step towards developing better treatments, and ultimately prevention.

What then determines whether a cell reaching the bone will grow into a clinically important metastasis? According to the century-old theory proposed by Paget, a disseminated cancer cell will act like a seed, growing only if it finds a suitable "soil" at a secondary site (Paget, 1889). The seed-and-soil theory has been invoked to explain why specific organs typically harbor metastases from one type of cancer but not another. Support for this idea comes from the observation that the target organ of metastasis is typically better than non-target organs in stimulating growth of cancer cells *in vitro* (Nicolson, 1988). For example, researchers have shown that bone marrow, but not various other organs, strongly stimulates prostate cancer cell growth *in vitro*, while having little or no effect on cancer cells that metastasize to non-bone organs (Chackal-Roy et al., 1989). Similar correlations have been made for cancer cells *in vivo*: in a study of mammary cancer sublines displaying different patterns of metastasis, the preferred organ of metastasis in each case was the organ allowing the most rapid growth of the cancer cells (Aslakson et al., 1991).

A traditional alternative to the seed-and-soil argument, known as the "anatomical-mechanical" hypothesis, challenges the importance of the "soil" in regulating cancer cell growth. It argues instead that metastasis will occur in the organ of any capillary bed in which a disseminated cancer cell becomes mechanically lodged (Nicolson, 1988). Consistent with this hypothesis, Batson noted in the 1940's that specific veins draining the prostate encountered their first capillary bed in the lumbar spine, a common site of prostate cancer metastasis (Nishijima et al., 1992). Nevertheless, despite occasional successes (Lindberg, 1972), the anatomical-mechanical theory fails to account for several observations that are entirely consistent with the seed-and-soil hypothesis (Nicolson, 1988). For example, following injection into the mouse circulation, cancer cells arrest within minutes in multiple organs throughout the body; however, despite this promiscuous dissemination, subsequent colonization most often occurs in only one specific organ, and altering the site of injection in many cases has no effect on the pattern of metastatic growth (Fidler, 1970; Potter et al., 1983). Moreover, the initial arrest of the cancer cells in capillary beds may only be temporary, and even after several days of residency in an organ's microvasculature, cells appear to recirculate before arresting at a new site (Fidler, 1970; Hart et al., 1981). Particularly compelling are studies that introduce target organ tissue at new sites in the mouse body- for example, bone implanted into subcutaneous tissue, or lung engrafted onto liver. In many of these cases, circulating cancer cells still colonize the ectopic target tissue (but not implanted tissue controls) despite its altered anatomical location (Hart and Fidler, 1980; Nemeth et al., 1999). Thus, although vascular anatomy likely helps direct disseminated cancer cells towards potential target organs, the microenvironment encountered at the secondary site appears to have the "final say" on whether overt metastases will develop (Fidler, 2001; Radinsky, 1995).

The role of the bone microenvironment on cancer cell survival and metastatic growth.

Disseminated cancer cells in the bone are exposed to a complex system of differentiated cells and signals that regulate bone composition and structure. Metastatic cells encountering this environment tend to affect the bone primarily by inducing one of two responses. An osteoblastic response is characterized by an increase in bone density resulting from increased osteoblast activity. Alternatively, an osteolytic response, or bone destruction, is mediated by lytic activity of increased osteoclast activity, cancer cells themselves and/or tumor infiltrated macrophages (Athanasou and Quinn, 1992; Gao et al., 1997; Quinn and Athanasou, 1992). However, a mixed response is common, with one type predominating. While prostate cancer bone metastasis tends to form osteoblastic lesions, other cancers, including breast cancer and myeloma tend to form osteolytic lesions

(Mundy, 2002). The specific mechanisms of how the presence of cancer cells in the bone directs the stimulation of osteoclasts, osteoblasts or both is not well understood. Insight in this regard would be an important advancement.

In addition to cellular components, bone is rich in growth factors, including Transforming Growth Factor β (TGFβ), Bone Morphogenic Protein (BMPs), Fibroblast Growth Factor (FGFs), Platelet Derived Growth Factor (PDGFs), and Insulin-Like Growth Factor (IGFs) I and II. This list continues to grow. Many of these secreted proteins have been shown to alter tumor cell phenotypes. Specifically, IGF-I and II function to stimulate osteoblastic differentiation, growth and matrix deposition, and can stimulate the *in vitro* growth of cell lines derived from breast, prostate, and colorectal cancers (Orr et al., 1995). In addition, pro-angiogenic bFGF stimulates the *in vitro* growth of the prostate cancer derived cell line LNCaP and assists in the formation of tumors in athymic, nude mice (Gleave et al., 1991). *In vitro* studies using the co-culture of bone cells and cancer cells, or treating cancer cells with bone cell conditioned media argue that bone cells have a proliferative effect on cancer cells (Lang et al., 1995). While known growth factors account for some of this effect, novel factors are likely to contribute as well (Lee et al., 2003). The bone environment can have a variety of effects on cancer cells depending on receptor and signaling pathway expression patterns.

A few specific pathways describing interplay between bone cells and cancer cells have been described. TGFβ is produced and secreted by osteoclasts, which signals in a paracrine manner to breast cancer cells expressing the TGFβ receptors. TGFβ receptor activation in breast cancer results in production and secretion of PTH-rp, a protein which stimulates osteoclast lytic activity and further TGFβ production, thus establishing a positive feedback loop (Mundy, 1997). This phenomenon has been studied *in vivo* using the MDA-MB-231 breast cancer model. Interestingly, inhibition of this feedback loop either by anti-PTHrP antibody treatment or by expression of a dominant negative TGFβ receptor type I on MDA-MB-231 cells reduces osteolytic bone lesions and tumor burder (Guise et al., 1996).

REGULATORY FACTORS IN METASTASIS

The cellular and molecular processes involved in regulating metastatic growth are quite diverse. Correspondingly, regulatory molecules and factors in metastasis have varied cellular functions. The best characterized of these fall into the following categories.

MMPs and Serine Proteinases

The matrix metalloproteinases (MMPs) (described in detail in Chapter 8) are a family of at least 26 enzymes that degrade extracellular matrix and basement membrane components. They are expressed as pro-proteins requiring cleavage as well as zinc (and/or calcium) for activation. Substrate specificity defines MMP subsets: collagenases, stomelysins, and gelatinases (Chambers and Matrisian, 1997). MMPs have been extensively studied in metastasis. Based on their function, it was originally thought that their primary role in metastasis was in promoting invasion of the primary tumor through basement membrane degradation. Further studies have revealed that MMPs have a complex functional role in metastasis. In addition to promoting invasion, they are critical for the maintenance of appropriate environmental conditions (Chambers and Matrisian, 1997). Inhibition of MMP activity inhibits bone matrix turnover and bone colonization of the metastatic prostate cancer cell line PC3, suggesting that MMP activity is needed to create a bone environment conducive to cancer cell growth (Nemeth et al., 2002).

Angiogenesis induction and regulation

Angiogenesis is defined as the recruitment of blood vessels to form new vessels, a process which requires the coordinated action of angiogenic factors on endothelial cells. Angiogenesis became a major focus after it was shown that cancers can promote their own growth through promotion of angiogenesis. Stimulators of angiogenesis include the secreted growth factors bFGF and vascular endothelial growth factor (VEGF), while inhibitors include the extracellular matrix protein cleavage products angiostatin and endostatin. These and additional angiogenesis regulators are reviewed in Liekens et al. (Liekens et al., 2001), and Hagedorn and Bikfalvi (Hagedorn and Bikfalvi, 2000).

Angiogenesis regulates metastasis in primarily two ways. First, intravasation of cancer cells is more productive if more vessels are present in a primary tumor, and thus angiogenesis within the primary lesion results in a promotion of metastasis. Secondly, at the secondary site, metastatic lesions will require a blood supply to grow, and hence it has been proposed that dormancy of micrometastases may be due to a lack of angiogenesis (Zetter, 1998).

The striking phenomenon in which malignant melanoma cells form blood carrying vessels themselves, without the involvement of endothelial cells has been termed vasculogenic mimicry (Maniotis et al., 1999). Vasculogenic mimicry may give some tumors an advantage by providing an additional blood supply. These exciting findings, first observed in melanoma, have now been observed in additional cancer types suggesting that this may be another mechanism used by tumors to develop needed blood supplies.

Adhesion molecules are critical for proper tissue organization. In addition, many adhesion molecules are now known to act as sensors of environmental features including basement membrane composition. Of particular interest to bone metastasis is the finding that osteoblasts can alter expression of adhesion molecules on endothelium and cancer cells by secreting Interleukin-1. The four major families of adhesion molecules, grouped by structural and functional characteristics, are the immunoglobulin superfamily, the cadherins, the integrins, and the selectins. Each family is briefly described with respect to its role in metastasis; more extensive reviews can be found in Zetter (Zetter, 1993), Miyasaka (Miyasaka, 1995), and Okegawa (Okegawa et al., 2002).

Immunoglobulin (IG) Superfamily

Members of this family contain variable numbers of Ig-like motifs within their ligand binding domain, and fibronectin like repeats within the intracellular, transmembrane and extracellular domains (Okegawa et al., 2002) A potential role for the ICAM-1 and N-CAM family members in metastasis has been described. ICAM-1 facilitates an interaction between tumor cells and lymphocytes, and misregulation of ICAM-1 may help the tumor cell evade immune mediated killing (Nouri et al., 1996). Abrogation of N-CAM expression increased the incidence of metastasis in a pancreatic β cell transgenic tumor model, suggesting that N-CAM adhesion interactions inhibit metastatic ability (Perl et al., 1999).

Cadherins

E-cadherin has a well accepted role in suppressing primary tumor invasion. However, only limited studies have demonstrated this effect *in vivo*. One study demonstrated that E-cadherin expression in a murine mammary tumor line (NM-f-ras-TD-CAM5) resulted in tumors with a more differentiated appearance (Vleminckx et al., 1991). Another demonstrated that interfering with E-cadherin function resulted in acquisition of a metastatic phenotype (Perl et al., 1999). Clinically, downregulation of E-cadherin frequently occurs in advanced prostate cancers and correlates with poor patient outcome (Paul et al., 1997).

Selectins (P-, E, L-)

Selectins, calcium-dependent transmembrane adhesion molecules, are characterized by an extracellular domain which consists of three specific subdomains. The three family members are cell type specific; L-selectin is expressed in lymphocytes, P-selectin is expressed in platelets and endothelial cells, while E-selectin is expressed solely by activated endothelial cells (Laferriere et al., 2002). Several studies have suggested that colon cancer cell interaction with E-selectin on endothelium promotes metastasis by promoting intravasation through the endothelium into the target tissue (Sawada et al., 1994; Mannori et al., 1997).

Integrins

Integrins are bidirectional transmembrane signaling complexes (Mizejewski, 1999). Heterodimeric integrin pairs recognize specific extracellular matrix components and relay signals into the cell. Integrin mediated signals include diverse cellular functions such as cell movement, proliferation, and survival signaling. It is likely that the dynamic misregulation of integrin signaling can give a metastatic tumor cell an advantage (Mizejewski, 1999). It has been proposed that the interaction between $\alpha v \beta 3$ integrin and vitronectin helps tumor cells extravasate into secondary organs (Lafrenie et al., 1992). Additionally, pro- and anti-angiogenic signaling may require integrins (Beckner, 1999). Detailed reviews on integrins and metastasis are found in Mercurio et al. (Mercurio et al., 2001) and Fornaro et al. (Fornaro et al., 2001).

Chemokines

Chemokines, secreted signaling molecules and their receptors, function to direct movement of cells expressing specific chemokine receptors towards a gradient of chemokine ligands. Metastatic cells can exploit this signaling network. Although it is not yet fully understood how this occurs, chemokines may have multiple regulatory functions in metastasis, altering migration, angiogenesis, immune response suppression, and survival signaling (Balkwill, 2003). In breast cancer metastasis, the chemokine receptors CXCR4 and CCR7 are highly expressed. Disrupting the interaction of these receptors with their ligands inhibited metastasis of the MDA-MB-231 breast cancer line in a mouse model, suggesting that chemokine- receptor interactions are important mediators of metastases (Muller et al., 2001).

Rho family GTPases

Multiple steps of metastasis are associated with major changes in cell shape, including migration into and out of vessels, movement within vessels and within the primary and secondary organ sites. Cellular migration and dynamic adhesion requires constant reorganization of the actin cytoskeleton. While there are a plethora of proteins involved in this process, the Rho family GTPases are of particular interest. A member of this family, RhoC, was found to be upregulated in highly metastatic derivative lines of human A375 and mouse B16F0 melanoma cells. Furthermore, expression of RhoC in poorly metastatic lines promoted their metastatic ability, thus demonstrating an example of Rho-mediated control of metastasis (Clark et al., 2000). The role of RhoC in metastasis is currently under further investigation (Debies and Welch, 2001).

Metastasis Suppressor Genes

Metastasis suppressor genes are defined by their ability to suppress the *in vivo* development of metastases. They are distinguished from tumor suppressor genes in that they suppress metastases without affecting growth of the primary tumor. Although metastasis suppressor genes are potentially involved in all steps of metastasis, it is clear that they are involved in the control of metastatic colonization. Using functional approaches a number of laboratories have identified either novel metastasis-suppressor genes or a novel function of a known gene in metastasis suppression. At this time metastasis suppressor activities for Nm23 (Leone et al., 1991), KAI-1 (Dong et al., 1995), CD44 (Gao et al., 1997), Kiss-1 (Goldberg et al., 1999), TXNIP (Goldberg et al., 2003), CRSP3 (Goldberg et al., 2003), MKK4 (Yoshida et al., 1999), BRMS1 (Shevde et al., 2002), SSeCKS (Xia et al., 2001), RhoGD12 (Seraj et al., 2000), Drg-1 (Guan et al., 2000) have been demonstrated and the list of metastasis suppressors is growing.

Recent comprehensive reviews on metastasis suppressor genes are provided by Kauffman et al., (Kauffman et al., 2003), Steeg (Steeg, 2003), and Shevde and Welch (Shevde and Welch, 2003).

Scatter Factors and Semaphorin Receptors

Scatter factors, the best characterized of which is HGF, are secreted proteins that interact with cell surface tyrosine kinase receptors of the Met family. Signaling from the Met receptor induces changes that result in promoting invasiveness. Met activation can alter the transcription, cellular localization, and/or protein activity of MMP's, cadherins, and integrins (Trusolino and Comoglio, 2002). Interestingly, prostate cancer cells secrete HGF, recruits osteoclasts and initiate bone remodeling, suggesting that HGF/Met is involved in the osteolytic prostate cancer phenotype.

CONCLUSION

Understanding the biology of metastasis regulation has vast translational and clinical implications; for both the design of appropriate metastasis studies as well as application of these findings to clinical disease. The field of drug design for cancer treatment has benefited from metastasis research; drugs targeting MMP's and angiogenesis are currently in clinical trials (Folkman, 2002). However, successes in discovering new, effective treatments for metastasis are rare. The complexity of the metastatic process has made the development of valid *in vivo* metastasis models and informative mechanistic studies challenging. It is hoped that technological advancements and the convergence of mechanistic biology and metastasis research will yield a more clear understanding of the complex molecular regulation of metastasis.

ACKNOWLEDGMENTS

This work is supported by NCI/NIH Predoctoral Cancer Biology Training Grant 5 T32 CA 09594 (V.L.R.)

The University of Chicago RESCUE Fund (C.W.R-S)

NCI 1 RO1 CA 89569 (C.W.R-S.)

DOD Prostate Cancer Research Award DAMD17-01-1-0700 (V.L.R., C.W. R-S)

Fletcher Scholar Award (C.W.R.-S.)

REFERENCES

Al-Mehdi, A.B., Tozawa, K., Fisher, A.B., Shientag, L., Lee, A. and Muschel, R.J. (2000) Intravascular origin of metastasis from the proliferation of endothelium-attached tumor cells: a new model for metastasis. *Nature Medicine*, **6**, 100-102.

Aslakson, C.J., Rak, J.W., Miller, B.E. and Miller, F.R. (1991) Differential influence of organ site on three subpopulations of a single mouse mammary tumor at two distinct steps in metastasis. *International Journal of Cancer*, **47**, 466-472.

Athanasou, N.A. and Quinn, J.M. (1992) Human tumour-associated macrophages are capable of bone resorption. *British Journal of Cancer*, **65**, 523-526.

Balkwill, F. (2003) Chemokine biology in cancer. Seminars in Immunology, **15**, 49-55.

Beckner, M.E. (1999) Factors promoting tumor angiogenesis. *Cancer Investigation*, **17**, 594-623.

Bockmann, B., Grill, H.J. and Giesing, M. (2001) Molecular characterization of minimal residual cancer cells in patients with solid tumors. *Biomolecular Engineering*, **17**, 95-111.

Chackal-Roy, M., Niemeyer, C., Moore, M. and Zetter, B.R. (1989) Stimulation of human prostatic carcinoma cell growth by factors present in human bone marrow. *Journal of Clinical Investigation*, **84**, 43-50.

Chambers, A.F., Groom, A.C. and MacDonald, I.C. (2002) Dissemination and growth of cancer cells in metastatic sites. *Nature Reviews Cancer*, **2**, 563-572.

Chambers, A.F., MacDonald, I.C., Schmidt, E.E., Morris, V.L. and Groom, A.C. (2000) Clinical targets for anti-metastasis therapy. *Advances in Cancer Research*, **79**, 91-121.

Chambers, A.F. and Matrisian, L.M. (1997) Changing views of the role of matrix metalloproteinases in metastasis. *Journal of the National Cancer Institute*, **89**, 1260-1270.

Cher, M.L., de Oliveira, J.G., Beaman, A.A., Nemeth, J.A., Hussain, M. and Wood, D.P., Jr. (1999) Cellular proliferation and prevalence of micrometastatic cells in the bone marrow of patients with clinically localized prostate cancer. *Clinical Cancer Research*, **5**, 2421-2425.

Christiano, A.P., Yoshida, B.A., Dubauskas, Z., Sokoloff, M. and Rinker-Schaeffer, C.W. (2000) Development of markers of prostate cancer metastasis. Review and perspective. *Urological Oncology*, **5**, 217-223.

Clark, E.A., Golub, T.R., Lander, E.S. and Hynes, R.O. (2000) Genomic analysis of metastasis reveals an essential role for RhoC. *Nature*, **406**, 532-535.

Corey, E., Arfman, E.W., Oswin, M.M., Melchior, S.W., Tindall, D.J., Young, C.Y., Ellis, W.J. and Vessella, R.L. (1997) Detection of circulating prostate cells by reverse transcriptase-polymerase chain reaction of human glandular kallikrein (hK2) and prostate-specific antigen (PSA) messages. *Urology*, **50**, 184-188.

Debies, M.T. and Welch, D.R. (2001) Genetic basis of human breast cancer metastasis. *Journal of Mammary Gland Biology and Neoplasia*, **6**, 441-451.

Deguchi, T., Yang, M., Ehara, H., Ito, S., Nishino, Y., Takahashi, Y., Ito, Y., Shimokawa, K., Tanaka, T., Imaeda, T., Doi, T. and Kawada, Y. (1997) Detection of micrometastatic prostate cancer cells in the bone marrow of patients with prostate cancer. *British Journal of Cancer*, **75**, 634-638.

Dong, J.T., Lamb, P.W., Rinker-Schaeffer, C.W., Vukanovic, J., Ichikawa, T., Isaacs, J.T. and Barrett, J.C. (1995) KAI1, a metastasis suppressor gene for prostate cancer on human chromosome 11p11.2. *Science*, **268**, 884-886.

Ellis, W.J., Vessella, R.L., Corey, E., Arfman, E.W., Oswin, M.M., Melchior, S. and Lange, P.H. (1998) The value of a reverse transcriptase polymerase chain reaction assay in preoperative staging and followup of patients with prostate cancer. *Journal of Urology*, **159**, 1134-1138.

Fidler, I.J. (1970) Metastasis: guantitative analysis of distribution and fate of tumor embolilabeled with 125 I-5-iodo-2'-deoxyuridine. *Journal of the National Cancer Institute*, **45**, 773-782.

Fidler, I.J. (2001) Seed and soil revisited: contribution of the organ microenvironment to cancer metastasis. *Surgical Oncology Clinical N Am*, **10**, 257-269, vii-viiii.

Folkman, J. (2002) Role of angiogenesis in tumor growth and metastasis. *Seminars in Oncology*, **29**, 15-18.

Fornaro, M., Manes, T. and Languino, L.R. (2001) Integrins and prostate cancer metastases. *Cancer Metastasis Reviews*, **20**, 321-331.

Funke, I. and Schraut, W. (1998) Meta-analyses of studies on bone marrow micrometastases: an independent prognostic impact remains to be substantiated. *Journal of Clinical Oncology*, **16**, 557-566.

Gao, A.C., Lou, W., Dong, J.T. and Isaacs, J.T. (1997) CD44 is a metastasis suppressor gene for prostatic cancer located on human chromosome 11p13. *Cancer Research*, **57**, 846-849.

Gleave, M., Hsieh, J.T., Gao, C.A., von Eschenbach, A.C. and Chung, L.W. (1991) Acceleration of human prostate cancer growth in vivo by factors produced by prostate and bone fibroblasts. *Cancer Research*, **51**, 3753-3761.

Goldberg, S.F., Harms, J.F., Quon, K. and Welch, D.R. (1999) Metastasis-suppressed C8161 melanoma cells arrest in lung but fail to proliferate. *Clinical Experimental Metastasis*, **17**, 601-607.

Goldberg, S.F., Miele, M.E., Hatta, N., Takata, M., Paquette-Straub, C., Freedman, L.P. and Welch, D.R. (2003) Melanoma metastasis suppression by chromosome 6: evidence for a pathway regulated by CRSP3 and TXNIP. *Cancer Research*, **63**, 432-440.

Guan, R.J., Ford, H.L., Fu, Y., Li, Y., Shaw, L.M. and Pardee, A.B. (2000) Drg-1 as a differentiation-related, putative metastatic suppressor gene in human colon cancer. *Cancer Research*, **60**, 749-755.

Guise, T.A., Yin, J.J., Taylor, S.D., Kumagai, Y., Dallas, M., Boyce, B.F., Yoneda, T. and Mundy, G.R. (1996) Evidence for a causal role of parathyroid hormone-related protein in the pathogenesis of human breast cancer-mediated osteolysis. *Journal of Clinical Investigation*, **98**, 1544-1549.

Hagedorn, M. and Bikfalvi, A. (2000) Target molecules for anti-angiogenic therapy: from basic research to clinical trials. *Critical Reviews in Oncology Hematology*, **34**, 89-110.

Hart, I.R. and Fidler, I.J. (1980) Role of organ selectivity in the determination of metastatic patterns of B16 melanoma. *Cancer Research*, **40**, 2281-2287.

Hart, I.R., Talmadge, J.E. and Fidler, I.J. (1981) Metastatic behavior of a murine reticulum cell sarcoma exhibiting organ-specific growth. *Cancer Research*, **41**, 1281-1287.

Hermanek, P. (1999) Disseminated tumor cells versus micrometastasis: definitions and problems. *Anticancer Research*, **19**, 2771-2774.

Jauch, K.W., Heiss, M.M., Gruetzner, U., Funke, I., Pantel, K., Babic, R., Eissner, H.J., Riethmueller, G. and Schildberg, F.W. (1996) Prognostic significance of bone marrow micrometastases in patients with gastric cancer. *Journal of Clinical Oncology*, **14**, 1810-1817.

Jemal, A., Thomas, A., Murray, T. and Thun, M. (2002) Cancer statistics, 2002. CA *Cancer Journal for Clinicians*, **52**, 23-47.

Kauffman, E.C., Robinson, V.L., Stadler, W.M., Sokoloff, M.H. and Rinker-Schaeffer, C.W. (2003) Metastasis suppression: the evolving role of metastasis suppressor genes for regulating cancer cell growth at the secondary site. *Journal of Urology*, **169**, 1122-1133.

Kuo, T.H., Kubota, T., Watanabe, M., Furukawa, T., Teramoto, T., Ishibiki, K., Kitajima, M., Moossa, A.R., Penman, S. and Hoffman, R.M. (1995) Liver colonization competence governs colon cancer metastasis. *Proceedings of the National Academy of Sciences U S A*, **92**, 12085-12089.

Laferriere, J., Houle, F. and Huot, J. (2002) Regulation of the metastatic process by E-selectin and stress-activated protein kinase-2/p38. *Annals of the New York Academy of Sciences*, **973**, 562-572.

Lafrenie, R.M., Podor, T.J., Buchanan, M.R. and Orr, F.W. (1992) Up-regulated biosynthesis and expression of endothelial cell vitronectin receptor enhances cancer cell adhesion. *Cancer Research*, **52**, 2202-2208.

Lang, S.H., Miller, W.R. and Habib, F.K. (1995) Stimulation of human prostate cancer cell lines by factors present in human osteoblast-like cells but not in bone marrow. *Prostate,* **27**, 287-293.

Lee, H.L., Pienta, K.J., Kim, W.J. and Cooper, C.R. (2003) The effect of bone-associated growth factors and cytokines on the growth of prostate cancer cells derived from soft tissue versus bone metastases in vitro. *International Journal of Oncology*, **22**, 921-926.

Leone, A., Flatow, U., King, C.R., Sandeen, M.A., Margulies, I.M., Liotta, L.A. and Steeg, P.S. (1991) Reduced tumor incidence, metastatic potential, and cytokine responsiveness of nm23-transfected melanoma cells. *Cell*, **65**, 25-35.

Liekens, S., De Clercq, E. and Neyts, J. (2001) Angiogenesis: regulators and clinical applications. *Biochemical Pharmacology*, **61**, 253-270.

Lindberg, R. (1972) Distribution of cervical lymph node metastases from squamous cell carcinoma of the upper respiratory and digestive tracts. *Cancer,* **29**, 1446-1449.

Lindemann, F., Schlimok, G., Dirschedl, P., Witte, J. and Riethmuller, G. (1992) Prognostic significance of micrometastatic tumour cells in bone marrow of colorectal cancer patients. *Lancet*, **340**, 685-689.

Luzzi, K.J., MacDonald, I.C., Schmidt, E.E., Kerkvliet, N., Morris, V.L., Chambers, A.F. and Groom, A.C. (1998) Multistep nature of metastatic inefficiency: dormancy of solitary cells after successful extravasation and limited survival of early micrometastases. *American Journal of Pathology*, **153**, 865-873.

Maniotis, A.J., Folberg, R., Hess, A., Seftor, E.A., Gardner, L.M., Pe'er, J., Trent, J.M., Meltzer, P.S. and Hendrix, M.J. (1999) Vascular channel formation by human melanoma cells in vivo and in vitro: vasculogenic mimicry. *American Journal of Pathology*, **155**, 739-752.

Mannori, G., Santoro, D., Carter, L., Corless, C., Nelson, R.M. and Bevilacqua, M.P. (1997) Inhibition of colon carcinoma cell lung colony formation by a soluble form of E-selectin. *American Journal of Pathology*, **151**, 233-243.

Melchior, S.W., Corey, E., Ellis, W.J., Ross, A.A., Layton, T.J., Oswin, M.M., Lange, P.H. and Vessella, R.L. (1997) Early tumor cell dissemination in patients with clinically localized carcinoma of the prostate. *Clinical Cancer Research*, **3**, 249-256.

Mercurio, A.M., Bachelder, R.E., Rabinovitz, I., O'Connor, K.L., Tani, T. and Shaw, L.M. (2001) The metastatic odyssey: the integrin connection. *Surgical Oncology Clinical N Am, 10, 313-328, viii-ix.*

Miyasaka, M. (1995) Cancer metastasis and adhesion molecules. *Clinical Orthopaedics*, 10-18.

Mizejewski, G.J. (1999) Role of integrins in cancer: survey of expression patterns. *Proceedings of the Society for Experimental Biology and Medicine*, **222**, 124-138.

Morris, V.L., Koop, S., MacDonald, I.C., Schmidt, E.E., Grattan, M., Percy, D., Chambers, A.F. and Groom, A.C. (1994) Mammary carcinoma cell lines of high and low metastatic potential differ not in extravasation but in subsequent migration and growth. *Clinical Experimental Metastasis*, **12**, 357-367.

Muller, A., Homey, B., Soto, H., Ge, N., Catron, D., Buchanan, M.E., McClanahan, T., Murphy, E., Yuan, W., Wagner, S.N., Barrera, J.L., Mohar, A., Verastegui, E. and Zlotnik, A. (2001) Involvement of chemokine receptors in breast cancer metastasis. *Nature*, **410**, 50-56.

Mundy, G.R. (1997) Mechanisms of bone metastasis. *Cancer*, **80**, 1546-1556.

Mundy, G.R. (2002) Metastasis to bone: causes, consequences and therapeutic opportunities. *Nature Reviews Cancer*, **2**, 584-593.

Naumov, G.N., MacDonald, I.C., Chambers, A.F. and Groom, A.C. (2001) Solitary cancer cells as a possible source of tumour dormancy? *Seminars in Cancer Biology*, **11**, 271-276.

Nemeth, J.A., Harb, J.F., Barroso, U., Jr., He, Z., Grignon, D.J. and Cher, M.L. (1999) Severe combined immunodeficient-hu model of human prostate cancer metastasis to human bone. *Cancer Research*, **59**, 1987-1993.

Nemeth, J.A., Yousif, R., Herzog, M., Che, M., Upadhyay, J., Shekarriz, B., Bhagat, S., Mullins, C., Fridman, R. and Cher, M.L. (2002) Matrix metalloproteinase activity, bone matrix turnover, and tumor cell proliferation in prostate cancer bone metastasis. *Journal of the National Cancer Institute*, **94**, 17-25.

Nicolson, G.L. (1988) Cancer metastasis: tumor cell and host organ properties important in metastasis to specific secondary sites. *Biochimica Biophysica Acta*, **948**, 175-224.

Nishijima, Y., Uchida, K., Koiso, K. and Nemoto, R. (1992) Clinical significance of the vertebral vein in prostate cancer metastasis. *Advances in Experimental Medicine and Biology*, **324**, 93-100.

Nouri, A.M., Hussain, R.F., Dos Santos, A.V. and Oliver, R.T. (1996) Defective expression of adhesion molecules on human bladder tumour and human tumour cell lines *Urology Internationalis*, **56**, 6-12.

Okegawa, T., Li, Y., Pong, R.C. and Hsieh, J.T. (2002) Cell adhesion proteins as tumor suppressors. *Journal of Urology*, **167**, 1836-1843.

Orr, F.W., Sanchez-Sweatman, O.H., Kostenuik, P. and Singh, G. (1995) Tumor-bone interactions in skeletal metastasis. *Clinical Orthopaedics*, 19-33.

Paul, R., Ewing, C.M., Jarrard, D.F. and Isaacs, W.B. (1997) The cadherin cell-cell adhesion pathway in prostate cancer progression. *British Journal of Urology*, **79 Suppl 1**, 37-43.

Perl, A.K., Dahl, U., Wilgenbus, P., Cremer, H., Semb, H. and Christofori, G. (1999) Reduced expression of neural cell adhesion molecule induces metastatic dissemination of pancreatic beta tumor cells. *Nature Medicine*, **5**, 286-291.

Poste, G. and Fidler, I.J. (1980) The pathogenesis of cancer metastasis. *Nature*, **283**, 139-146.

Potter, K.M., Juacaba, S.F., Price, J.E. and Tarin, D. (1983) Observations on organ distribution of fluorescein-labelled tumour cells released intravascularly. *Invasion and Metastasis*, **3**, 221-233.

Quinn, J.M. and Athanasou, N.A. (1992) Tumour infiltrating macrophages are capable of bone resorption. *Journal of Cell Science*, **101 (Pt 3)**, 681-686.

Radinsky, R. (1995) Modulation of tumor cell gene expression and phenotype by the organ-specific metastatic environment. *Cancer Metastasis Reviews*, **14**, 323-338.

Riethmuller, G. and Klein, C.A. (2001) Early cancer cell dissemination and late metastatic relapse: clinical reflections and biological approaches to the dormancy problem in patients. *Seminars in Cancer Biology*, **11**, 307-311.

Rusciano, D., Welch, D. R., Burger, M. M. (2000) "Laboratory Techniques in Biochemistry and Molecular Biology; Cancer Metastasis" In *Vitro and In Vivo Experimental Approaches*. Edited by P.C. van der Vliet and S. Pillai. Elsevier Press.

Sawada, R., Tsuboi, S. and Fukuda, M. (1994) Differential E-selectin-dependent adhesion efficiency in sublines of a human colon cancer exhibiting distinct metastatic potentials. *Journal of Biological Chemistry*, **269**, 1425-1431.

Seraj, M.J., Harding, M.A., Gildea, J.J., Welch, D.R. and Theodorescu, D. (2000) The relationship of BRMS1 and RhoGDI2 gene expression to metastatic potential in lineage related human bladder cancer cell lines. *Clinical and Experimental Metastasis*, **18**, 519-525.

Shevde, L.A., Samant, R.S., Goldberg, S.F., Sikaneta, T., Alessandrini, A., Donahue, H.J., Mauger, D.T. and Welch, D.R. (2002) Suppression of human melanoma metastasis by the metastasis suppressor gene, BRMS1. *Experimental Cell Research*, **273**, 229-239.

Shevde, L.A., and Welch, D.R. (2003) Metastasis suppressor pathways- an evolving paradigm. *Cancer Letters*, In Press.

Sokoloff, M.H., Tso, C.L., Kaboo, R., Nelson, S., Ko, J., Dorey, F., Figlin, R.A., Pang, S., deKernion, J. and Belldegrun, A. (1996) Quantitative polymerase chain reaction does not improve preoperative prostate cancer staging: a clinicopathological molecular analysis of 121 patients. *Journal of Urology*, **156**, 1560-1566.

Steeg, P.S. (2003) Metastasis suppressors alter the signal transduction of cancer cells. *Nature Reviews Cancer*, **3**, 55-63.

Su, S.L., Boynton, A.L., Holmes, E.H., Elgamal, A.A. and Murphy, G.P. (2000) Detection of extraprostatic prostate cells utilizing reverse transcription-polymerase chain reaction. *Seminars in Surgical Oncology*, **18**, 17-28.

Thorban, S., Roder, J.D., Nekarda, H., Funk, A., Pantel, K. and Siewert, J.R. (1996) Disseminated epithelial tumor cells in bone marrow of patients with esophageal cancer: detection and prognostic significance. *World Journal of Surgery*, **20**, 567-572; discussion 572-563.

Trusolino, L. and Comoglio, P.M. (2002) Scatter-factor and semaphorin receptors: cell signalling for invasive growth. *Nature Reviews Cancer*, **2**, 289-300.

Varghese, H.J., Davidson, M.T., MacDonald, I.C., Wilson, S.M., Nadkarni, K.V., Groom, A.C. and Chambers, A.F. (2002) Activated ras regulates the proliferation/apoptosis balance and early survival of developing micrometastases. *Cancer Research*, **62**, 887-891.

Vleminckx, K., Vakaet, L., Jr., Mareel, M., Fiers, W. and van Roy, F. (1991) Genetic manipulation of E-cadherin expression by epithelial tumor cells reveals an invasion suppressor role. *Cell*, **66**, 107-119.

Weiss, L. (1990) Metastatic inefficiency. *Advances in Cancer Research*, **54**, 159-211.

Wood, D.P., Jr. and Banerjee, M. (1997) Presence of circulating prostate cells in the bone marrow of patients undergoing radical prostatectomy is predictive of disease-free survival. *Journal of Clinical Oncology*, **15**, 3451-3457.

Wood, D.P., Jr., Banks, E.R., Humphreys, S., McRoberts, J.W. and Rangnekar, V.M. (1994) Identification of bone marrow micrometastases in patients with prostate cancer. *Cancer*, **74**, 2533-2540.

Wood, D.P., Jr., Beaman, A., Banerjee, M., Powell, I., Pontes, E. and Cher, M.L. (1998) Effect of neoadjuvant androgen deprivation on circulating prostate cells in the bone marrow of men undergoing radical prostatectomy. *Clinical Cancer Research*, **4**, 2119-2123.

Xia, W., Unger, P., Miller, L., Nelson, J. and Gelman, I.H. (2001) The Src-suppressed C kinase substrate, SSeCKS, is a potential metastasis inhibitor in prostate cancer. *Cancer Research*, **61**, 5644-5651.

Yoshida, B.A., Dubauskas, Z., Chekmareva, M.A., Christiano, T.R., Stadler, W.M. and Rinker-Schaeffer, C.W. (1999) Mitogen-activated protein kinase kinase 4/stress-activated protein/Erk kinase 1 (MKK4/SEK1), a prostate cancer metastasis suppressor gene encoded by human chromosome 17. *Cancer Research*, **59**, 5483-5487.

Yoshida, B.A., Sokoloff, M.M., Welch, D.R. and Rinker-Schaeffer, C.W. (2000) Metastasis-suppressor genes: a review and perspective on an emerging field. *Journal of the National Cancer Institute*, **92**, 1717-1730.

Zetter, B.R. (1993) Adhesion molecules in tumor metastasis. *Seminars in Cancer Biology*, **4**, 219-229.

Zetter, B.R. (1998) Angiogenesis and tumor metastasis. *Annual Reviews in Medicine*, **49**, 407-424.

Chapter 2

CLINICAL ASPECTS OF BONE METASTASES IN PROSTATE CANCER

Shi-Ming Tu[1] and Sue-Hwa Lin[1,2]
[1]*Department of Genitourinary Medical Oncology and* [2]*Molecular Pathology, The University of Texas, M.D. Anderson Cancer Center, Houston, TX 77030*

INTRODUCTION

Bone is the second most common site of metastases in human cancer. At least two-thirds of the approximately 553,400 Americans who die from cancer each year have bone metastases (Greenlee et al., 2001). Prostate, breast, and lung cancers account for at least 80% of the skeletal metastases. Tumors arising in the prostate and breast are particularly prone to disseminate to bone; up to 85% of patients with these cancers have evidence of bone metastases at autopsy. Carcinomas of the lung, thyroid, and kidney also commonly spread to the bone (30-40%). However, tumors of the gastrointestinal tract rarely metastasize to the bone (5%) (Galasko, 1986).

Treatment of bone metastasis is a major challenge in oncology. Bone metastases from various cancers present different properties and patterns of progression, suggesting distinct biological mechanisms. This chapter will emphasize the clinical aspects of prostate cancer bone metastasis; however, bone metastases from other cancers will be mentioned when relevant.

INCIDENCE OF PROSTATE CANCER BONE METASTASIS

The incidence of bone metastases at the time of prostate cancer diagnosis has decreased markedly in recent years, from about 20% in 1986 to 11% in 1993 (Mettlin et al., 1996). In contrast, the incidence of clinically palpable prostate cancer increased from 19% to 49% during the same time period. This shifting trend is believed to be a result of increased awareness and early detection. The incidence of bone metastases in prostate cancer is influenced by the clinical stage, histologic grade, and prostate specific antigen (PSA) level (Table 1).

Table 1. Frequency of bone metastases according to clinical T stage, Gleason histologic grading, and serum PSA level

Newly diagnosed, untreated (Chybowski et al): overall 14%					
PSA (ng/ml)	<10 0%	10-20 1%	20-50 7%	50-100 38%	>100 71%
Clinical Stage	A1, A2 0% 19%	B1, B2 1%, 9%	C1, C2 29%, 54%		
Tumor Grade (Mayo	1 0%	2 6%	3 25%	4 38%	
After watchful waiting at 15 years (Johansson et al): overall 13%					
Tumor Grade (WHO)	I 8%	II 18%	III 67%		
After radical prostatectomy at 7 years (Pound et al): overall 5%					
Tumor Grade (Gleason	5-7 38%*	8-10 71%*			
After Radiotherapy at 5 years (Zagars et al): overall 6%					
PSA (ng/ml)	≤ 4 2%	4-20 5%	>20 16%		
Clinical Stage	T1-T2 1%	T3-T4 44%			
Tumor Grade (Gleason)	2-6 5%	7-10 9%			

For those patients who developed PSA recurrence

In men with newly diagnosed and untreated prostate cancer, the chance of diagnosing bone metastases was about 14% (Chybowski et al., 1991). The probability of having bone metastases increased with PSA levels. Similarly, higher clinical stage and tumor grade were associated with increased incidence of bone metastases. Interestingly, stage A2 tumors were more highly associated with bone metastases than stages B1/B2 tumors, consistent with the fact that stage A2 tumors were reported to be more aggressive than stage B tumors (Oesterling et al., 1987). The rate of developing bone metastases for prostate cancer patients who chose watchful waiting was about 13% (Johansson et al., 1997). The frequency of bone metastases was greater for higher-grade tumors (Chodak et al., 1994; Johansson et al., 1997). Recently, a randomized study showed that 27% of the patients who were conservatively managed developed bone metastases after 8 years of follow-up compared with 13% of the patients who underwent radical prostatectomy (Holmberg et al., 2002). According to Pound et al. (1999), about 5% of patients developed bone metastases after radical prostatectomy, with median time to bone metastases after PSA recurrence of 8 years. In another study of men who received radiation therapy to the prostate, about 6% of the patients developed bone metastases (Zagars et al., 1995). Again, the chance of developing bone metastases after radiation therapy increases with higher PSA level, clinical stage, and Gleason score before treatment.

SIGNIFICANCE OF BONE METASTASIS

The extent of osseous involvement is directly correlated with patient survival. The median survival of men with androgen-dependent prostate cancer and bone metastases is 30 to 35 months. The 2-year survival rate was 96% for men with fewer than 6 lesions, 76% for men with 6-20 lesions, 62% for men with more than 20 lesions, and 43% for men with a superscan on the bone scan (Soloway et al., 1988). After androgen ablation, a PSA increase was the first evidence of progression in 88% of patients (Newling et al., 1993). Progression in bone metastases occurred in 9% of patients before the PSA increase. After androgen ablation and with PSA recurrence, bone metastases became detectable within 2.5 years; among those patients who already had bone metastases, progression of bone metastases with appearance of new bone lesions usually occurred within a year. The median survival time of patients with advanced androgen-independent prostate cancer (AIPCa) and progressive bone metastases was 4 months (Pollen et al., 1981).

CLINICAL FEATURES

A hallmark of prostate cancer is osteoblastic metastasis: about 65% of the bone metastasis is osteoblastic, 23% is mixed, and 12% is osteolytic (Berruti et al., 2000). Because of osteosclerosis, certain complications of bone metastases, such as pathologic fracture and hypercalcemia, are less common in prostate cancer than expected. The axial skeleton is the earliest and most frequent site of osseous metastases in men with prostate cancer. The bones that are most frequently involved by metastases in prostate cancer are the ileum (83%), ischium (78%), lumbar sacral spine (71%), and thoracic spine (60%) (Byar, 1977). Hence, the distribution of bone metastases follows that of the hematopoietic marrow sites in the axial skeleton. Although some tumors do invade the bone itself, the principle site of bone metastases is the bone marrow rather than the bone tissue per se (Arguello et al., 1990).

Bone pain

Bone metastasis is the most common cause of pain from cancer. Bone pain is often poorly localized. It is usually described as a deep boring ache accompanied by intermittent stabbing discomfort. Initially, the pain is episodic and unrelated to activity. Eventually, the pain becomes continuous and unrelenting and may be aggravated by movement or changes in body position or posture. However, many metastatic foci detected by bone scintigraphy do not cause pain. Bone pains arise from either mechanical or chemical stimulation of pain receptors in the periosteum or endosteum. Mechanical stimulation may result from an expanding tumor mass, skeletal instability, formation of microfractures, or development of pathologic fractures. Chemical stimulation may arise from cytokine release from the tumors.

Bone metastases at different sites elicit distinct pain syndromes. For example, metastases at the base of the skull may cause head, neck, or facial pain. Lower cervical and upper thoracic spine lesions may elicit pain in the interscapular region. Rib fractures are a common cause of chest pains and may be pleuritic in nature. Involvement of nerve root causes radicular and neuropathic pain. Sometimes, referred pain from thoracic spine lesions may be difficult to distinguish from that of angina pectoris or peptic ulcer. Pain from a lower spine and pelvic lesion may be felt in the groin, thigh, or knee. In prostate cancer, lumbar plexus pains are uncommon.

Pathologic fractures

Despite the high frequency and increased incidence of bone metastases, pathologic fracture is relatively uncommon in men with prostate cancer. Pathologic fracture is likely to occur if more than 50% of the cortex is destroyed. Of the pathologic fractures involving the femur or humerus, 56% of the patients had breast cancer, 11% kidney cancer, and only 4% had prostate cancer (Habermann et al., 1982).

The overall incidence of bone fractures after lutenizing hormone-releasing hormone (LHRH) agonist treatment for prostate carcinoma was about 9% (Townsend et al., 1997). More than half of the cases were considered to be osteoporotic fractures, with only one of 11 cases attributed to a pathologic fracture. Similarly, the incidence of bone fracture after orchiectomy for prostate cancer was 26% (Daniell, 1997). Osteoporotic fracture was about 10 times more common than either pathologic fracture or major trauma. Using bone fracture as an endpoint for skeletal complication in prostate cancer can be misleading, since it is difficult to distinguish bone fractures resulting from cancer (i.e., pathologic) from those contributed by androgen ablative therapy (i.e., osteoporotic).

The possibility of a compression fracture needs to be considered for patients whose pain does not improve despite an apparent response (e.g., decline in the PSA) to various therapies (e.g., castration or chemotherapy). In such cases, the pain is usually localized and is frequently accompanied by a radicular component because of compression of spinal nerve roots. In contrast to pathologic fracture of the long bones or compression fracture of the spinal cord, rib fracture may be distressing but does not entail serious sequelae. Rib fractures tend to be localized by palpation. They can be treated with analgesics and a single fraction of radiotherapy.

Base of skull syndromes

Cranial nerve palsies commonly occur in prostate cancer metastases that involve the base of the skull (Ransom et al., 1990). Orbital and parasellar lesions may cause proptosis and/or diplopia. Sphenoid and ethmoid lesions may cause feelings of head fullness, nasal stuffiness, or diplopia. Jugular foramen involvement often produces dysfunction of the ninth, tenth, and eleventh cranial nerves, leading to hoarseness, dysarthria, and dysphagia. Middle fossa and foramen ovale involvement produces facial and trigeminal neuropathy, resulting in sensory loss in the tongue, face, and chin and in facial weakness. Clivial and hypoglossal nerve involvement causes dysphagia, dysarthria, and tongue weakness.

Patients with base of skull syndrome require prompt intervention with high-dose steroids and radiation therapy to prevent or reverse serious and permanent neurological disability. Although the median survival of patients with advanced AIPCa and base of skull syndrome is estimated to be 4-5 months, appropriate treatments may alleviate morbid symptoms and improve quality of life.

Spinal cord compression

The most serious complication of bone metastases is secondary epidural compression of the spinal cord or cauda equina. This constitutes a medical emergency and requires prompt recognition and immediate treatment. Neurologic recovery is markedly diminished if the spinal compression is not relieved within 24-48 hours. Patients who complain of increasing and intractable back pain must be immediately evaluated for this complication. Early cord compression is heralded by increasing local spinal and radicular pain followed by neurologic compromise, such as lower extremity weakness, sensory loss, and autonomic dysfunction as manifested by bladder or bowel incontinence.

Prostate cancer ranks third (after breast and lung cancers) in producing spinal cord compression (Gilbert et al., 1978). The importance of early diagnosis and treatment and its favorable impact on eventual clinical outcome is highlighted by a study of patients with breast cancer (Hill et al., 1993). Of those patients who were ambulatory before treatment, 96% preserved the ability to walk. However, of those who were unable to walk, only 45% regained ambulation. Radiotherapy and surgery were equally effective in accomplishing this objective, and median survival following cord compression was 4 months. The most important predictor of survival was the ability to ambulate after treatment.

RADIOGRAPHIC EVALUATION OF BONE METASTASIS

Plain radiography

Prostate cancer typically develops osteoblastic metastases that can be detected on plain radiographs. The osteoblastic component represents the reaction of bone to the metastatic cancer. The amount and pattern of sclerosis indicate the growth rate of the tumor: the denser the pattern, the slower the growth rate. If the growth rate is fast, a mixed dense and lytic pattern is seen. Therefore, increasing sclerosis (especially during therapy) may not represent progression of metastasis but may be a sign of repair.

Given the low sensitivity of plain radiography, bone survey is not routinely ordered for patients with asymptomatic prostate cancer. However, plain radiography can help evaluate a localized complaint or focal abnormality detected on a screening bone scintigraph. Metastasis to the distal extremities (e.g, radius, tibia, carpal or tarsal bones, and terminal phalanges) is unusual for prostate carcinoma. Bronchogenic or renal cell carcinomas are more likely origins of such metastases. In the case of a solitary osseous abnormality in an atypical site (e.g., skull, scapula), it may be difficult to distinguish prostate cancer from other malignant or benign entities. A biopsy is needed to confirm the nature of these lesions.

Bone scintigraphy

Bone scanning using technetium-99m (^{99m}Tc)-labeled methylene diphosphonate (MDP) is the most widely used method to screen and diagnose osseous metastases in prostate cancer. In general, bone scans will detect metastatic lesions between 2 to 18 months before they become apparent on plain radiographs (Galasko, 1986). Even though bone scan is more sensitive than plain radiography, the specificity is not sufficiently high because positive scans may occur in metabolically hyperactive bones, including sites of inflammation, healing fractures, osteoarthritis, and Paget's disease. Hence, for patients with known cancer and solitary foci, only 50% of the lesions represent metastases (Rosenthal, 1997). The nature of such lesions needs to be evaluated by plain radiography.

Serum PSA level can be used to select asymptomatic patients who may benefit from a staging bone scan. Since the probability of bone metastases for patients whose serum PSA is $\leq$20 ng/ml is very low ($\leq$1%), performing a bone scan in these patients seems not warranted (Chybowski et al., 1991). A bone scan may provide early diagnosis of bone metastasis for men whose PSA is >20 ng/ml, because the probability of bone metastases for this group of patients is greater (see Table 1). However, for patients who have progressed (with a rising PSA) after local therapy (i.e., radiotherapy, radical prostatectomy) or hormonal ablative therapy, the usefulness of PSA levels in selecting patients for bone scan is not known.

Uptake of (^{99m}Tc)MDP in bone scanning is dependent on local osteoblastic activity. Hence, purely osteolytic diseases without any significant osteoblastic activity (e.g., multiple myeloma) may not be detected by bone scintigraphy. When skeletal metastasis is extensive, a bone scan may appear "normal" at first glance because the lesions have become confluent. On such a "superscan," the soft tissues, including the kidneys, are inconspicuous or invisible because of the increased uptake of (^{99m}Tc)MDP into the skeleton. During the course of disease, the development of new lesions indicates progression of bone metastases. However, the development of new lesions on a bone scan within 6 months of treatment may indicate a flare phenomenon from an osteoblast response as a result of healing. A flare response may indicate improved clinical outcome. The mean interval from positivity on bone scan to overt symptoms of bone metastases is 6 months (Merrick et al., 1985).

Computed tomography (CT) and magnetic resonance imaging (MRI)

CT is useful for the evaluation of "hot" spots on a bone scan (and a normal plain radiograph) to confirm the presence of metastatic or other disease. MRI accurately images the medullary (marrow) component of the bone and is therefore ideal for the early detection of bone metastases. The ability of MRI to detect metastases is due to the high signal intensity (brightness) of the mostly fatty content of the normal marrow. The increased cellularity of an infiltrating metastasis has higher water content and will appear as a darker area on T1-weighted images and often has a rim (a halo sign) around the bright signal on T2-weighted images. However, MRI results should be confirmed with other studies, because infection, infarction, and other entities can also cause a decreased signal.

Positron emission tomography (PET)

Currently, there is no established role for the use of PET in the detection of bone metastases. Fluorodeoxyglucose (FDG)-PET detects prostate cancer metastases to the bone with moderate sensitivity (65%) and high specificity (98%) (Shrieve et al., 1996) and may helpdifferentiate bone metastases from Paget's disease and other benign bone lesions (Dehdashti et al., 1996).

Radiography for treatment evaluation

Accurate radiographic assessment of responses in bone metastases is difficult. Osteoblastic lesions often remain osteosclerotic even after a positive response to therapy. Healing response of an osteolytic or mixed lesion may manifest as new sclerotic foci, which is considered to be a sign of progression for patients who are not receiving or responding to treatment. In addition, an osteosclerotic response of lytic lesions may take 3 to 6 months to become evident on a plain radiograph after the start of therapy.

Laboratory Evaluation of Bone Metastasis

Because of the limitations of radiographic methods, markers of bone turnover are increasingly being used to determine the presence and extent of bone metastases as well as to monitor treatment response or progression. Laboratory evaluation for the detection of bone disease includes measurement of serum calcium, phosphorus, and alkaline phosphatase levels. However, none of these tests are specific for osseous metastases. Hypercalcemia is rare and occurs in less than 2% of men with prostate cancer (Smith et al., 1992). A majority of these cases are associated with the presence of neuroendocrine or small cell carcinoma in the tumor.

Other laboratory tests monitor the rate of formation or degradation of the bone matrix. This is determined by measuring specific enzymatic activity of bone-forming cells (osteoblasts) or bone-resorbing cells (osteoclasts) or by measuring bone matrix components released into the circulation during bone formation or degradation.

Markers of bone formation

Proteins produced by osteoblasts at different stages of development and differentiation are potential markers for bone formation. Serum type I collagen C-terminal propeptide (PICP) bone-specific alkaline phosphatase (BAP), and osteocalcin are produced by osteoblasts during early proliferation, matrix maturation, and late bone formation, respectively. Among these, BAP is the most sensitive and specific marker. Several studies have shown that there is a significant correlation between BAP and the presence of bone metastases and the extent of skeletal involvement (Maeda et al., 1997). Both osteocalcin and PICP are not sensitive enough for the early detection of bone metastases. In addition, osteocalcin does not correlate well with the extent of bone metastases.

Markers of bone degradation

N-Telopeptide (NTX) and deoxypyridinoline (DPD), both breakdown products from collagen cross-links, may reflect activity of bone degradation. Costa et al. (2002) and Demers et al. (1995) reported that NTX and DPD were the best predictors for the presence of bone metastases among collagen cross-links. Although bone metastases from prostate cancer are mainly osteoblastic, it was reported that the level of collagen cross-links in urine correlated with the extent of bone metastases better than did serum PSA level (Ikeda et al., 1996; Takeuchi et al., 1996; Maeda et al., 1997). Serial urinary DPD levels correlated with clinical progression (PSA increase) of prostate cancer before detection of new bone lesions by bone scintigraphy (Takeuchi et al., 1996). Serial urinary DPD also correlated with response to treatment in prostate cancer (Ikeda et al., 1996). There are reports that the bone markers have prognostic significance for skeletal-related events (Berruti et al., 2000) or survival (Kylmala et al., 1993).

BIOLOGY OF BONE METASTASES

Unlike other cancer types, prostate cancer typically spreads to the bone and not other organ sites. Among prostate cancer patients with metastasis, about two thirds have only bone metastases. The predominantly axial distribution of bone metastasis in prostate cancer led Batson (1940) to postulate that prostate cancer cells are preferentially deposited in bone through a hemodynamic mechanism. Recently, Paget's "seed-and-soil" theory has gained favor to account for the biological basis of bone tropism in prostate cancer. Bone-homing chemokines produced by bone cells induce prostate cancer cells to metastasize to the bone and promote their growth and survival within the bone (Taichman et al., 2002). The osteomimetic theory (Koeneman et al., 1999) hypothesized that the prostate cancer ("seed") acquires an "osteoblastic" phenotype, which allows it to thrive in the bone environment ("soil").

Bone-epithelial interaction

Paracrine interaction between tumor and bone stromal cells contributes to the development of osteoblastic metastases in prostate cancer (Chung, 1993; Chung, 1995; Olumi et al., 1999; Keller et al., 2001). The paracrine interaction between prostate cancer and bone stromal cells is expected to be different and distinct from the interaction between prostate cancer and lymph node stromal cells. This may account for the fact that bone metastasis compared with lymph node metastasis has a clinically more lethal and therapeutically resistant phenotype. The paracrine interaction between prostate cancer and bone stromal cells may also determine whether micrometastases will eventually become established as bone metastases (Wood et al., 1997). Paracrine factors induce proliferation of both tumor cells and osteoblasts, leading to an osteosclerotic reaction in the bone. Putative paracrine factors with osteoblast-stimulating activity include insulin-like growth factor-1 (IGF-1), transforming growth factor-β, and endothelin-1 (ET-1) (Glotzman, 1997). However, the precise identity of the osteoblastic-stimulating factors remains unknown.

Osteoclastogenesis versus osteoblast-stimulating factors

Since osteoblast function is influenced by testosterone (Colvard et al., 1989), there is a decrease in osteoblastic activity in both the tumor-free bone and within the bone metastases after androgen ablative therapy. Androgen ablation also promotes osteoclastic activity and increases the level of certain cytokines (such as interleukin-6;IL-6) that facilitate osteoporosis (Jilka et al., 1992). It remains unclear whether the osteoclastogenetic effects of androgen ablation render a favorable environment for bone metastases and promote the development of bone metastases in prostate cancer (Thalmann et al., 1994).

Despite the osteoblastic phenotype of prostate cancer bone metastases, biochemical and histomorphological analyses indicated that significant osteoclastic activity also takes place in these metastases (Percival et al., 1987; Clarke et al., 1992; Taube et al., 1994). The lytic component in a predominance of osteosclerotic metastases in prostate cancer can also be detected by CT (Coleman, 1991). In fact, Vinholes et al. (1997) reported that the level of bone resorption markers is higher for patients with prostate cancer than for patients with breast and other cancers that produce predominantly lytic bone metastases. However, the basic mechanism underlying the development of osteoblastic metastases is still unknown, as is the role of bone resorption in the midst of osteosclerosis in prostate cancer.

Percival et al. (1987) reported that bone resorption is increased in the area of bone not directly involved with osseous metastases and actually occurs at a higher rate in the tumor-free bone than in the tumor-infiltrated bone. It has been postulated that there are soluble factors that induce osteoblast proliferation in vicinity of the tumor-infiltrated bone (Jacobs et al., 1979; Simpson et al., 1985; Koutsilieris et al., 1987). Thus, it is likely that the predominant osteoblastic growth with osteolytic components in prostate cancer bone metastasis arises from soluble factors that induce a pervasive bone resorptive activity in both the tumor-free and tumor-infiltrated bones and the osteoblast-stimulating factors in the tumor-infiltrated bone.

According to Galasko (1976), osteoclasts are initially involved in the bone resorption of osseous metastases. Subsequently, the osteoclasts become depleted at the sites of bone metastases and the tumor cells become predominantly and directly involved in bone resorption. Hence, following bisphosphonate treatment, bone erosion is suppressed in tumor-free bone but is maintained in areas of tumor infiltration, suggesting that bone resorption is directly mediated by tumor (Clarke et al., 1992). Similarly, collagen cross-link levels increased after the first month of bisphosphonate treatment despite sustained suppression of osteoclastic activity (for at least 6 months), indicating that the tumor is directly involved in bone resorption (Kylmala et al., 1993; Taube et al., 1994). Therefore, the increased levels of collagen cross-link observed in osteoblastic metastases are derived from the bone resorptive activity of both osteoclasts and prostate cancer cells.

THERAPY OF BONE METASTASIS

Radiation therapy

Radiation is an effective treatment for bone metastases. Goals of treatment include pain relief, improved activity, and control of local tumor growth. Effective treatment substantially reduces or eliminates the need for narcotic use. For those patients with a solitary site of symptomatic bone metastasis, radiation therapy may render them disease-free and symptom-free for a prolonged period. For patients with extensive, multifocal disease, systemic treatments such as hormonal therapy, chemotherapy, or radioisotope use may be preferable.

Approximately 80% of patients receiving radiation therapy for painful bone metastases will experience partial pain relief, and at least 25% will have complete relief (Gaze et al., 1997). A significantly higher percentage of patients with metastases from prostate (and breast) cancer achieved complete pain relief compared with patients with lung cancer and other primaries (Tong et al., 1982). Most patients begin to experience some pain relief 10 to 14 days after start of treatment, 70% experience pain relief by 2 weeks after completion of treatment, and 90% have relief within 1 to 3 months. The time to achieve pain relief following treatment tends to be longer with slowly proliferating tumors, such as prostate cancer. The median duration of pain relief after treatment is 3 months. Seventy percent of patients did not develop recurrent pain in the treatment area. Interestingly, the bone metastases did not recur in the previously irradiated field of some prostate cancer patients (Jacobsson et al., 1991).

For patients with advanced AIPCa and limited life expectancy, the goal is to deliver effective treatment with minimal toxicity and over the shortest duration of time. One study suggested that protracted fractionation schemes might be more efficacious (Blitzer, 1985). However, prospective randomized controlled studies have failed to show any significant advantage for more prolonged and higher-dose radiation schedules (Gaze et al., 1997; Nielsen et al., 1998).

Surgery

In general, the presence of a pathologic fracture, impending fracture, or painful lesion in a long bone despite radiotherapy should be considered for surgical intervention. The goals of surgery include palliation of pain and improvement of mobility and function. Surgery should be performed with the intent to provide benefit that will outlast the patient's anticipated survival.

An important objective in the management of bone metastases is prophylactic surgical fixation of a bone deemed to be at high risk of fracture. There is greater difficulty and increased morbidity in stabilizing an established fracture compared with an impending fracture. Factors that predict pathologic fracture include intractable pain aggravated by function and lytic lesions greater than two-thirds of the diameter of the involved long bone. Impending spinal cord compression after prior radiotherapy at the same site of disease is also an indication for surgical intervention. For compression fractures of the spine, vertebroplasty provides immediate pain control and spinal stability.

Androgen ablation

The discovery over a half century ago that prostate cancer is dependent on certain hormonal factors provided the foundation for an effective treatment for advanced prostate cancer. Androgen ablative therapy is more effective in inducing regression of the primary tumor and soft tissue metastases than in inducing regression of bone metastases. Hence, 84% of patients with local and soft tissue diseases responded to androgen ablation (37% had a complete response), compared with only 27% of patients with bone metastases (15% had a complete remission) (Goldenberg et al., 1988). The relapse rate after androgen ablative therapy was far greater in the bone (85%) than in non-skeletal sites (23%) (Goldenberg et al., 1988).

The most widely used approach to achieve androgen ablation is the use of LHRH agonists (e.g., leuprolide, goserelin) and bilateral orchiectomy. During the first 2 weeks of treatment, LHRH agonist causes a surge in testosterone levels that can exacerbate bone pains and impending cord compression. This can be prevented by the combined use of an anti-androgen (e.g., flutamide, bicalutamide, nilutamide), which blocks the effect of testosterone on the prostate cancer cells. In an emergent situation when immediate castration is needed (impending cord compression, base of skull syndrome, or disseminated intravascular coagulation), ketoconazole can be used without causing a testosterone surge (Lowe et al., 1987). Ketoconazole inhibits testicular and adrenal steroid synthesis by blocking cytochrome p-450-dependent 14-demethylation, thereby preventing conversion of lanosterol to cholesterol. Serum testosterone begins to decline within 30 minutes after treatment and reaches a 90% reduction by 48 hours (Trachtenberg et al., 1983).

Estrogen

Unlike LHRH agonists and orchiectomy, estrogen suppresses androgen levels without causing bone loss and decreased bone mineral density. Consequently, estrogen may potentially retard the development of bone metastases by reducing osteoclastogenesis. Estrogen may also provide a superior clinical outcome by affecting both androgen-dependent and -independent cells (Robertson et al., 1996). Despite the well-known risk for thromboembolic complications, some studies suggested improved survival for patients with prostate cancer who received estrogens compared with orchiectomy and LHRH agonist treatments (Haapiainen et al., 1986; Osborne et al., 1990). It is of interest that certain selective estrogen receptor modulators (SERM) may be developed for their androgen suppressive effect while preserving their favorable bone effects without the cardiovascular risks.

Radioisotope

Bone-targeted radiotherapy is suitable for multifocal bone pain. Response to targeted radiotherapy is dependent on osteoblastic activity in the bone. Consequently, radioisotopes may not alleviate the bone pain caused by osteolytic metastases. Repeated and combination treatments with chemotherapy can be given in appropriate cases.

Strontium-89 (^{89}Sr) and samarium-153 (^{153}Sm) are radioisotopes approved by the Food and Drug Administration for the treatment of osteoblastic bone metastases. [89]Sr is a pure beta emitter with a long half-life (50.5 days) and a short range of penetrance in bone (3-8 mm). It is incorporated into the mineral structure of the bone by virtue of its similarity to calcium. [89]Sr provides an overall response rate of about 75% and duration of response of 6 months. Although 33% of patients who received ^{89}Sr had a complete pain relief, radiographic improvement on the bone scan or biochemical decrease of serum alkaline phosphastase or PSA levels was uncommon. [89]Sr can delay progression of bone pain as measured by sites of new pain or requirement for radiotherapy (Porter et al., 1993). Fewer patients developed new painful sites after ^{89}Sr treatment compared with local or hemibody radiation therapy (Quilty et al., 1994). In a selected group of patients with advanced AIPCa who responded to induction chemotherapy and received consolidation ^{89}Sr plus doxorubicin, there was improved time to progression and overall survival (Tu et al., 2001) (Figure 1). The results suggest for the first time that bone-targeted therapy may provide a survival advantage even in the presence of systemic metastasis.

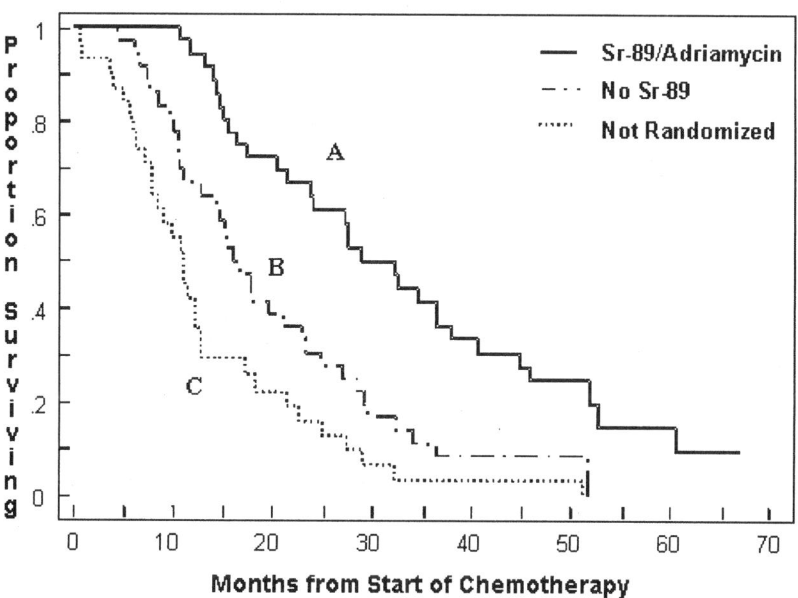

Figure 1. Survival curve of men with androgen-independent prostate cancer who responded to induction chemotherapy followed by consolidation therapy consisting of 6 weekly treatments of doxorubicin with (A) or without (B) one dose of strontium-89 and compared with patients who were not randomized (C).

[153]Sm has a half-life of 46.8 hours. It actively seeks out bone invaded by tumor by bridging the hydroxyapatite. [153]Sm provided some pain relief in up to 72% of patients and complete pain relief in 31% of patients at 4 weeks after treatment. Onset of pain relief was noted between 1 and 2 weeks after treatment began. Pain relief lasted 16 weeks in 43% of the patients (Serafini et al., 1998).

Bisphosphonate

The value of bisphosphonate in the treatment of osteolytic metastases is well established (Berenson et al., 1996; Hortobagyi et al., 1996). However, the role of bisphosphonates in the treatment of osteoblastic metastases is still unresolved. A phase III trial using pamidronate for the treatment of metastatic prostate cancer did not reduce the incidence of skeletal-related events (Lipton et al., 2002). Patients with prostate cancer and bone metastases who received zoledronic acid had a delay in the median time to first skeletal event (pathologic and vertebral fractures). However, time to tumor progression or overall survival was not increased (Saad et al., 2002).

Targeted Therapies

Therapies targeting molecules and their signal transduction mechanisms that participate in the metastatic progression in bone should provide specificity and efficacy and result in less side effects. Several factors that are implicated in metastatic progression of prostate cancer in bone have been considered as targets for therapy.

Endothelin-1 (ET-1)

ET is a potent vasoconstrictor produced by prostate cancer cells and may mediate osteoblastic response of bone to prostate cancer metastases. The plasma ET-1 level is significantly elevated in men with metastatic prostate cancer (Nelson et al., 1995). Recently, treatment using an ET-1 antagonist (Atrasentan) has been shown to delay PSA progression in patients with AIPCa (Nelson et al., 2001).

Insulin like growth factor (IGF-1) and insulin-like growth factor binding protein-3 (IGFBP-3) are potential targets in the treatment of advanced prostate cancer with bone metastases. IGF-1 is increased and IGFBP-3 decreased in the blood of patients with prostate cancer and bone metastases (Shariat et al., 2002). Suramin (Sartor et al., 1994) and vitamin D-3 analogues (Boyle et al., 2001) may lower IGF-1 production or induce IGFBP-3 expression. Dexamethasone decreases the bioavailability of IGF-1 at the site of bone metastases by inhibiting urokinase plaminogen activator expression and decreasing the cleavage of IGFBP-3 by urokinase plaminogen kinase (Koutsilieris et al., 1997). Dexamethasone provides a PSA response rate of 79% and radiographic regression rate of 35% in patients with AIPCa (Storlie et al., 1995).

Platelet-Derived Growth Factors (PDGFs)—The receptor for PDGFs, i.e., PDGF-α, is the most consistently expressed receptor protein tyrosine kinase in the bone metastases of patients with AIPCa (Chott et al., 1999). Recently, PDGF has become an attractive target for the treatment of bone metastases in prostate cancer, in part because of the availability of novel agents (such as suramin and imanitib) that may antagonize its actions or effects. However, SU101, a potent and specific PDGF-α and -β inhibitor, provided a PSA or measurable response in only 8% of patients who received the treatment (Ko et al., 2001).

Receptor activator of NFkB ligand (RANKL)--The RANK axis provides potential novel targets for osteoclast inhibition (Keller et al., 2001). RANKL is a key factor in osteoclast formation and acts by way of its receptor RANK. Osteoprotegerin (OPG) is an inhibitory decoy receptor that competes for RANKL and attenuates osteoclast functions. Hence, OPG analogues may be useful in the treatment of the osteolytic metastases or the bone resorptive component of osteoblastic metastases. Drugs (e.g., the proteosome inhibitor PS-341) that affect targets downstream of the RANKL/RANK pathway (i.e., NFkB) may also be effective in the treatment of osteolytic bone diseases (Richardson et al., 2002). The clinical value of OPG analogues and PS-341 in the treatment of prostate cancer bone metastases requires further investigation.

Considering the heterogeneity of prostate cancer and the redundancies of multiple intricate pathways that may be involved in bone metastases, it is likely that targeting a single factor may not be sufficient to halt the metastatic progression of prostate cancer in bone. Instead, combination treatments designed to affect disparate targets may improve clinical results. Indeed, strategies to enhance the effects of IGF-1 lowering agents (Xie et al., 1999) with chemotherapy, e.g., calcitriol with docetaxel (Beer et al., 2003), have already been implemented. Combining PDGF antagonists with cytotoxic agents or with alternative targeting agents may also increase its therapeutic efficacy. In many ways, suramin is a paradigm of a combination therapy because it inhibits the binding of multiple growth factors to their respective receptors on the cancer cell. Unfortunately, studies using suramin alone (Small et al., 2000) or combining suramin with chemotherapy have shown only modest clinical benefits (Tu et al., 1998).

The unique relationship between prostate cancer and bone metastasis suggests that bone-targeted therapy will play a pivotal role in a new breakthrough for prostate cancer treatment. An important clinical challenge is to devise strategies to identify pertinent targets and to devise methods to validate potential targets in the proper clinical context so that they can be used for therapeutic purposes. Elucidation of the basic mechanism of bone metastasis will expedite the discovery of pertinent targets and improve the current treatment of bone metastases in prostate and other cancers.

REFERENCES

Arguello, F., Baggs, R.B. Duerst, R.E., et al. (1990) Pathogenesis of vertebral metastases and epidural spinal cord compression. *Cancer*, **65**, 98-106.

Batson, O.V. (1940) The function of the vertebral veins and their role in the spread of metastasis. *Annals of Surgery*, **112**, 138-139.

Beer, T.M., Eilers, K.M., Garzotto, M., Egorin, M.J., Lowe, B.A. and Henner, W.D. (2003) Weekly high-dose calcitriol and docetaxel in metastatic androgen-independent prostate cancer. *Journal of Clinical Oncology*, **21**, 123-128.

Berenson, J.R., Lichtenstein, A., Porter, L., Dimopoulos, M.A., Bordoni, R., George, S., Lipton, A., Keller, A., Ballester, O., Kovacs, M.J., Blacklock, H.A., Bell, R., Simeone, J., Reitsma, D.J., Heffernan, M., Seaman, J. and Knight, R.D. (1996) Efficacy of pamidronate in reducing skeletal events in patients with advanced multiple myeloma. *New England Journal of Medicine*, **334**, 488-493.

Berruti, A., Dogliotti, L., Bitossi, R., Fasolis, G., Gorzegno, G., Bellina, M., Torta, M., Porpiglia, F., Fontana, D. and Angeli, A. (2000) Incidence of skeletal complications in patients with bone metastatic prostate cancer and hormone refractory disease: predictive role of bone resorption and formation markers evaluated at baseline. *Journal of Urology*, **164**, 1248-1253.

Blitzer, P.H. (1985) Reanalysis of the RTOG study of the palliation of symptomatic osseous metastasis. *Cancer*, **55**, 1468-1472.

Boyle, B.J., Zhao, X.-Y., Cohen, P. and Feldman, D. (2001) Insulin-like growth factor binding protein-3 mediates 1α, 25-dihydroxyvitamin D_3 growth inhibition in the LNCaP prostate cancer cell line through p21/WAF1. *Journal of Urology*, **165**, 1319-1324.

Byar, D.P. (1977). *VACURG studies on prostate cancer and its treatment*. Philadelphia, Lea and Febiger.

Chodak, G.W., Thisted, R.A., Gerber, G.S., Johansson, J.E., Adolfsson, J., Jones, G.W., Chisholm, G.D., Moskovitz, B., Livne, P.M. and Warner, J. (1994) Results of conservative management of clinically localized prostate cancer. *New England Journal of Medicine*, **330**, 242-248.

Chott, A., Sun, Z., Morganstern, D., Pan, J., Li, T., Susani, M., Mosberger, I., Upton, M.P., Bubley, G.J. and Balk, S.P. (1999) Tyrosine kinases expressed in vivo by human prostate cancer bone marrow metastases and loss of the type I insulin-like growth factor receptor. *American Journal of Pathology*, **155**, 1271-1279.

Chung, L., W.K. (1993) Implications of stromal-epithelial interaction in human prostate cancer growth, progression and differentiation. *Seminars in Cancer Biology*, **4**, 183-192.

Chung, L. W.K. (1995) The role of stromal-epithelial interaction in normal and malignant growth. *Cancer Surveys*, **23**, 33-42.

Chybowski, F.M., Keller, J.J.L. and Bergstrahl, E.J. (1991) Predicting radionuclide bone scan findings in patients with newly diagnosed, untreated prostate cancer: prostate specific antigen is superior to all other clinical parameters. *Journal d Urologie*, **145**, 313-318.

Clarke, N.W., McClure, J. and George, N.J.R. (1992) Disodium pamidronate identifies differential osteoclastic bone resorption in metastatic prostate cancer. *British Journal of Urology*, **69**, 64-70.

Coleman, R.E. (1991). *Bone metastases: Diagnosis and Treatment*. London, Springer-Verlag.

Colvard, D.S., Eriksen, E.F., Keeting, P.E., Wilson, E.M., Lubahn, D.B., French, D.B., Riggs, B.L. Spelsberg, T.C. (1989) Identification of androgen receptors in normal human osteoblast-like cells. *Proceedings of National Academy of Sciences USA*, **86**, 854-857.

Costa, L., Demers, L.M., Gouveia-Oliveira, A., Schaller, J., Costa, E.B., de Moura, M.C. and Lipton, A. (2002) Prospective evaluation of the peptide-bound collagen type I cross-links N-telopeptide and C-telopeptide in predicting bone metastases status. *Journal of Clinical Oncology*, **20**, 850-856.

Daniell, H.W. (1997) Osteoporosis after orchiectomy for prostate cancer. *Journal of Urology*, **157**, 439-444.

Dehdashti, F., Siegel, B.A., Griffeth, L.K., Fusselman, M.J., Trask, D.D., McGuire, A.H. and McGuire, D.J. (1996) Benign versus malignant intraosseous lesions: discrimination by means of PET with 2-[F-18]fluoro-2-deoxy-D-glucose. *Radiology*, **200**, 243-247.

Demers, L.M., Costa, L., Chinchilli, V.M., Gaydos, L., Curley, E. and Lipton, A. (1995) Biochemical markers of bone turnover in patients with metastatic bone disease. *Clinical Chemistry*, **41**, 1489-1494.

Galasko, C.S. (1986b) Skeletal metastases. *Clinical Orthopaedics Related Research*, **210**, 18-30.

Galasko, C.S.B. (1976) Mechanisms of bone destruction in the development of skeletal metastases. *Nature*, **263**, 507-508.

Galasko, C.S.B. (1986a). *Incidence and distribution of skeletal metastases*. Cambridge, Butterworths Co.

Gaze, M.N., Kelly, C.G., Kerr, G.R., Cull, A., Cowie, V.J., Gregor, A., Howard, G.C.W. and Rodger, A. (1997) Pain relief and quality of life following radiotherapy for bone metastases: a randomised trial of two fraction schedules. *Radiotherapy and Oncology*, **45**, 109-116.

Gilbert, R.W., Kim, J.H. and Posner, J.B. (1978) Epidural spinal cord compression from metastatic tumor: diagnosis and treatment. *Annals of Neurology*, **3**, 40-51.

Glotzman, D. (1997) Mechanisms of the development of osteoblastic metastasis. *Cancer* [suppl], **80**, 1581-1587.

Goldenberg, S.L., Bruchovsky, N., Rennie, P.S. and Coppin, C.M. (1988) The combination of cyproterone acetate and low dose diethylstilbestrol in the treatment of advanced prostatic carcinoma. *Journal of Urology*, **140**, 1460-1465.

Greenlee, R.T., Hill-Harmon, M.B., Murray, T. and Thun, M. (2001) Cancer statistics, 2001. *CA: A Cancer Journal for Clinicians*, **51**, 15-36.

Haapiainen, R., Rannikko, S. and Alfthan, O. (1986) Comaprison of primary orchiectomy with oestrogen therapy in advanced prostatic cancer. *British Journal of Urology*, **58**, 528-533.

Habermann, E.T., Sachs, R., Stern, R.E., Hirsh, D.M. and Anderson, W.J.J. (1982) The pathology and treatment of metastatic disease of the femur. *Clinical Orthopaedics and Related Research*, **169**, 70-82.

Hill, M.E., Richards, M.A., Gregory, W.M., Smith, P. and Rubens, R.D. (1993) Spinal cord compression in breast cancer: a review of 70 cases. *British Journal of Cancer*, **68**, 969-973.

Holmberg, L., Bill-Axelson, A., Helgesen, F., Salo, J.O., Folmerz, P., Haggman, M. andersson, S.-O., Spangberg, A., Busch, C., Nordling, S., Palmgren, J., Adami, H.O., Johansson, J.E. and Norlen, B.J. (2002) A randomized trial comparing radical prostatectomy with watchful waiting in early prostate cancer. *New England Journal of Medicine*, **347**, 781-789.

Hortobagyi, G.N., Theriault, R.L., Porter, L., Blayney, D., Lipton, A., Sinoff, C., Wheeler, H., Simeone, J.F., Seaman, J. and Knight, R. D. (1996) Efficacy of pamidronate in reducing skeletal complications in patients with breast cancer and lytic bone metastases. *New England Journal of Medicine*, **335**, 1785-1791.

Ikeda, I., Miura, T. and Kondo, I. (1996) Pyridinium cross-links as urinary markers of bone metastasesnin patients with prostate cancer. *British Journal of Urology*, **77**, 102-106.

Jacobs, S.C., Pikna, D. and Lawson, R.K. (1979) Prostatic osteoblastic factor. *Investigational Urology*, **17**, 195-198.

Jacobsson, H. Naslund, I. (1991) Reduced incidence of bone metastases in irradiated areas after external radiation therapy of prostatic carcinoma. *International Journal of Radation Oncology Biological Physics*, **20**, 1297-1303.

Jilka, R.L., Hangoc, G., Girasole, G., Passeri, G., Williams, D. C., Abrams, J.S., Boyce, B., Broxmeyer, H. and Manolagas, S.C. (1992) Increased osteoclast development after estrogen loss: mediation by interleukin-6. *Science,* **257**, 88-91.

Johansson, J.-E., Holmberg, L., Johansson, S., Bergstrom, R. and Adami, H.-O. (1997) Fifteen-year survival in prostate cancer: a prospective, population-based study in Sweden. *Journal of the American Medical Association*, **277**, 467-471.

Keller, E.T., Zhang, J., Cooper, C.R., Smith, P.C., McCauley, L.K., Pienta, K.J. and Taichman, R. S. (2001) Prostate carcinoma skeletal metastases: cross-talk between tumor and bone. *Cancer and Metastasis Reviews*, **20**, 333-349.

Ko, Y,-J., Small, E.J., Kabbinavar, F., Chachoua, A., Taneja, S., Reese, D., DePaoli, A., Hannah, A., Balk, S.P. and Bubley G. J. (2001) A multi-institutional phase II study of SU101, a platelet-derived growth factor receptor inhibitor, for patients with hormone-refractory prostate cancer. *Clinical Cancer Research*, **7**, 800-805.

Koeneman, K.S., Yeung, F. and Chung, L.W.K. (1999) Osteomimetic properties of prostate cancer cells: a hypothesis supporting the predilection of prostate cancer metastasis and growth in the bone environment. *Prostate*, **39**, 246-261.

Koutsilieris, M., Rabbini, S.A., Bennett, H.P.J. and Goltzman, D. (1987) Characteristics of prostate-derived growth factors for cells of the osteoblast phenotype. *Journal of Clinical Investigation,* **80**, 941-946.

Koutsilieris, M., Reyes-Moreno, C., Sourla, A., Dimitriadou, V. and Choki, I. (1997) Growth factors mediate glucocorticoid receptor function and dexamethasone-induced regression of osteoblastic lesions in hormone refractory prostate cancer. *Anticancer Research*, **17**, 1461-1465.

Kylmala, T., Tammela, T., Risteli, L., Risteli, J., Taube, T. and Elomaa, I. (1993) Evaluation of the effects of oral clodronate on skeletal metastases with type 1 collagen metabolites. A controlled trial of the Finnish Prostate Cancer Group. *European Journal of Cancer*, **29A**, 821-825.

Lipton, A., Small, E., Saad, F., Gleason, D., Gordon, D., Smith, M., Rosen, L., Kowalski, M. O., Reitsma, D. and Seaman, J. (2002) The new bisphosphonate, Zometa (zoledronic acid), decreases skeletal complications in both osteolytic and osteoblastic lesions: a comparison to pamidronate. *Cancer Investigation*, **20**, 45-54.

Lowe, F.C. and Somers, W. J. (1987) The use of ketoconazole in the emergency management of disseminated intravascular coagulation due to metastatic prostate cancer. *Journal of Urology*, **137**, 1000-1002.

Maeda, H., Koizumi, M., Yoshimura, K., Yamauchi, T., Kawai, T. and Ogata, E. (1997) Correlation between bone metabolic markers and bone scan in prostate cancer. *Journal of Urology*, **157**, 539-543.

Merrick, M.V., Ding, C.L., Chisholm, G.D. and Elton, R.A. (1985) Prognostic significance of alkaline and acid phosphatase and skeletal scintigraphy in carcinoma of the prostate. *British Journal of Urology*, **57**, 715-720.

Mettlin, C.J., Murphy, G.P., Ho, R. and Menck, H. R. (1996) The national cancer data base report on longitudinal observations on prostate cancer. *Cancer*, **77**, 2162-2166.

Nelson, J.B., Carducci, M.A., Padley, R.J., Janus, T., Humerickhouse, R. and Hippensteel, R. (2001). The endothelin-A receptor antagonist Atrasetan (ABT-627) reduces skeletal remodeling activity in men with advanced, hormone refractory prostate cancer. *Proceedings of the American Society of ClinicalOncology*, San Francisco, CA.

Nelson, J.B., Hedican, S.P., George, D.J., Reddi, A.H., Piantadosi, S., Eisenberger, M.A. and Simons, J.W. (1995) Identification of endothelin-1 in the pathophysiology of metastatic adenocarcinoma of the prostate. *Nature Med*, **1**, 944-949.

Newling, D.W.W., Denis, L. and Vermeylen, K. (1993) Orchiectomy versus goserelin and flutamide in the treatment of newly diagnosed metastatic prostate cancer. *Cancer*, **72**, 3793-3798.

Nielsen, O.S., Bentzen, S.M., Sandberg, E., Gadeberg, C.C. and Timothy, A.R. (1998) Randomized trial of single dose versus fractionated palliative radiotherapy of bone metastases. *Radiotherapy and Oncology*, **47**, 233-240.

Oesterling, J.E., Brendler, C.B., Epstein, J.I., Kimball, A.W.J. and Walsh, P.C. (1987) Correlation of clinical stage, serum prostatic acid phosphatase and preoperative Gleason grade with final pathological stage in 275 patients with clinically localized adenocarcinoma of the prostate. *Journal of Urology*, **138**, 92-98.

Olumi, A.F., Grossfeld, G.D., Hayward, S.W., Carroll, P.R., Tlsty, T.D. and Cunha, G. R. (1999) Carcinoma-associated fibroblasts direct tumor progression of initiated human prostatic epithelium. *Cancer Research*, **59**, 5002-5011.

Osborne, C.K., Blumenstein, B., Crawford, E.D., Coltman, C. J., Smith, A.Y., Lambuth, B.W. and Chapman, R.A. (1990) Combined versus sequential chemo-endocrine therapy in advanced prostate cancer: final results of a randomized Southwest Oncology Group study. *Journal of Clinical Oncology*, **8**, 1675-1682.

Percival, R.C., Urwin, G.H., Harris, S., Yates, A.J., Williams, J.L. and Beneton, M.E.A. (1987) Biochemical and histological prostate is associated with increased bone resorption. *European Journal of Surgical Oncology*, **13**, 41-49.

Pollen, J.J., Gerber, K., Ashburn, W.L. and Schmidt, J.D. (1981) Nuclear bone imaging in metastatic cancer of the prostate. *Cancer*, **47**, 2585-2594.

Porter, A.T., McEwan, A.J.B., Powe, J.E., Reid, R., McGowan, D.G., Lukka, H., Sathyanarayana, J.R., Yakemchuk, V.N., Thomas, G.M., Erlich, L.E., Crook, J., Gulenchyn, K.Y., Hong, K.E., Wesolowski, C. and Yardley, J. (1993) Results of a randomized phase III trial to evaluate the efficacy of strontium-89 adjuvant to local field external beam irradiation in the management of endocrine resistant metastatic prostate cancer. *International Journal of Radiation Oncology Biological Physics*, **25**, 805-813.

Pound, C.R., Partin, A.W., Eisenberger, M.A., Chan, D.W., Pearson, J.D. and Walsh, P.C. (1999) Natural history of progression after PSA elevation following radical prostatectomy. *Journal of the American Medical Association*, **281**, 1591-1597.

Quilty, P. M., Kirk, D., Bolger, J. J., Dearnaley, D. P., Lewington, V. J., Mason, M. D., Reed, N.S., Russell, J.M. and Yardley, J. (1994) A comparison of the palliative effects of strontium-89 and external beam radiotherapy in metastatic prostate cancer. *Radiotherapy and Oncology*, **31**, 33-40.

Ransom, D.T., Dinapoli, R.P. and Richardson, R.L. (1990) Cranial nerve lesions due to base of the skull metastases in prostate carcinoma. *Cancer*, **65**, 586-589.

Richardson, P.G., Barlogie, B., Berenson, J., Traynor, A., Singhal, S., Jagannath, S., Irwin, D., Rajkumar, V., Srkalovic, G., Alsina, M., Alexanian, R., Siegel, D., Orlowski, Z., Kuter, D., Limentani, S., Esseltine, D., Kauffman, M., Adams, J., Schenkein, D. and Anderson, K.C. (2002). Phase II study of the proteasome inhibitor PS-341 in multiple myeloma patients with relapsed/refractory disease. *Proceedings of the American Society of Clinical Oncology*, Orlando, FL.

Robertson, C.N., Roberson, K.M., Padilla, G.M., O'Brien, E.T., Cook, M., Kim, C.S. and Fine, R.L. (1996) Induction of apoptosis by diethylstilbestrol in hormone-insensitive prostate cancer cells. Journal of the National Cancer Institute, **88**, 908-917.

Rosenthal, D.I. (1997) Radiologic diagnosis of bone metastases. *Cancer*, **80**, 1595-1607.

Saad, F., Gleason, D.M., Murray, R., Tchekmedyian, S., Venner, P., Lacombe, L., Chin, J.L., Vinholes, J.J., Goad, J.A. and Chen, B. (2002) A randomized, placebo-controlled trial of zoledronic acid in patients with hormone-refractory metastatic prostate carcinoma. *Journal of the National Cancer Institute*, **94**, 1458-1468.

Sartor, O., Cooper, M.R., Khleif, S.N. and Myers, C.E. (1994) Suramin decreases circulating levels of insulin-like growth factor-1. *American Journal of Medicine*, **96**, 390.

Serafini, A.N., Houston, S.J., Resche, I., Quick, D.P., Grund, F.M., Ell, P.J., Bertrand, A., Ahmann, F.R., Orihuela, E., Reid, R.H., Lerski, R.A., Collier, B.D., McKillop, J.H., Purnell, G.L., Pecking, A.P., Thomas, F.D. and Harrison, K.A. (1998) Palliation of pain associated with metastatic bone cancer using samarium-153 lexidronam: a double-blind placebo-controlled clinical trial. *Journal of Clinical Oncology*, **16**, 1574-1581.

Shariat, S.F., Lamb, D.J., Kattan, M.W., Nguyen, C., Kim, J., Beck, J., Wheeler, T.M. ans Slawin, K.M. (2002) Association of preoperative plasma levels of insulin-like growth factor I and insulin-like growth factor binding proteins-2 and -3 with prostate cancer invasion, progression, and metastasis. *Journal of Clinical Oncology*, **20**, 833-841.

Shreve, P.D., Grossman, H.B., Gross, M.D. and Wahl, R.L. (1996) Metastatic prostate cancer: initial findings of PET with 2-deoxy-2-[F-18] fluoro-D-glucose. Radiology, **199**, 751-756.

Simpson, E., Harrod, J. and Eilan, G. e. a. (1985) Identification of a messenger ribonucleic acid fraction in human prostatic cancer cells coding for a novel osteoblast-stimulating factor. *Endocrinology*, **117**, 1615-1620.

Small, E.J., Meyer, M. Marshall, M.E., et al. (2000) Suramin therapy for patients with symptomatic hormone-refractory prostate cancer: results of a randomized phase III trial comparing suramin plus hydrocortisone to placebo plus hydrocortisone. *Journal of Clinical Oncology*, **18**, 1440-1450.

Smith, D.C., Tucker, J.A. and Trump, D.L. (1992) Hypercalcemia and neuroendocrine carcinoma of the prostate: a report of three cases and a review of the literature. *Journal of Clinical Oncology*, **10**, 499-505.

Soloway, M.S., Hardeman, S.W., Hickey, D., Raymond, J., Todd, B., Soloway, S. and Moinuddin, M. (1988) Stratification of patients with metastatic prostate cancer based on extent of disease on initial bone scan. *Cancer*, **61**, 195-202.

Storlie, J.A., Buckner, J.C., Wiseman, G.A., Burch, P.A., Hartmann, L.C. and Richardson, R.L. (1995) Prostate specific antigen levels and clinical response to low dose dexamethasone for hormone-refractory metastatic prostate carcinoma. *Cancer*, **76**, 96-100.

Taichman, R.S., Cooper, C., Keller, E.T., Pienta, K.J., Taichman, N.S. and McCauley, L.S. (2002) Use of the stromal cell-derived factor-1/CXCR4 pathway in prostate cancer metastasis to bone. *Cancer Research*, **62**, 1832-1837.

Takeuchi, S.-i., Arai, K., Saitoh, H., Yoshida, K.-i. and Miura, M. (1996) Urinary pyridinoline and deoxypyridinoline as potential markers of bone metastasis in patients with prostate cancer. *Journal of Urology*, **156**, 1691-1695.

Taube, T., Kylmala, T., Lamberg-Allardt, C., Tammela, T.L.J. and Elomma, I. (1994) The effect of clodronate on bone in metastatic prostate cancer. Histomorphometric report of a double-blind randomised placebo-controlled study. *European Journal of Cancer*, **30A**, 751-758.

Thalmann, G.N., Anezinis, P.E., Chang, S., Zhau, H.E., Kim, E., Hopwood, V.L., Pathak, S., von Eschenbach, A.C. and Chung, L.W.K. (1994) Androgen-independent cancer progression and bone metastasis in the LNCaP model of human prostate cancer. *Cancer Research*, **54**, 2577-2581.

Tong, D., Gillick, L. and Hendrickson, F.R. (1982) The palliation of symptomatic osseous metastases: final results of the Study by the Radiation Therapy Oncology Group. *Cancer*, **50**, 893-899.

Townsend, M.F., Sanders, W.H., Northway, R.O. and Graham, S.D.J. (1997) Bone fractures associated with luteinizing hormone-releasing hormone agonists used in the treatment of prostate carcinoma. *Cancer*, **79**, 545-550.

Trachtenberg, J., Halpern, N. and Pont, A. (1983) Ketoconazole: a novel and rapid treatment for advanced prostate cancer. *Journal of Urology*, **130**, 152-153.

Tu, S.-M., Millikan, R.E., Mengistu, B., Delpassand, E.S., Amato, R.J., Pagliaro, L.C., Daliani, D., Papandreou, C.N., Smith, T.L., Kim, J., Podoloff, D.A. and Logothetis, C.J. (2001) Bone-targeted therapy for advanced androgen-independent carcinoma of the prostate: a randomized phase II trial. *Lancet*, **357**, 336-341.

Tu, S.-M., Pagliaro, L.C., Banks, M.E., Amato, R.J., Millikan, R.E., Bugazia, N.A., Madden, T., Newman, R.A. and Logothetis, C.J. (1998) Phase I study of suramin combined with doxorubicin in the treatment of androgen-independent prostate cancer. *Clinical Cancer Research*, **4**, 1193-1201.

Vinholes, J.J.F., Purohit, O.P., Abbey, M.E. and Coleman, R.E. (1997) Relationships between biochemical and symptomatic response in a double-blind randomised trial of pamidronate for metastatic bone disease. *Annals of Oncology*, **8**, 1243-1250.

Wood, D.P. and Banerjee, M. (1997) Presence of circulating prostate cells in the bone marrow of patients undergoing radical prostatectomy is predictive of disease-free survival. *Journal of Clinical Oncology*, **15**, 3451-3457.

Xie, S.P., Pirianov, G. and Colston, K.W. (1999) Vitamin D analogues suppress IGF-1 signalling and promote apoptosis in breast cancer cells. *European Journal of Cancer*, **35**, 1717-1723.

Zagars, G.K., Pollack, A. and von Eschenbach, A.C. (1995) Prostate cancer and radiation therapy - message conveyed by serum prostate-specific antigen. *International Journal of Radiation Oncology, Biology, Physics*, **33**, 23-35.

Chapter 3

ANIMAL MODELS OF BONE METASTASIS

Thomas J. Rosol[1], Sarah H. Tannehill-Gregg[1], Stephanie Corn[1], Abraham Schneider[2], and Laurie K. McCauley[2]
[1]*Department of Veterinary Biosciences, The Ohio State University, Columbus, OH;* [2]*Department of Periodontics, Prevention, and Geriatrics, University of Michigan, Ann Arbor, MI*

INTRODUCTION

Animal models are important tools to investigate the pathogenesis and develop treatment strategies for bone metastases as they occur in humans. However, there are few spontaneous models of bone metastasis despite the fact that rodents (rats and mice) and other animals, such as dogs and cats, often spontaneously develop cancer. Therefore, most experimental models of bone metastasis in rodents require injection or implantation of neoplastic cells into orthotopic locations, bones, or the left ventricle of the heart.

Ideal animal models of human cancers that metastasize to bone would be those that reproduce the genetic and phenotypic changes that occur with human cancers. These include invasion, vascular spread to bone, and proliferation and survival in the bone marrow microenvironment with subsequent modifications of bone structure. In addition, such models would be reproducible and progress rapidly to permit timely investigations. Based on the pathogenesis of cancer in rodents and smaller mammals, this ideal may represent an unrealistic and impractical goal. However, animal models of bone metastasis that mimic selected aspects of human disease have been utilized and refinements to the models will continue to be developed.

Since spontaneous bone metastasis in animals is uncommon, most animal models of bone metastasis must be experimentally derived. This limitation has resulted in the development of specific models that represent unique stages of human bone metastasis, and thorough characterization of these animal models is therefore required to permit their appropriate use as a representation of human disease. This concise review will include information on the infrequent spontaneous bone metastasis in animals with mammary and prostate cancer, the current uses of these and other animal models of bone metastasis, and recent developments that will serve to better model human disease. There is a role for animal models in the study of bone metastasis as well as a need for refinement of these models to advance our understanding of this important manifestation of oncogenesis.

Cancer progression with resulting bone metastases requires genetic changes that permit tissue invasion at the site of the primary tumor, entry into the vasculature, localization in bone, exit from the vasculature, survival and proliferation in the bone marrow microenvironment, and modification of bone structure and function (Yoneda et al., 1999b; Cher, 2001). The genetic changes include metastasis-enhancing and suppressing genes and many of these are currently being identified and characterized using animal models. Bone metastasis-enhancing (and suppressing) genes are associated with multiple cellular processes that occur normally during mammalian development, and include genes that regulate cell shape and migration, interactions with extracellular matrix and stroma, angiogenesis, apoptosis, proliferation, and proteins that are usually associated with normal bone function (such as bone matrix proteins and hormones/cytokines that regulate bone cell activity). Although genes associated with bone metastasis can be readily identified by screening techniques, such as gene arrays, the validation and characterization of these genes will require sophisticated animal models that closely mirror the pathophysiology of bone metastasis in humans.

Because of the relatively artificial nature of animal models of bone metastasis it is necessary to define what is considered a bone metastasis. End-stage lesions are readily identifiable and usually reveal tumor cell proliferation in bone that modifies bone structure. These would be comparable to clinically significant bone metastases in humans. Such overt lesions can be identified by radiography or histopathology in animals. However, quantification of metastases with these insensitive techniques likely underestimate the actual number of bone metastases. For example, radiography will only detect severe lesions and will not measure all bone metastases. In addition, radiography will not detect bone metastases that fail to induce severe bone lysis or induce formation of mineralized matrix. In contrast, overestimation may result from newer highly sensitive imaging techniques or PCR detection of tumor cells in bone. These methods may detect cells that are arrested in blood vessels or quiescent cells in the bone marrow that may or may not develop into metastases (Sung et al., 1997; van der Pluijm et al., 2001). Therefore, morphological assessment is necessary to confirm the incidence and nature of bone metastases in each animal model.

Animal models of metastasis have supported drug development, and have been useful for identification of metastasis suppressor and promoter genes as targets for the development of novel therapies. Further refinement of these models will involve spatiotemporal analysis of the metastatic process by imaging, and use of image data to stage disease and guide tissue sampling for gene expression profiling via gene array technology. In the future, integrated analyses of these models will be needed to understand the complexities of this important disease process.

MODELS OF BONE METASTASIS-GENERAL

Animal models of bone metastasis include spontaneous tumors that arise in rodents or small mammals (such as dogs and cats), syngeneic transplantation of spontaneously occurring rodent cancers, chemical induction of cancers in selected strains of rats and mice, newly developed transgenic mouse models, and xenografts of tumors or cell lines derived from human cancers into immunodeficient rodents (such as nude mice and rats and SCID mice) (Figure 1).

local injection of cancer cells near the viable bone substrate (Nemeth et al., 1999; Yonou et al., 2001).

Subcutaneous Ossicles: Subcutaneous bone nodules or ossicles can be generated from the differentiation of human bone marrow stromal cells (BMSCs) seeded in gelatin sponges (Figure 2). Following transplantation into immunodeficient mice, BMSCs form self-contained, highly vascularized, mineralized bone/bone marrow organs that consists in cortical and trabecular bone surrounding a marrow cavity with fat and active hematopoiesis (Schneider et al., 2003). Osseous responses characteristic of end-stage metastatic lesions can be studied by mixing BMSCs with cancer cells at the time of surgical implantation or by injecting cancer cells into the ossicles once they are fully formed (Schneider et al., 2002). This model system also provides a potential tool for elucidating the role of specific osteoblastic-related gene products in metastatic tumor growth and survival by implanting or injecting cancer cells into ossicles derived from BMSCs obtained from genetically modified mice.

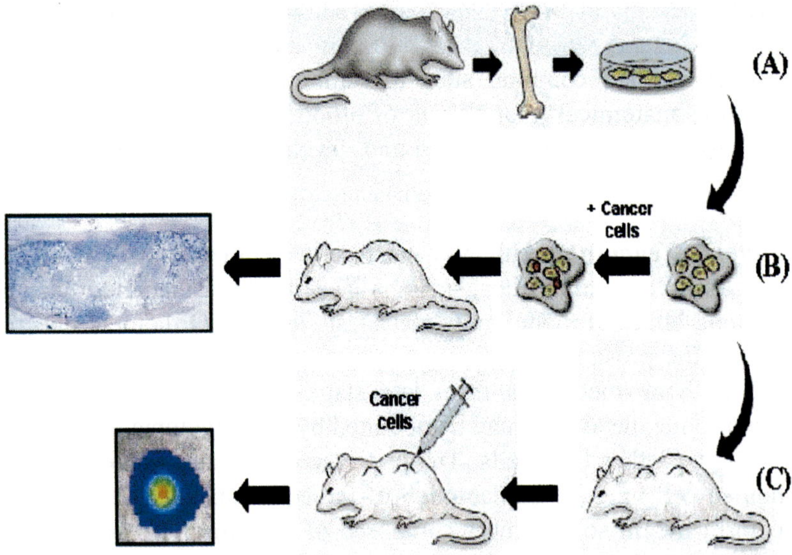

Figure 2. (A) Subcutaneous ossicles are produced from ex vivo expanded bone marrow stromal cells (BMSCs) obtained from wild-type mice. Cancer cell/bone cell interactions can be studied by (B) cotransplanting BMSCs with cancer cells seeded into gelatin sponges or (C) by injecting cancer cells into fully developed ossicles.(Continued on next page).

(Fig. 2 continued). Intraossicle infection of luciferase-expressing cancer cells provides a novel strategy to serially and non-invasively monitor tumor growth by quantifying photon emission through bioluminescence optical imaging.

MODELS OF BONE METASTASIS – MAMMARY CANCER

Spontaneous Mammary Cancer in Animals

Rats and mice frequently develop benign and malignant mammary neoplasms with the incidence dependent on the strain. Unfortunately these may not be good models for human disease. Most spontaneous mammary cancers in mice and rats do not metastasize and have mild local tissue invasion (Seely et al., 1999). There is a low incidence of spontaneous metastasis to regional lymph nodes or the lungs, and bone metastasis is very rare. In addition, most adenocarcinomas in rodents rapidly lose their estrogen responsiveness and may not be good models of estrogen-responsive neoplasms in humans. Spontaneous development of mammary neoplasms in mice are due, in some cases, to a retrovirus, mouse mammary tumor virus (MMTV), but the role of retroviruses in the pathogenesis of human mammary cancer is uncertain. Proviral DNA, similar to MMTV, has nonetheless been detected in a high percentage of human mammary cancers (Liu et al., 2001). It is for these reasons that other models have been developed in rodents.

Dogs frequently develop benign and malignant mammary neoplasia with an incidence similar to that observed in humans (Misdorp, 2002). Dogs develop hyperplasia, ductular carcinoma in situ, complex neoplasms with epithelial and myoepithelial components, and mixed neoplasms with cartilaginous and osseous differentiation of myoepithelial cells. Spontaneous mammary neoplasia in dogs has been imaged using indocyanin green (ICG) as an optical contrast agent (Hawrysz et al., 2000); ICG is a red fluorescent dye with emission that is ideal for imaging in mammals and it has been approved for human use. Approximately 50% of the carcinomas metastasize to regional lymph nodes and the lungs; however, bone metastases are infrequent. Cats also have a high incidence of spontaneous mammary neoplasia. In cats, the neoplasms are typically invasive adenocarcinomas or ductular carcinomas that have a very high incidence of recurrence after surgical removal with metastasis to regional lymph nodes and the lungs.

Bone metastases in cats are also infrequent. Benign mammary tumors are rare in cats.

Experimental Models of Mammary Cancer and Bone Metastasis

Syngeneic Models: Many syngeneic models of mammary cancer in rats and mice do not readily metastasize to bone. However, sublines of the cancers can be selected in vivo that have an increased incidence of bone metastasis after orthotopic or intracardiac administration. For example, the 4T1.2 subclone of the 4T1 subline of a spontaneous mammary gland carcinoma from a Balb/cfC3H mouse has been demonstrated to have an increased incidence of metastasis to bone after injection into the mammary fat pad (orthotopic) or left ventricle of the heart (Lelekakis et al., 1999). Mice with xenografts of the 4T1 cells or its sublines often die of the primary tumors or lung metastases before overt bone metastases develop.

Chemical Induction of Mammary Cancer in Rats and Mice: Mammary neoplasia can be induced in rats by administration of dimethylbenzanthracene, methylnitrosourea (MNU), and N-ethyl-N-nitrosourea (ENU) (Ip, 1996). ENU-induced mammary adenocarcinomas in Sprague-Dawley rats may metastasize to the lungs, and the rats often develop mild hypercalcemia, but bone metastases do not occur spontaneously (Stoica et al., 1983; Stoica et al., 1984).

Transgenic Induction of Mammary and Prostate Cancer in Mice: Oncogene expression can be targeted to the mammary glands using tissue selective promoters (Cardiff et al., 2000; Huss et al., 2001). The whey acidic protein (WAP), C(3)1, and mouse mammary tumor virus promoters are often used for the mammary gland. The advantages of transgenic models of cancer include their predictability and the autochthonous development of cancer (i.e., originating where normally found). A consensus report for the pathology of mammary carcinomas in genetically modified mice concluded that transgenes usually induced characteristic phenotypes and some of the neoplasms developed morphological similarities to human mammary cancer (Cardiff et al., 2000). The disadvantage of the transgenic models is the low incidence of metastasis, especially bone metastases, often due to rapid progression of the primary neoplasm.

Human Mammary Cancer Xenografts: Intracardiac and Orthotopic Models: A widely used and successful model of human breast cancer bone metastases uses left ventricular injection of the MDA-MB-231 cells

(Yoneda, 1997; Yoneda, 2000; Guise et al., 2002). This model has produced success in multiple laboratories and has been used to investigate the roles of specific molecules using transfected genes and other techniques. Additional human mammary cancer lines used to induce bone metastases include LCC-15 (Figure 3) and MDA-MB-435. Most mammary cancer cell lines induce osteolytic lesions, but some cell lines have induced osteoblastic or mixed osteolytic/osteoblastic metastases. Human mammary cancer cell lines (ZR-75-1 and MCF-7/Neu) have been used to model osteoblastic metastases in vivo, and have demonstrated important roles of PDGF BB and endothelin-1 in the pathogenesis of osteoblastic metastases (Mohammad et al., 2001; Yi et al., 2002). Orthotopic injection of human mammary cancer cell lines has been used less frequently to induce bone metastases. However, this technique has been used with hybrid mouse/human tissue using human MDA-MB-435 cells, which resulted in bone metastases after implantation of tumor tissue in the mammary glands of nude mice (Hoffman, 1999).

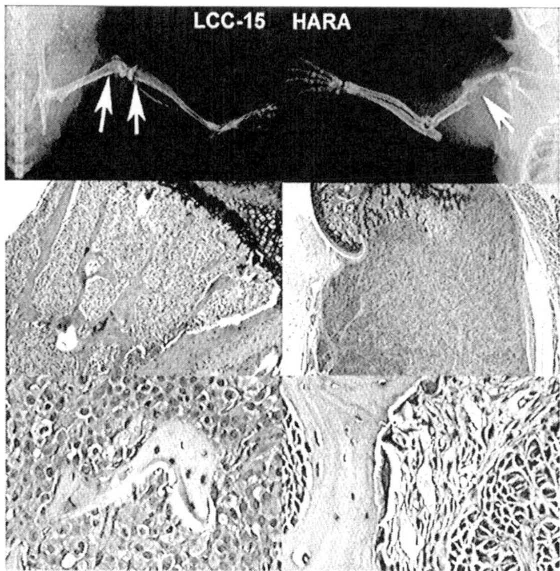

Figure 3. Human breast (LCC-15) and lung (HARA) metastases in nude mice after injection of cancer cells into the left ventricle of the heart. The LCC-15 metastases in the distal femur and proximal tibia do not induce much osteoclastic resorption of bone. In contrast the HARA cells induce marked lysis and osteoclastic resorption of bone.

MODELS OF BONE METASTASIS – PROSTATE CANCER

Prostate cancer is among the most common cancers in men, affecting approximately 1 in 11 men in the United States (Landis et al., 1998). Bone metastases are common and have been reported in 65-75% of advanced cases (Coleman, 1997). Bone metastases typically induce new woven bone ('osteoblastic metastases'), which cause significant morbidity through spinal cord and nerve compression. Most metastases have new bone formation and osteoclastic bone resorption (osteoblastic/osteolytic), but in late lesions the osteoblastic component often predominates. The development of animal models that accurately depict osteoblastic and mixed osteolytic/osteoblastic metastases is critical to understanding the pathophysiology of these metastases. Unfortunately, most animal models of prostate cancer do not induce osteoblastic lesions. It is essential to accurately assess the pathology of animal models of bone metastasis, especially the models that are used to reproduce osteoblastic lesions. If a cancer results in severe lysis of cortical bone or induces pathologic fractures, then an intense proliferation of periosteal woven bone (Codman's Triangle) is expected. It is important not to interpret this reaction as an osteoblastic lesion (Blomme et al., 1999). Osteoblastic metastases of human prostate cancer typically induce new woven bone on the surface of pre-existing medullary trabecular bone. The most accurate models will reproduce this phenomenon. It is also possible that tumor induction of woven bone on the periosteum by cancer cells could mimic the pathogenesis of osteoblastic metastases if the bone proliferation is not secondary to disruption of the cortex.

Spontaneous Prostate Cancer in Animals

Animals have a very low incidence of prostate cancer compared to humans. Spontaneous prostate cancer occurs most commonly in dogs and is rare in rodents and other animals, including nonhuman primates. Dogs also develop spontaneous skeletal metastasis in 22% of cases (Cornell et al., 2000). Rodent models include transgenic mice that have genetic mutations that predispose them to the development of prostate cancer, human tumor xenografts in immunodeficient mice, and rat strains that have increased rates of prostate cancer. Few of the rodent models develop skeletal metastasis. Some strains of rats have been developed that have an increased incidence of prostate neoplasia, and transgenic mouse models of prostate cancer have also been described (below).

There are important anatomical differences between the prostate glands of rodents and humans. Humans have a single gland with multiple regions, which include the transitional zone near the urethra, the central zone, the peripheral zone, and the anterior fibromuscular zone. Benign prostatic hyperplasia is most common in the transitional zone and prostate cancer is most common in the peripheral zone. Rats and mice have four distinct lobes to the prostate gland (Figure 4). The anterior prostate (coagulating gland) extends rostrally along the ventral aspect of the seminal vesicle. The dorsal, lateral, and ventral prostate gland lobes extend around the base of the penis near the neck of the urinary bladder. The prostate gland in rodents is composed of compound ductules that lack the true acini that exist in humans, and each lobe has a unique branching pattern (Cunha et al., 1987). Rats and mice have a very low incidence of spontaneous proliferative lesions that develop in the prostate glands as they age (Suwa et al., 2001; Suwa et al., 2002). Secondary neoplasms, such as lymphoma, occur more commonly in aged rodents compared to primary prostate neoplasms. There is no known rodent equivalent of prostate-specific antigen (PSA) to correlate with tumor progression.

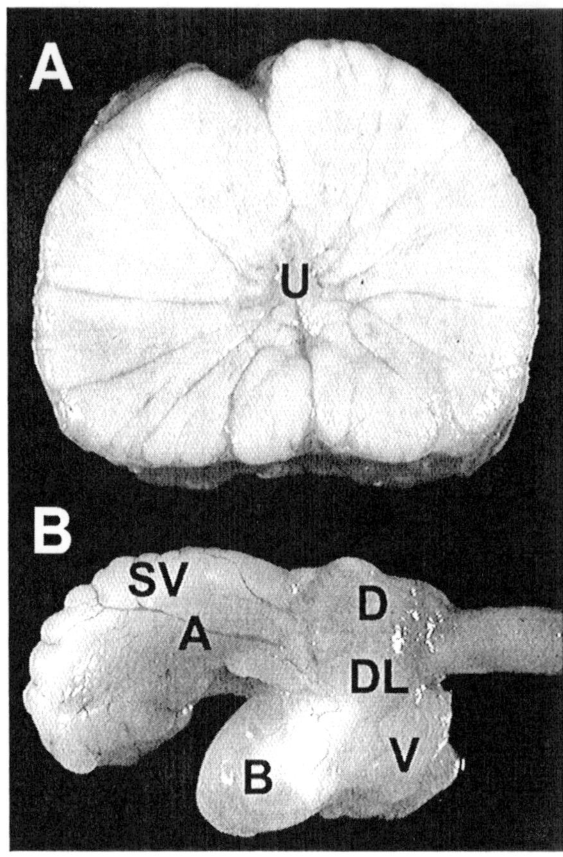

Figure 4. A. Cross-section of dog prostate gland. The urethra is in the middle of the gland (U) and the lobules containing acini radiate from the urethra and periurethral ducts. B. Rat prostate gland and bladder (B) demonstrating the dorsal (D), dorsolateral (DL), ventral (V), and anterior (A) lobules. The seminal vesicles (SV) are dorsal to the anterior prostate lobes (coagulating glands).

Spontaneous Prostate Cancer in Rats: Specific strains of rats have been bred to have an increased incidence of prostate neoplasms, including the Lobund Wistar rat and ACI/seg rats. Up to 30% of aged (>20-months-old) Lobund Wistar rats develop prostate cancer in the anterior prostate/seminal vesicle complex (Pollard, 1998b). Administration of methynitrosourea (MNU) and testosterone will increase the incidence and reduce the age of cancer development so that up to 90% of rats will develop prostate cancer by 12 months-of-age (Pollard et al., 1989). Lobund Wistar rats have high circulating concentrations of testosterone, which may predispose to the development of prostate cancer. Initially the carcinomas are testosterone-dependent, but as they progress they become testosterone-independent. The carcinomas eventually expand into the dorsolateral lobes of the prostate gland and will metastasize to lymph nodes and the lungs. Development of the prostate carcinomas can be suppressed by diet restriction, testosterone ablation, dihydrotestosterone, diets with soy protein containing isoflavones, tamoxifen, and a vitamin D analogue (Pollard, 1998a; Pollard, 1999). Cell lines have been developed from the prostate carcinomas, such as PA-I, II, III, and IV. The PA-III cell line has been shown to induce both osteoblastic and osteolytic bone lesions when the carcinoma is transplanted adjacent to the calvarium or scapula (Koutsilieris, 1992). The ACI/Seg strain of rats develop a high incidence (80%) of microscopic prostate neoplasia in the ventral lobes at 36 months-of-age and a moderate incidence (16%) of grossly evident prostate cancer at the same age (Varma et al., 1990). In contrast, Copenhagen rats have a 10% incidence of microscopic prostate cancer and <1% incidence of grossly evident prostate carcinomas at 36 months-of-age (Isaacs, 1984).

Spontaneous Prostate Cancer in Dogs: Dogs have a single-lobed prostate gland similar to humans, but it does not have different anatomic regions (Figure 4). The prostatic urethra traverses through the gland and is surrounded by ducts that quickly arborize into branched alveolar glands. All intact male dogs will develop simple (glandular) and complex (glandular and stromal) forms of benign prostatic hyperplasia as they age (Leav et al., 2001b). Both intact and castrated male dogs have a similar incidence of prostate cancer (the incidence in neutered dogs may be slightly greater), but dogs do not have the high incidence of prostate cancer that occurs in humans. Most cases of prostate cancer in dogs are androgen-independent and expression of the testosterone receptor is uncommon. Prostate cancer in dogs is initially confined to the gland and can result in dysuria, hematuria, or constipation. Many cancers will eventually invade the urinary bladder, the pelvic cavity, lumbar vertebrae and pelvis, and some will metastasize to distant bones or organs. In some cases the initial presenting feature is lameness due to a bone metastasis (Figure 5). The bone metastases are typically a mixture of osteoblastic and osteolytic changes, although the osteoblastic component can be the predominant pattern.

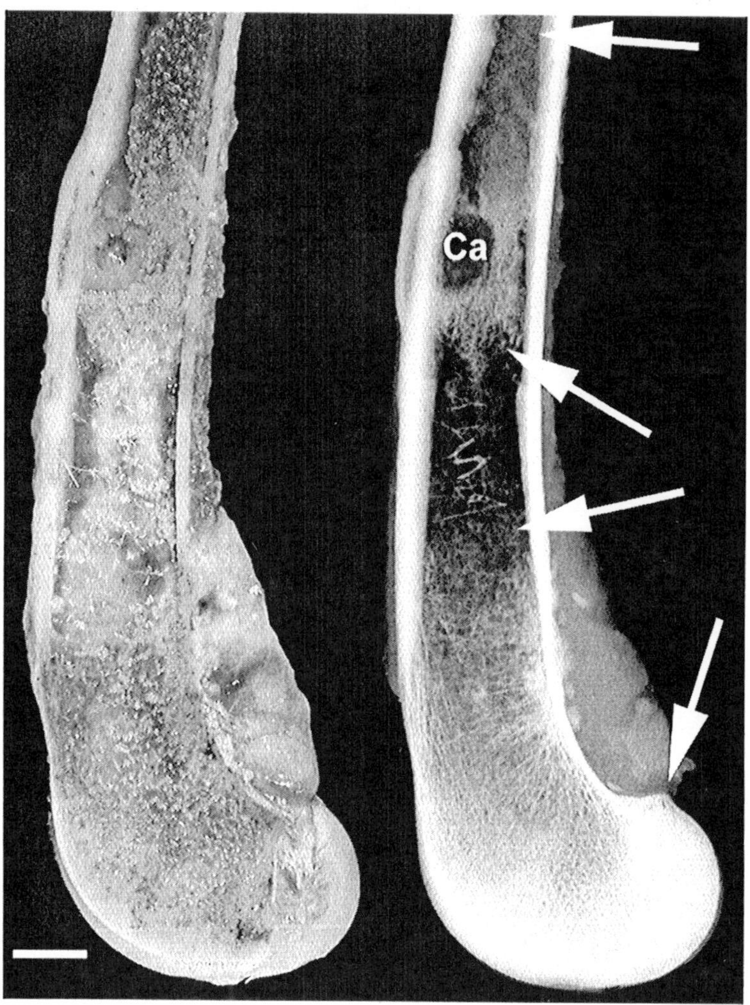

Figure 5.   Metastatic prostate cancer in the dog femur (gross photograph and Faxitron radiograph).   Two predominantly osteoblastic and partially osteolytic bone metastases of prostate cancer in the diaphysis (ca) and metaphysis/epiphysis. Notice the extensive proliferation of new woven bone trabeculae in the diaphysis and metaphysis induced by the prostate cancer (regions between the arrows).

Prostate carcinomas in dogs have multiple morphologic patterns that include adenocarcinoma, intra-alveolar carcinoma, papillary carcinoma, cribiform pattern, anaplastic carcinoma, and transitional cell-like carcinoma (Cornell et al., 2000; Leav et al., 2001b). Multiple patterns often exist in the same carcinoma. The cell of origin of prostate carcinoma in the dog has not been definitively determined, but immunohistochemical studies have led to the conclusion that the neoplasms arise from ductal cells (Leav et al.,

2001a). It is possible that the carcinomas arise from the ductal epithelium and then differentiate into ductal, glandular, and transitional cell patterns. Prostatic intraepithelial neoplasia (PIN) has been reported in dogs, but most cases occurred in dogs with overt carcinoma, so it has not been proven that PIN is a preneoplastic lesion in dogs (Waters et al., 1997). The incidence of PIN in aged, intact and castrated dogs without carcinoma is unknown. PIN occurred in 3% of aged military working dogs without prostate cancer and in 72% of the dogs (n = 25) that had prostate cancer (Aquilina et al., 1998).

Prostate specific antigen (PSA) cannot be used as a marker for prostate cancer in dogs, since dogs do not express this specific serine protease (Clements, 1989). The dog homolog to PSA is canine prostate-specific arginine esterase (AE), which has 58% homology to PSA and has similar enzymatic activity as PSA on natural protein substrates. PSA has chymotrypsin-like activity and AE has trypsin-like activity on synthetic substrates. Canine AE is produced under androgen control by prostate glandular epithelial cells. Therefore, PSA and AE are related, but distinct enzymes.

When prostate cancer invades through the prostate gland capsule and infiltrates the pelvic cavity in dogs, the neoplastic tissue induces marked new woven bone production from the periosteum of the lumbar vertebrae and pelvis. Eventually the tumor will invade into the medullary cavity of the bones. In addition, prostate cancer in dogs will metastasize directly to the medullary cavity of bones in the appendicular or axial skeleton. Intramedullary bone metastases are typically osteoblastic or a combination of osteoblastic/osteolytic lesions (Figure 5). Normal dog prostate tissue is also capable of inducing new bone formation in vivo. Prostate gland tissue was implanted adjacent to the calvarium of nude mice and periosteal new bone proliferation was induced and increased the thickness of the calvarium by 70% in two weeks (Figure 6) (LeRoy et al., 2002). The bone formation was dependent on the presence of tissue containing both glands and stroma, since cultured epithelial or stromal cells alone did not induce the periosteal new bone formation. These data demonstrated that new bone formation induced by prostate cancer in vivo may represent an inherent characteristic of prostate tissue and may not be dependent on the cancer phenotype. It is likely that the new bone formation is due to growth factors secreted by the prostate epithelial and/or stromal cells, and may be dependent on paracrine interactions between the two cell types.

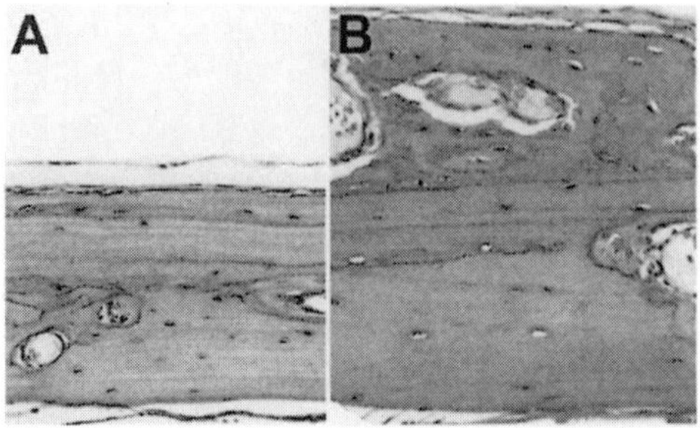

Figure 6. Mouse calvaria. Control calvarium (A). Calvarium (B) has marked periosteal new bone proliferation on the convex surface induced by implantation of normal canine prostate in the subcutis (not demonstrated in the photograph) for two weeks.

Experimental Models of Prostate Cancer and Bone Metastasis

Syngeneic Models: Several strains of rats have an increased incidence of spontaneous prostate cancer (as described above). However, most of these strains develop tumors that do not metastasize to bone and have a long latency period before development (Lucia et al., 1998). Sublines of the cancers can be selected in vivo that have an increased incidence of bone metastasis after orthotopic or intracardiac administration. A transplantable cell line, prostate adenocarcinoma-III (PA-III), was derived from a spontaneous prostate tumor in a Lobund-Wistar rat and causes a mixed osteolytic/osteoblastic reaction when implanted over the calvarium or scapula (Koutsilieris, 1992).

The Dunning model was developed from a spontaneous prostate cancer in a Copenhagen rat and sublines were developed following serial transplantation of the initial tumor (Tennant et al., 2000). Cells from these tumors grow well in vitro and can be transfected, making them useful for imaging studies (Lucia et al., 1998). The Dunning sublines vary in rate of growth, ability to metastasize, location of the metastases, and androgen dependence (Tennant et al., 2000). One of the sublines, MatLyLu, which was initially characterized by its consistent metastases to lung and lymph node, has been injected into the left ventricle of rats to produce osteolytic metastases (Blomme et al., 1999). The MatLyLu androgen-insensitive subline of the rat Dunning prostate carcinoma (R3327) has been used as reliable model for bone metastasis in vivo (Tennant et al., 2000). Copenhagen rats develop hind limb paralysis 2 to 3 weeks after left ventricular injection of MatLyLu cells due to metastases in the lumbar vertebrae (Blomme et al., 1999). The bone metastases are osteolytic and do not mimic the osteoblastic or mixed osteolytic/osteoblastic metastases of human prostate cancer.

A canine prostate cancer cell line (DPC-1) has been successfully transplanted in the prostate of an aged dog that was immunosuppressed with cyclosporine (Anidjar et al., 2001). The prostate carcinoma grew in the normal prostate gland and invaded into the pelvic cavity and regional iliac lymph nodes. Although bone metastases were not observed, the study demonstrated the potential for using dogs to investigate the pathogenesis and treatment of transplantable prostate cancer in a large animal model.

Chemical Induction of Prostate Cancer in Rats: Prostate and seminal vesicle adenocarcinomas can be induced in Noble rats with testosterone/estradiol or MNU/testosterone combinations. An increased incidence of prostate adenocarcinomas can be induced in Lobund Wistar rats with MNU and testosterone (Pollard et al., 2000). These tumors uncommonly metastasize to lymph nodes and the lungs, and do not metastasize to bone.

Transgenic Induction of Prostate Cancer in Mice: Oncogene expression can be targeted to the prostate glands using tissue selective promoters (Huss et al., 2001). The C(3)1, probasin, and prostate-specific antigen promoters are used for the prostate gland. The advantages of transgenic models of cancer include their predictability and the autochthonous development of cancer. The disadvantage of the transgenic models is the low incidence of metastasis, especially bone metastases, often due to rapid progression of the primary neoplasm. Sublines of a spontaneous bone metastasis from a prostate carcinoma in a TRAMP mouse (transgenic mouse with the rat probasin promoter and expression of the SV40 early genes) have been developed that will permit investigations on bone metastasis in this transgenic model (Foster et al., 2001).

Human Prostate Cancer Xenografts: Human prostate cancer cell lines have been transplanted orthotopically in mice and utilized to successfully represent different stages of cancer progression in vivo ranging from androgen-dependent growth, androgen independence, androgen insensitivity, androgen repression, and metastatic behavior, including lymph node, lung, and bone metastases (Stearns et al., 1998; Zhau et al., 2000). Some of the most commonly used human xenograft cell lines are PC-3, LuCaP, and LNCaP. The PC-3 cell line was one of the earliest cell lines developed and grows well *in vitro* and *in vivo* (Kaighn et al., 1979). After implantation in nude mice, PC-3 forms an androgen-independent, poorly differentiated adenocarcinoma and will metastasize to bone after intravenous injection with vena cava occlusion (Shevrin et al., 1988; Wang et al., 1991). PC-3 cells have also been injected directly into the tibia to mimic bone metastasis. Both bone metastases and direct intraosseous implantation result in osteolytic lesions rather than the more typical osteoblastic lesions seen in humans (Corey et al., 2002). PC-3 cells do not produce PSA (Ellis et al., 1996).

The LuCaP xenograft was developed from lymph node and liver metastases and produces PSA, but the cells must be maintained in vivo as xenografts and do not grow in vitro (Ellis et al., 1996). LuCaP cells also are initially androgen-sensitive and then will progress to androgen insensitivity after androgen deprivation, recapitulating the progression of prostate carcinoma in humans (Ellis et al., 1996). When injected into the tibia, the LuCaP xenograft initially produces a mixed osteolytic/osteoblastic lesion that progresses to an osteoblastic lesion (Corey et al., 2002).

LNCaP xenograft cells can be propagated *in vitro* and secrete PSA. LNCaP tumors in mice are initially androgen-dependent and progress to androgen independence after castration (Thalmann et al., 2000). Sublines of LNCaP cells that have a higher incidence of bone metastasis after subcutaneous or orthotopic implantation have been successfully selected (Thalmann et al., 2000). Intratibial injection of LNCaP cells produce tumors with osteolytic morphology (Corey et al., 2002). Intracardiac injections of LNCaP cells have failed to produce bone metastases (Wu et al., 1998).

A severe combined immunodeficient (SCID)-human model has been developed to evaluate these xenografts in human fetal bones that have been implanted in SCID mice. PC-3 and LNCaP cells injected intravenously into mice with human bone implants selectively grew in the human implanted bone at a much higher rate than in mouse tissues. PC-3 tumors had a predominantly osteolytic morphology, and LNCaP tumors had mixed osteolytic/osteoblastic morphology (Nemeth et al., 1999). Another study has recently reported similar results with human adult bone (Yonou et al., 2001).

Dog Prostate Cancer Xenograft: We have developed a prostate cancer cell line (ACE-1) isolated from a dog with a spontaneous prostate carcinoma and bone metastases. The ACE-1 cells invade locally and into the spine when transplanted in the dorsal subcutis of nude mice and metastasize to lymph nodes and the lungs. The cells grow in vitro and will induce mixed osteolytic and osteoblastic lesions in the tibias of nude mice.

MODELS OF BONE METASTASIS – LUNG CANCER

Lung cancer is the third most common type of malignancy to metastasize to bone. Metastatic lung cancer often localizes to the spine, ribs, pelvis, and long bones, and has a unique predilection for the hand and foot (one-half of all metastases to the hand are from the lung and 15% of metastases to the feet are from the lung). One investigation compared the incidence of bone metastases at postmortem and found a 36% incidence associated with lung cancer (Galasko, 1981a). Metastatic lung cancer has a poor prognosis, with a median post-diagnosis survival time of 6 months, and a 5-year survival rate of less than 5% (Rubens et al., 1995). The development of animal models of lung cancer that metastasize to bone is important to investigate the mechanisms of disease and improve the prognosis. Use of lung cancer models lags behind models for human breast and prostate cancer; however, several models using the rat and mouse have been described.

Primary lung tumors in most animals are uncommon or rare. This is consistent with the fact that approximately 85% of lung tumors in humans are associated with cigarette use (Malkinson, 2001). The development of spontaneous primary lung tumors in inbred mice is strain-dependent, with "A" (A/J, ACR, etc) and SWR strains being the most sensitive. The lung tumors in these strains are usually adenomas with few metastases compared to lung cancer in humans (Jackson et al., 2003). Charles River Laboratories reported an incidence from 0-25% for spontaneous pulmonary adenomas and 0-3.3% for spontaneous carcinomas in 24-month male $B6C3F_1/CrlBR$ mice, and 48% for spontaneous adenomas and 0.8% for carcinomas in 24-month male CD rats. The low incidence of spontaneous carcinomas and bone metastasis makes utilization of mice and rats as natural models for lung cancer metastases to bone impractical. Chemical induction of primary lung tumors in laboratory mice and rats is a common procedure; however, bone metastases are not routinely measured in these studies.

Spontaneous lung cancer in domestic animals, such as dogs and cats, is uncommon. However, bronchial carcinomas in the cat have a predisposition to metastasize to the bones of the digit (Gottfried et al., 2000; Linde-Sipman et al., 2000), similar to bronchogenic carcinomas in humans (Vaezy et al., 1978; Galmarini et al., 1998; Cohen, 2001). Bronchogenic carcinomas that metastasize to the digits in cats often affect multiple digits (especially the third phalanx), and the first clinical sign is usually lameness rather than respiratory disease associated with the primary neoplasm (Hahn et al., 1997). The cat represents an ideal spontaneous animal model for this syndrome in humans since cats are: (1) outbred, (2) allowed to live a normal lifespan, and

(3) exposed to similar environmental factors as humans. A disadvantage to this model is that primary lung cancers are infrequent in the cat (Hahn et al., 1997).

Orthotopic Lung Cancer Models and Bone Metastasis: There have been few investigations on metastasis of human cancers after intrapulmonary administration of tumor cells or tissue, but this technique may have utility as a model for human lung cancer (Hoffman, 1999). The mouse has a complete mediastinum, which permits intrathoracic surgery without positive-pressure ventilation of the lungs. Unilateral xenotransplantation of tumor tissue will permit growth of a large primary tumor and may allow enough time for metastasis to occur before tumor cachexia results.

The nude rat and mouse have been used in these orthotopic models of lung cancer with development of bone metastases. The models involve a left thoracotomy and implantation of solid pieces of primary tumor or tumor grown subcutaneously in nude mice onto the pleural surface of the left lung lobe, or direct injection of tumor cells in suspension into the lung. Introduction of the lung cancer tissue or cells into the lung permits the cells to interact with pulmonary epithelial cells and stroma. The injection of tumor cells in suspension is less desirable since this works only with established cell lines and has a lower rate of metastasis compared to tumor implantation (Hoffman, 1999). The maintenance of the tissue architecture in the solid tumor implants improves the rate of metastasis and more readily mimics the natural disease by encouraging implanted tumor growth, invasion, and metastasis (Hoffman, 1999).

Implantation models that induce bone metastasis include the NCI-H460 large cell carcinoma in the rat (Johnston et al., 2001) and the NCI-H460 (Yang et al., 1998; Hoffman, 2001), SBC-5 small-cell carcinoma, and ANIP 973 adenocarcinoma in mice (Hoffman, 1998; Miki et al., 2000). Injection of cell suspensions in the lung with subsequent bone metastasis has been reported in the mouse with the A549 adenocarcinoma (Hastings et al., 2000). In addition, hybrid nude rat/human lung cancer tissue was implanted into the lungs of nude rats using an endotracheal cannula, which resulted in a 75% incidence of bone metastases (Howard et al., 1999). A disadvantage to intrapulmonary tumor transplantation is the technical difficulty of the procedure. After growth in the lung, the resultant tumor is chimeric since it contains mouse-derived blood vessels and fibroblasts, which could lead to challenging problems when analyzing human-specific gene or protein expression. Some xenotransplanted tumors may grow quickly and result in dyspnea before metastases can develop. Advantages of the intrapulmonary tumor models include similarities to the clinical course of disease in humans, retention of more normal tumor architecture, a high rate of metastasis (especially with solid tumor implantation) (Kuo et al., 1993), usefulness for drug discovery, ability to use patient-derived primary tumors, and the ability to serially passage tumors in mice with a stable phenotype (Hoffman, 1999).

Intracardiac Injection and Lung Cancer Metastasis: Left ventricular injection of lung cancer cells has been used to induce bone metastases with cell lines, such as the HARA squamous cell carcinoma (Iguchi et al., 1996) (Figure 3) and the RWGT2 cells (Iwasaki et al., 2002). Intracardiac injection does not replicate the development of bone metastasis as closely as orthotopic implantation of solid tissue. The injected cells do not undergo the early stages of metastasis including escape from the primary tumor, migration through surrounding stroma, and entrance into blood vessels. This method is considered to be an improvement compared to direct injection of cancer cells into bone since it allows for cells to localize preferentially in bone compared to soft tissues. Several published models of intracardiac injection of lung cancer cells to evaluate bone metastases exist. Lung cancer cells can also be injected directly into the tibias of immunodeficient mice or rats.

Human Fetal Bone and Lung Cancer Metastasis: For studies involving bone metastasis of lung cancer cells, human fetal bone (18-22 weeks gestational age) was implanted subcutaneously into SCID mice (Namikawa et al., 1999). Human small cell lung cancer cells were injected into the tail vein after 7-8 weeks. Controls consisted of SCID mice implanted with newborn mouse bone. One SCLC line (N4BM) developed human bone metastases in 65% of the mice, while only 22% of the implanted mouse bones developed metastases. This demonstrated species-specificity of the injected lung cancer cells.

MODELS OF BONE METASTASIS – MALIGNANT MELANOMA

Malignant melanoma of the skin is a common tumor in humans, with 53,600 new cases and 7,400 new deaths predicted for 2003. It is the 5th most common tumor for men and 6th for women. The five-year survival rate for localized malignant melanoma is 96%; however, in patients with distant metastasis (including bone metastasis) this rate is reduced to 12% (American cancer society, 2003). During the 1970's the incidence of malignant melanoma increased rapidly (at approximately 4% per year) making it the fastest rising cancer (Centers for Disease Control, 1995). The most common sites of metastasis for malignant melanoma are lymph nodes, brain, and lung. In one study of 190 patients with malignant melanoma, 4% developed bone metastases as the site of initial distant metastasis (Cohn-Cedermark et al., 1999). Clinical studies of malignant melanoma in humans have reported that 11-17% of patients had bone metastases and 23-49% of autopsy patients had bone metastases (Meyers et al., 1998).

Spontaneous melanomas in the mouse and rat are extremely rare and may be strain related. For example, spontaneous malignant melanoma occurs in 4% of aging male BN/Bi rats (Zurcher et al., 1989; Kanno, 1989). The incidence of bone metastasis in spontaneous malignant melanoma of rodents is not readily available. Experimentally induced models of malignant melanoma include topical application of chemical carcinogens such as DMBA (Kligman et al., 2001) and use of UV irradiation (Klein-Szanto et al., 1994). Numerous transgenic rodent models for malignant melanoma exist. Bone metastases have not been a characteristic of any of these models.

Malignant melanoma is common in the dog. Most of the cases arise in the oral cavity, with approximately 10% involving haired skin, and 8% occurring in the nail bed (subungual malignant melanoma). The subungual and oral melanomas tend to be locally invasive and destructive of bone, however metastases occur most commonly to the lungs and regional lymph nodes (Goldschmidt et al., 2002).

Numerous xenograft models of malignant melanoma and bone metastases exist. These include left ventricular injection of LOX cells in nude rats, and B16 cells, green fluorescent protein (GFP)-expressing B16 cells, and A375 cells in nude mice (Arguello et al., 1988; Kjonniksen et al., 1990; Hiraga et al., 1995; Yang et al., 1999; Nemoto et al., 2001). Early detection of tumor growth and metastases in vivo has been reported using GFP-transfected cells.

MODELS OF BONE METASTASIS – RENAL CELL CARCINOMA

The American Cancer Society estimates 31,900 new cases of renal cell carcinoma in 2003, with 11,900 deaths. The 5-year survival rate for all stages is 62%; however, this rate is only 9% in patients with distant metastases (American Cancer Society, 2003). Renal cell carcinomas often metastasize to bone. In a retrospective study of renal carcinoma, the clear cell subtype (the most common subtype), metastasized in 137/283 patients (48.4%), with 30/137 (21.9%) patients developing bone metastases (Mai et al., 2001). The incidence of bone metastases at postmortem was reported to be 35% in patients with renal cancer (Galasko, 1981b). Transitional cell carcinomas (of the urinary bladder) will metastasize to bone with low frequency and typically induce osteolytic or mixed osteolytic/osteoblastic lesions (Evison et al., 1981).

Spontaneous renal carcinomas in rodents are rare. In NTP carcinogenicity studies with 1351 B6C3F1mice, 0.1% of male and female mice developed renal tubular carcinomas (Haseman et al., 1999). Incidences in rats are reported to be 0.3-0.6% in F344, 0.3% in Osborne-Mendel rats, and 0.1-1.2% in Sprague-Dawley rats (Arnold et al., 1991), and bone metastases are not reported (Chandra et al., 1993). Long-Evans Cinnamon rats develop an increasing incidence of renal cell tumors with age (up to 58% after 188 days); however, they are not reported to develop bone metastases (Izumi et al., 1994). Ekers rats are commonly used for renal carcinoma studies, but they are not reported to develop bone metastases (Everitt et al., 1992).

Experimentally induced models of renal cell carcinoma with bone metastases are uncommon. One model utilizes the RBM1 cell line developed from a bone metastasis of a patient with renal cell carcinoma. The cells were injected intratibially into nude mice and bone lesions similar to those of the patient developed. The cell line demonstrated cytogenetic abnormalities common to renal cell carcinomas, and the production of cytokines (parathyroid hormone-related protein, IL-6, and macrophage colony-stimulating factor) induced bone lysis (Weber et al., 2002). Other models of renal carcinoma, such as the rabbit VX-2 and RENCA tumors do not produce bone metastases (Young et al., 1976; Maurer-Gebhard et al., 1999). The VX2 carcinoma was derived from a Shope papilloma virus-induced neoplasm in a domestic rabbit. Injection of VX2 cells into the tibia or ileum of rabbits will induce mixed osteolytic and osteoblastic lesions (Galasko, 1982).

Renal carcinomas in domestic animals are rare, but are reported most commonly in the dog and cat (Meuten, 2002). Bone metastases of renal carcinomas in domestic animals have been reported (Arai et al., 1991); however, they are considered to be rare (Lucke et al., 1976).

MODELS OF BONE METASTASIS – MULTIPLE MYELOMA

Multiple myeloma almost always involves the bone, with osteolytic bone destruction (Bataille, 1996). Osteolysis of bones causes the major clinical manifestations of multiple myeloma, including pain, pathologic fracture, and hypercalcemia (Osterborg et al., 1996). The American Cancer society predicts 14,600 new cases of multiple myeloma in 2003, with 10,900 new deaths (American Cancer Society, 2003). Multiple myeloma accounts for approximately 10% of all hematological malignancies in humans, and 1% of all human cancers (Gado et al., 2001).

The development of spontaneous multiple myeloma in rodents is rare. C57BL/KaLwRij aged mice (>2-years-old) develop multiple myeloma (frequency 0.5%) and demonstrate lesions typical of the human disease including disseminated growth and bone lesions (Gado et al., 2001). Cells derived from these mice are often used in animal models of multiple myeloma (see below), however the low frequency of tumor development makes them inefficient as spontaneous models.

There are multiple mouse models of multiple myeloma, some of which involve bone lesions. Experimental mouse models of multiple myeloma that affect bone include the 5T and ARH-77 models. The 5T model was developed from spontaneous myeloma in aging inbred C57 black mice (C57BL/KaLwRij substrain), which exhibits classic characteristics of the disease with marrow involvement and osteolytic lesions. These cells, when transferred to young syngeneic mice by tail vein or marrow inoculation, result in the development of myeloma bone disease with similar characteristics to the human disease (including a monoclonal gammopathy, replacement of bone marrow, multifocal osteolysis, hind limb paralysis, and hypercalcemia). The cells demonstrate an absence of structural c-myc abnormalities, similar to the disease in humans (Croese et al., 1987; Radl et al., 1990). The ARH-77 model involves intravascular injection of human ARH-77 leukemic plasma cells into irradiated SCID mice. The ARH-77 cells express $(Ig)G_\kappa$ and grow in many organs. The mice develop hind limb paralysis due to vertebral involvement within 39 days, and become hypercalcemic. Vertebrae and long bones develop marked osteolysis (Alsina et al., 1996). One disadvantage to this model is the ARH-77 cells are not dependent on IL-6 for growth, in contrast to most human myelomas. The KPMM2 line, developed from a primary human tumor, exhibits marked involvement of bone and osteolysis with hypercalcemia when injected intravenously in mice, and is also IL-6 dependent, and more closely mimics the human disease compared to the ARH-77 cells (Gado et al., 2001).

Models using human-derived myeloma cell lines and human fetal bone grafts in SCID mice permit the evaluation of interactions between human neoplastic cells and the human bone microenvironment. In one such model, investigators utilized 4 cell lines (ARH-77, OCI-My5, U-266, or RPMI-8226) and injected them directly into the marrow cavity of a fetal bone implant in irradiated SCID-hu mice. The cells successfully engrafted into the human fetal implant, and metastasized to a second implant after 12 weeks, without metastasis to the mouse bones. Monoclonal human IgG was detected in the mouse blood, and monoclonal Ig light chains were present in renal tubules of the mice (Urashima et al., 1997). These models have several advantages including the use of human cells in a partially humanized mouse system.

Several transgenic models of multiple myeloma exist, including the Eμ-IL-6/C57BL/6 model (which has IL-6 expression under the control of the murine major histocompatability class (H-2Ld) promoter). Although some marrow involvement is reported, extensive osteolytic bone lesions do not appear to be a major component of these models (Gado et al., 2001).

In domestic animals, multiple myeloma is rare and accounts for less than 1% of all malignant neoplasms, and 8% of hemolymphatic tumors. Domestic animals usually develop a similar clinical syndrome to humans with bone involvement and osteolysis, hypercalcemia, renal disease and hyperviscosity syndrome. The low incidence of spontaneous multiple myeloma in domestic animals will prevent them from being a natural animal model for this disease (Jacobs et al., 2002).

IMAGING, IN VIVO OF BONE METASTASES IN ANIMAL MODELS

The study of bone metastasis in small animal models has often relied on histological analyses, PCR amplification and radiography; however, such assays that utilize excised tissues are subject to sampling limitations and can not assess the overall extent of disease in a given animal subject (Edinger et al., 1999; Sweeney et al., 1999; Wetterwald et al., 2002; Tester et al., 2002). To overcome this limitation, in vivo detection of bone metastases using high resolution Faxitron radiography has been used in attempt to provide temporal information (Figure 3). Radiography has proven to be useful for the detection of large osteolytic lesions, but micrometastatic lesions are the desired target for therapeutic intervention and these are not detectable radiographically.

Newer imaging modalities based on optical detection of reporter genes promise to improve throughput and accuracy of quantitation in animal models of bone metastases (Edinger et al., 1999; Yang et al., 2000; Wetterwald et al., 2002). Transfection of tumor cells with fluorescent or luciferase reporter genes has enabled in vivo imaging and longitudinal studies to be performed. In vivo fluorescence imaging and in vivo bioluminescent imaging (BLI) are inherently different in that fluorescence requires that excitation light travel through tissue to the tumor and emitted fluorescent light travel back to the detector. In contrast, BLI requires that the chemical substrate, luciferin, be distributed systemically and only the light emitted from the labeled cells to travel out of the tissue. Autofluorescence of tissue reduces the signal to noise ratio (SNR) in fluorescent imaging, and the SNR is expected to be higher in BLI (Rice et al., 2001). Luciferase activity can be readily measured ex vivo using tissue extracts, and fluorescence can be assayed by microscopy in tissue sections as well as in dissociated cells via flow cytometry. Thus, combination reporter genes that are bioluminescent and fluorescent may offer the best of both approaches (Costa et al., 2001). Instrumentation for optical imaging typically employs imaging systems based on sensitive charge coupled device (CCD) detectors that are usually less expensive than the instrumentation required for some of the more conventional imaging modalities (e.g., magnetic resonance imaging; MRI). These optical techniques require that the cells stably express reporter genes.

In a xenograft model small numbers of human mammary carcinoma cells were detectable in the bone marrow of immunodeficient mice by BLI (Wetterwald et al., 2002). In this study, the BLI data was cross validated using radiography at different stages of disease. The bioluminescent signal was detectable much earlier in the disease than the radiographic detection of osteolytic lesions. We have used BLI to study human prostate cancer cells (PC-3M-luc) in a xenograft model after intracardiac injection of 100,000 cells in nude mice (Figure 7). Mice were imaged using the Xenogen IVIS Imaging System after injection of 3 μg of luciferin (Biosynth International Inc., Naperville, IL). Within 3 minutes, cancer cells were homogeneously distributed in all areas of the body (Figure 7). Subsequently, at 15 minutes, cancer cells were localized to specific organs such as the lungs, kidneys, long bones, bones of the head, and eyes. It is interesting that some organs with a clearly detectable signal at these early time points, such as the kidneys, rarely develop overt metastases. At 24 hours no viable tumor cells could be visualized demonstrating that most injected cells died (or were metabolically inactive) after intracardiac administration. At day 20, the first bone metastases in the long bones and the spine could be visualized. This is approximately 2 weeks prior to the detection of bone metastases by Faxitron radiography. In vivo imaging is also very useful to determine the immediate success of intracardiac injection, since some injections may result in tumor cell deposition into the pericardial or pleural cavities. Obviously bone marrow micrometastases can elude radiographic detection; however, using BLI these lesions were detectable. Detection of micrometastatic lesions and the ability to follow tumor growth at multiple tissue sites over time will greatly enhance the study of metastatic disease.

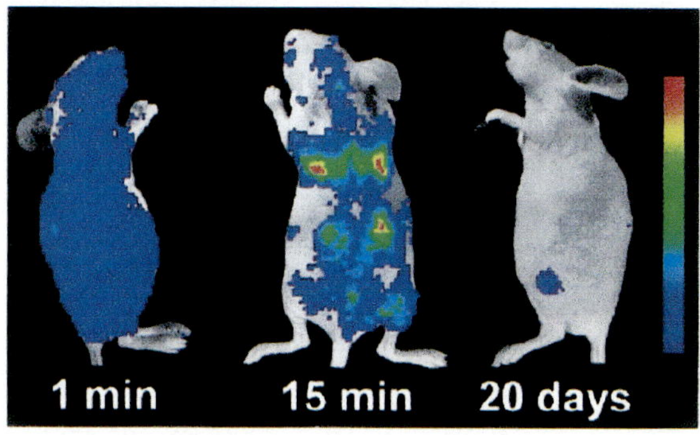

Figure 7. In vivo bioluminescent imaging of light emitted from luciferase in human PC-3M-luc prostate cancer cells in a nude mouse. At 3 min. after injection of 100,000 cells into the left ventricle of the heart cells were apparent throughout the body with very early localization in the kidney (light green focus). At 15 min. the signals from labeled cancer cells localized to the lungs, kidneys, bones (spine, long bones, and maxilla and mandible), and the eyes. At day 1 (not shown) there was no detectable signal indicating that most of the cancer cells died or were metabolically inactive. At day 20 initial metastases were evident in the long bones (blue focus) and spine. The scale bar on the right is the relative intensity of light, which is an indirect measure of cell number.

SUMMARY AND CONCLUSIONS

Animal models will continue to be indispensable to investigate the pathogenesis of bone metastasis in vivo, conduct preclinical chemotherapeutic, chemoprevention and genetic therapy studies, test gene delivery mechanisms, and identify metastasis suppressor and inducer genes. It is likely that the bone marrow microenvironment, such as the endothelial cells, stromal cells, hematopoietic cells, bone cells, and the intercellular matrix play important roles in the localization and clonal growth of cancer cells in bone. Given the complexity of bone metastasis, many genes are expected to be involved in the pathogenesis and few are likely indispensable. The use of genomic and proteomic approaches to study these animal models will identify key targets for therapeutic intervention. As we further refine these models and use imaging for real-time evaluation of cells, and eventually target genes, these models will more closely mirror human disease and will hopefully become more predictive of the human response to therapy.

ACKNOWLEDGMENTS

Financial support was received from the United State Public Health Service, National Institutes of Health grant numbers CA77911, CA100730, and RR00168 (TJR) and CA83766 (STG).

REFERENCES

Alsina, M., Boyce, B., Devlin, R. D., Anderson, J. L., Craig, F., Mundy, G. R. and Roodman, G. D. (1996). Development of an in vivo model of human multiple myeloma bone disease.

American Cancer Society. American Cancer Society Cancer Facts and Figures 2002. worldwide web . 2003. Ref Type: Electronic Citation

Anidjar, M., Villette, J. M., Devauchelle, P., Delisle, F., Cotard, J. P., Billotey, C., Cochand-Priollet, B., Copin, H., Barnoux, M., Triballeau, S., Rain, J. D., Fiet, J., Teillac, P., Berthon, P. and Cussenot, O. (2001) In vivo model mimicking natural history of dog prostate cancer using DPC-1, a new canine prostate carcinoma cell line. *The Prostate* **46**: 2-10.

Aquilina, J. W., McKinney, L., Pacelli, A., Richman, L. K., Waters, D. J., Thompson, I., Burghardt, W. F., Jr. and Bostwick, D. G. (1998) High grade prostatic intraepithelial neoplasia in military working dogs with and without prostate cancer. *The Prostate* **36**: 189-193.

Arai, C., Ono, M., Une, Y., Shirota, K., Watanabe, T. and Nomura, Y. (1991) Canine renal carcinoma with extensive bone metastasis. *Journal of Veterinary Medical Science* **53**: 495-497.

Arguello, F., Baggs, R. B. and Frantz, C. N. (1988) A murine model of experimental metastasis to bone and bone marrow. *Cancer Research* **48**: 6876-6881.

Arnold, J. and Eustis, S. L. 1991. "Tumor incidences in Fischer 344 rats: NTP historical data." In: Haseman, J. K. (ed.), *Pathology of the Fischer Rat*. Academic Press, pp. 555-564.

Bataille, R. 1996. "Human myeloma-induced bone changes" In: Gahrton, G. and Durie, B. G. M. (eds.), *Multiple Myeloma*. Arnold, pp. 51-54.

Blomme, E. A., Dougherty, K. M., Pienta, K. J., Capen, C. C., Rosol, T. J. and McCauley, L. K. (1999) Skeletal metastasis of prostate adenocarcinoma in rats: morphometric analysis and role of parathyroid hormone-related protein. *Prostate* **39**: 187-197.

Cardiff, R. D., Anver, M. R., Gusterson, B. A., Hennighausen, L., Jensen, R. A., Merino, M. J., Rehm, S., Russo, J., Tavassoli, F. A., Wakefield, L. M., Ward, J. M. and Green, J. E. (2000) The mammary pathology of genetically engineered mice: the consensus report and recommendations from the Annapolis meeting. *Oncogene* **19**: 968-988.

Centers for Disease Control (1995) Deaths from melanoma--United States,1973-1992. *MMWR Morbidity and Mortality Weekly Report* **44**: 337, 343-347.

Chandra, M., Riley, M. G. and Johnson, D. E. (1993) Spontaneous renal neoplasms in rats. *Journal of Applied Toxicology* **13**: 109-116.

Cher, M. L. (2001) Mechanisms governing bone metastasis in prostate cancer. *Current Opinions of Urology* **11**: 483-488.

Clements, J. A. (1989) The glandular kallikrein family of enzymes: tissue-specific expression and hormonal regulation. *Endocrine Reviews* **10**: 393-419.

Cohen, P. R. (2001) Metastatic tumors to the nail unit: subungual metastases. *Dermatology Surgery* **27**: 280-293.

Cohn-Cedermark, G., Mansson-Brahme, E., Rutqvist, L. E., Larsson, O., Singnomklao, T. and Ringborg, U. (1999) Metastatic patterns, clinical outcome, and malignant phenotype in malignant cutaneous melanoma. *Acta Oncology* **38**: 549-557.

Coleman, R. E. (1997) Skeletal complications of malignancy. *Cancer* **80**: 1588-1594.

Corey, E., Quinn, J. E., Bladou, F., Brown, L. G., Roudier, M. P., Brown, J. M., Buhler, K. R. and Vessella, R. L. (2002) Establishment and characterization of osseous prostate cancer models: intra-tibial injection of human prostate cancer cells. *Prostate* **52**: 20-33.

Cornell, K. K., Bostwick, D. G., Cooley, D. M., Hall, G., Harvey, H. J., Hendrick, M. J., Pauli, B. U., Render, J. A., Stoica, G., Sweet, D. C. and Waters, D. J. (2000) Clinical and pathologic aspects of spontaneous canine prostate carcinoma: a retrospective analysis of 76 cases. *Prostate* **45**: 173-183.

Costa, G. L., Sandora, M. R., Nakajima, A., Nguyen, E. V., Taylor-Edwards, C., Slavin, A. J., Contag, C. H., Fathman, C. G. and Benson, J. M. (2001) Adoptive immunotherapy of experimental autoimmune encephalomyelitis via T cell delivery of the IL-12 p40 subunit. *Journal of Immunology* **167**: 2379-2387.

Croese, J. W., Vas Nunes, C. M., Radl, J., Enden-Vieveen, M. H., Brondijk, R. J. and Boersma, W. J. (1987) The 5T2 mouse multiple myeloma model: characterization of 5T2 cells within the bone marrow. *British Journal of Cancer* **56**: 555-560.

Cunha, G. R., Donjacour, A. A., Cooke, P. S., Mee, S., Bigsby, R. M., Higgins, S. J. and Sugimura, Y. (1987) The endocrinology and developmental biology of the prostate. *Endocrine Reviews* **8**: 338-362.

Edinger, M., Sweeney, T. J., Tucker, A. A., Olomu, A. B., Negrin, R. S. and Contag, C. H. (1999) Noninvasive assessment of tumor cell proliferation in animal models. *Neoplasia* **1**: 303-310.

Ellis, W. J., Vessella, R. L., Buhler, K. R., Bladou, F., True, L. D., Bigler, S. A., Curtis, D. and Lange, P. H. (1996) Characterization of a novel androgen-sensitive, prostate-specific antigen-producing prostatic carcinoma xenograft: LuCaP 23. *Clinical Cancer Research* **2**: 1039-1048.

Everitt, J. I., Goldsworthy, T. L., Wolf, D. C. and Walker, C. L. (1992) Hereditary renal cell carcinoma in the Eker rat: a rodent familial cancer syndrome. *Journal of Urology* **148**: 1932-1936.

Evison, G., Pizey, N. and Roylance, J. (1981) Bone formation associated with osseous metastases from bladder carcinoma. *Clinical Radiology* **32**: 303-309.

Foster, B. A. and Greenberg, N. M. (2001) New model of bone metastasis for prostate cancer: Cell lines derived from a bone metastasis in TRAMP. Proceedings of the American Association for Cancer Research **42**: 140 (abstract).

Gado, K., Silva, S., Paloczi, K., Domjan, G. and Falus, A. (2001) Mouse plasmacytoma: an experimental model of human multiple myeloma. *Haematologica* **86**: 227-236.

Galasko, C. S. (1981a) Monitoring of bone metastases. *Schweiz. Med. Wochenschr.* **111**: 1873-1875.

Galasko, C. S. (1982) Mechanisms of lytic and blastic metastatic disease of bone. *Clin Orthop* **169**: 20-27.

Galasko, C. S. B. (1981b). "The anatomy and pathways of skeletal metastases" In: Weiss, L. and Gilbert, A. H. (eds.), *Bone Metastases*. GK Hall, pp. 49-63.

Galmarini, C. M., Kertesz, A., Oliva, R., Porta, J. and Galmarini, F. C. (1998) Metastasis of bronchogenic carcinoma to the thumb. *Medical Oncology* **15**: 282-285.

Goldschmidt, M. H. and Hendrick, M. J. 2002. "Tumors of the Skin and Soft Tissues" In: Meuten, D. J. (ed.), *Tumors in Domestic Animals* Iowa State Press, pp. 45-117.

Gottfried, S. D., Popovitch, C. A., Goldschmidt, M. H. and Schelling, C. (2000) Metastatic digital carcinoma in the cat: a retrospective study of 36 cats (1992-1998). *Journal of American Animal Hospital Association* **36**: 501-509.

Guise, T. A. (2000) Molecular mechanisms of osteolytic bone metastases. *Cancer* **88**: 2892-2898.

Guise, T. A., Yin, J. J., Thomas, R. J., Dallas, M., Cui, Y. and Gillespie, M. T. (2002) Parathyroid hormone-related protein (PTHrP)-(1-139) isoform is efficiently secreted in vitro and enhances breast cancer metastasis to bone in vivo. *Bone* **30**: 670-676.

Hahn, K. A. and McEntee, M. F. (1997) Primary lung tumors in cats: 86 cases (1979-1994). *Journal of American Veterinary Medical Association* **211**: 1257-1260.

Haseman, J. K., Elwell, M. R. and Hailey, J. R. (1999). "Neoplasm Incidences in B6C3F1 Mice: NTP Historical Data" In: Maronpot, R. R., Boorman, G. A. and Gaul, B. W. (eds.), *Pathology of the Mouse*. Cache River Press, pp. 679-689.

Hastings, R. H., Burton, D. W., Summers-Torres, D., Quintana, R., Biederman, E. and Deftos, L. J. (2000) Splenic, thymic, bony and lymph node metastases from orthotopic human lung carcinomas in immunocompromised mice. *Anticancer Research* **20**: 3625-3629.

Hawrysz, D. J. and Sevick-Muraca, E. M. (2000) Developments toward diagnostic breast cancer imaging using near-infrared optical measurements and fluorescent contrast agents. *Neoplasia.* **2**: 388-417.

Hiraga, T., Nakajima, T. and Ozawa, H. (1995) Bone resorption induced by a metastatic human melanoma cell line. *Bone* **16**: 349-356.

Hoffman, R. M. (1998) Orthotopic transplant mouse models with green fluorescent protein-expressing cancer cells to visualize metastasis and angiogenesis. *Cancer Metastasis Review.* **17**: 271-277.

Hoffman, R. M. (1999) Orthotopic metastatic mouse models for anticancer drug discovery and evaluation: a bridge to the clinic. *Investigating New Drugs* **17**: 343-359.

Hoffman, R. M. (2001) Visualization of GFP-expressing tumors and metastasis in vivo. *Biotechniques* **30**: 1016.

Howard, R. B., Mullen, J. B., Pagura, M. E. and Johnston, M. R. (1999) Characterization of a highly metastatic, orthotopic lung cance model in the nude rat. *Clinical Experimental Metastasis* **17**: 157-162.

Huss, W. J., Maddison, L. A. and Greenberg, N. M. (2001) Autochthonous mouse models for prostate cancer: past, present and future. *Semin. Cancer Biol*ogy **11**: 245-260.

Iguchi, H., Tanaka, S., Ozawa, Y., Kashiwakuma, T., Kimura, T., Hiraga, T., Ozawa, H. and Kono, A. (1996) An experimental model of bone metastasis by human lung cancer cells: the role of parathyroid hormone-related protein in bone metastasis. *Cancer Research* **56**: 4040-4043.

Ip, C. (1996) Mammary tumorigenesis and chemoprevention studies in carcinogen-treated rats. *Journal of Mammary Gland Biology Neoplasia* **1**: 37-47.

Isaacs, J. T. (1984) The aging ACI/Seg versus Copenhagen male rat as a model system for the study of prostatic carcinogenesis. *Cancer Research* **44**: 5785-5796.

Iwasaki, T., Yamashita, K., Tsujimura, T., Kashiwamura, S., Tsutsui, H., Kaisho, T., Sugihara, A., Yamada, N., Mukai, M., Yoneda, T., Okamura, H., Akedo, H. and Terada, N. (2002) Interleukin-18 inhibits osteolytic bone metastasis by human lung cancer cells possibly through suppression of osteoclastic bone-resorption in nude mice. *Journal of Immunotherapy* **25 Suppl 1**: S52-S60.

Izumi, K., Kitaura, K., Chone, Y., Tate, H., Nakagawa, T., Suzuki, Y. and Matsumoto, K. (1994) Spontaneous renal cell tumors in Long-Evans Cinnamon rats. *Japananese Journal of Cancer Research* **85**: 563-566.

Jackson, E. L. and Jacks, T. MMHC The mouse models of human cancers consortium. worldwide web . 2003. Ref Type: Electronic Citation

Jacobs, R. M., Messick, J. B. and Valli, V. E. (2002). "Tumors of the Hemolymphatic System" In: Meuten, D. J. (ed.), *Tumors in Domestic Animals* Iowa State Press, pp. 119-198.

Johnston, M. R., Mullen, J. B., Pagura, M. E. and Howard, R. B. (2001) Validation of an orthotopic model of human lung cancer with regional and systemic metastases. *Annals of Thoracic Surgery* **71**: 1120-1125.

Kaighn, M. E., Narayan, K. S., Ohnuki, Y., Lechner, J. F. and Jones, L. W. (1979) Establishment and characterization of a human prostatic carcinoma cell line (PC-3). *Invest Urology* **17**: 16-23.

Kanno, J. 1989. "Melanocytic tumors, skin, mouse" In: Jones, T. C. (ed.), *Integument and Mammary Glands* Springer-Verlag, pp. 63-69.

Kjonniksen, I., Nesland, J. M., Pihl, A. and Fodstad, O. (1990) Nude rat model for studying metastasis of human tumor cells to bone and bone marrow. *Journal of National Cancer Institute* **82**: 408-412.

Klein-Szanto, A. J., Silvers, W. K. and Mintz, B. (1994) Ultraviolet radiation-induced malignant skin melanoma in melanoma- susceptible transgenic mice. *Cancer Research* **54**: 4569-4572.

Kligman, L. H. and Elenitsas, R. (2001) Melanoma induction in a hairless mouse with short-term application of dimethylbenz[a]anthracene. *Melanoma Research* **11**: 319-324.

Koutsilieris, M. (1992) PA-III rat prostate adenocarcinoma cells (review). *In Vivo* **6**: 199-203.

Kuo, T. H., Kubota, T., Watanabe, M., Furukawa, T., Teramoto, T., Ishibiki, K., Kitajima, M. and Hoffman, R. M. (1993) Early resection of primary orthotopically-growing human colon tumor in nude mouse prevents liver metastasis: further evidence for patient-like hematogenous metastatic route. *Anticancer Research* **13**: 293-297.

Landis, S. H., Murray, T., Bolden, S. and Wingo, P. A. (1998) Cancer statistics, 1998. *CA Cancer J. Clin.* **48**: 6-29.

Leav, I., Schelling, K. H., Adams, J. Y., Merk, F. B. and Alroy, J. (2001a) Role of canine basal cells in postnatal prostatic development, induction of hyperplasia, and sex hormone-stimulated growth; and the ductal origin of carcinoma. *The Prostate* **48**: 210-224.

Leav, I., Schelling, S. H. and Merk, F. B. (2001b). "Age-related and sex hormone-induced changes in the canine prostate" In: Mohr, U., Carlton, W. W., Dungworth, D. L.,

Benjamin, SA., Capen, C. C. and Hahn, F. A. (eds.), *Pathobiology of the Aging Dog*. Iowa State Press, pp. 310-329.

Lelekakis, M., Moseley, J. M., Martin, T. J., Hards, D., Williams, E., Ho, P., Lowen, D., Javni, J., Miller, F. R., Slavin, J. and Anderson, R. L. (1999) A novel orthotopic model of breast cancer metastasis to bone. *Clinical Exp Metastasis* **17**: 163-170.

LeRoy, B. E., Bahnson, R. R. and Rosol, T. J. (2002) Canine prostate induces new bone formation in mouse calvaria: A model of osteoinduction by prostate tissue. *The Prostate* **50**: 104-111.

Linde-Sipman, J. S. and van den Ingh, T. S. (2000) Primary and metastatic carcinomas in the digits of cats. *Vet Q.* **22**: 141-145.

Liu, B., Wang, Y., Melana, S. M., Pelisson, I., Najfeld, V., Holland, J. F. and Pogo, B. G. (2001) Identification of a proviral structure in human breast cancer. *Cancer Research* **61**: 1754-1759.

Lucia, M. S., Bostwick, D. G., Bosland, M., Cockett, A. T., Knapp, D. W., Leav, I., Pollard, M., Rinker-Schaeffer, C., Shirai, T. and Watkins, B. A. (1998) Workgroup I: rodent models of prostate cancer. *Prostate* **36**: 49-55.

Lucke, V. M. and Kelly, D. F. (1976) Renal carcinoma in the dog. *Veterinary Pathology* **13**: 264-276.

Mai, K. T., Landry, D. C., Robertson, S. J., Commons, A. S., Burns, B. F., Thijssen, A. and Collins, J. (2001) A comparative study of metastatic renal cell carcinoma with correlation to subtype and primary tumor. *Pathology Research Pract.* **197**: 671-675.

Malkinson, A. M. (2001) Primary lung tumors in mice as an aid for understanding, preventing, and treating human adenocarcinoma of the lung. *Lung Cancer* **32**: 265-279.

Maurer-Gebhard, M., Schmidt, M., Azemar, M., Stocklin, E., Wels, W. and Groner, B. (1999) A novel animal model for the evaluation of the efficacy of drugs directed against the ErbB2 receptor on metastasis formation. *Hybridoma* **18**: 69-75.

Meuten, D. J. 2002. "Tumors of the Urinary System" In: Meuten, D. J. (ed.), *Tumors of Domestic Animals*. Iowa State Press, pp. 509-546.

Meyers, M. L. and Balch, C. M. 1998. "Diagnosis and treatment of metastatic melanoma." In: Balch, C. M., Houghton, A. N., Sober, A. J. and Soong, S. J. (eds.), *Cutaneous Melanoma*. Quality Medical Publishing, Inc., pp. 325-372.

Miki, T., Yano, S., Hanibuchi, M. and Sone, S. (2000) Bone metastasis model with multiorgan dissemination of human small-cell lung cancer (SBC-5) cells in natural killer cell-depleted SCID mice. *Oncology Research* **12**: 209-217.

Misdorp, W. 2002. "Tumors of the Mammary Gland" In: Meuten, D. J. (ed.), *Tumors in Domestic Animals*. Iowa State Press, pp. 575-606.

Mohammad, K. S., Yin, J. J., Grubbs, B. G., Cui, Y., Padley, R. and Guise, T. A. (2001) Endothelin-1 (ET-1) mediates pathological but not normal bone remodeling [Abstract]. *Journal of Bone and Mineral Research* **16 (Suppl. 1)**: S453.

Namikawa, R. and Shtivelman, E. (1999) SCID-hu mice for the study of human cancer metastasis. *Cancer Chemotherapy. Pharmacology* **43 Suppl**: S37-S41.

Nemeth, J. A., Harb, J. F., Barroso, U., Jr., He, Z., Grignon, D. J. and Cher, M. L. (1999) Severe combined immunodeficient-hu model of human prostate cancer metastasis to human bone. *Cancer Research* **59**: 1987-1993.

Nemoto, H., Rittling, S. R., Yoshitake, H., Furuya, K., Amagasa, T., Tsuji, K., Nifuji, A., Denhardt, D. T. and Noda, M. (2001) Osteopontin deficiency reduces experimental tumor cell metastasis to bone and soft tissues. *Journal of Bone and Mineral Research* **16**: 652-659.

Osterborg, A. and Mellstedt, H. (1996). "Clinical features and staging" In: Gahrton, G. and Durie, B. G. M. (eds.), *Multiple Myeloma*. Arnold, pp. 98-107.

Paget, S. (1889) The distribution of secondary growths in cancer of the breast. *Lancet* **1**: 571-573.

Pollard, M. (1998a) Dihydrotestosterone prevents spontaneous adenocarcinomas in the prostate-seminal vesicle in aging L-W rats. *The Prostate* **36**: 168-171.

Pollard, M. (1998b) Lobund-Wistar rat model of prostate cancer in man. *The Prostate* **37**: 1-4.

Pollard, M. (1999) Prevention of prostate-related cancers in Lobund-Wistar rats. *The Prostate* **39**: 305-309.

Pollard, M., Luckert, P. H. and Snyder, D. L. (1989) The promotional effect of testosterone on induction of prostate-cancer in MNU-sensitized L-W rats. *Cancer Letters* **45**: 209-212.

Pollard, M., Wolter, W. R. and Sun, L. (2000) Prostate-seminal vesicle cancers induced in noble rats. *The Prostate* **43**: 71-74.

Radl, J., Punt, Y. A., Enden-Vieveen, M. H., Bentvelzen, P. A., Bakkus, M. H., van den Akker, T. W. and Benner, R. (1990) The 5T mouse multiple myeloma model: absence of c-myc oncogene rearrangement in early transplant generations. *British Journal of Cancer* **61**: 276-278.

Rice, B. W., Cable, M. D. and Nelson, M. B. (2001) In vivo imaging of light-emitting probes. *Journal of Biomedical Opthamology* **6**: 432-440.

Rosol, T. J. (2000) Pathogenesis of bone metastases: Role of tumor-related proteins. *Journal of Bone and Mineral Research* **15**: 844-850.

Rubens, R. D. and Coleman, R. E. (1995). "Bone Metastases" In: Abeloff, M. D., Armitage, J. O., Lichter, A. S. and Niederhuber, J. E. (eds.), *Clinical Oncology*. Churchill Livingstone, pp. 643-665.

Schneider, A., Taboas, J. M., Krebsbach, P. H. and McCauley, L. K. (2002) An ectopic tissue engineered bone model to study hormonal responses in vivo [abstract]. Presented at the Third North American Symposium on Skeletal Complications of Malignancy, Bethesda, MD, April 25-27, 2002.

Seely, J. C. and Boorman, G. A. (1999). "Mammary Gland and Specialized Sebaceous Glands" In: Maronpot, R. R., Boorman, G. A. and Gaul, B. W. (eds.), *Pathology of the Mouse*. Cache River Press, pp. 613-636.

Shevrin, D. H., Kukreja, S. C., Ghosh, L. and Lad, T. E. (1988) Development of skeletal metastasis by human prostate cancer in athymic nude mice. *Clinical Exp. Metastasis* **6**: 401-409.

Stearns, M. E., Ware, J. L., Agus, D. B., Chang, C. J., Fidler, I. J., Fife, R. S., Goode, R., Holmes, E., Kinch, M. S., Peehl, D. M., Pretlow, T. G. and Thalmann, G. N. (1998) Workgroup 2: human xenograft models of prostate cancer. *The Prostate* **36**: 56-58.

Stoica, G., Koestner, A. and Capen, C. C. (1983) Characterization of N-ethyl-N-nitrosourea-induced mammary tumors in the rat. *American Journal of Pathology* **110**: 161-169.

Stoica, G., Koestner, A. and Capen, C. C. (1984) Neoplasms induced with high single doses of N-ethyl-N-nitrosourea in 30-day-old Sprague-Dawley rats, with special emphasis on mammary neoplasia. *Anticancer Research* **4**: 5-12.

Sung, V., Cattell, D. A., Bueno, J. M., Murray, A., Zwiebel, J. A., Aaron, A. D. and Thompson, E. W. (1997) Human breast cancer cell metastasis to long bone and soft organs of nude mice: a quantitative assay. *Clinical Experimental Metastasis* **15**: 173-183.

Suwa, T., Nyska, A., Haseman, J. K., Mahler, J. F. and Maronpot, R. R. (2002) Spontaneous lesions in control B6C3F1 mice and recommended sectioning of male accessory sex organs. *Toxicologic Pathology* **30**: 228-234.

Suwa, T., Nyska, A., Peckham, J. C., Hailey, J. R., Mahler, J. F., Haseman, J. K. and Maronpot, R. R. (2001) A retrospective analysis of background lesions and tissue accountability for male accessory sex organs in Fischer-344 rats. *Toxicologic Pathology* **29**: 467-478.

Sweeney, T. J., Mailander, V., Tucker, A. A., Olomu, A. B., Zhang, W., Cao, Y., Negrin, R. S. and Contag, C. H. (1999) Visualizing the kinetics of tumor-cell clearance in living animals. Proceedings of the National Academy of Science U S A **96**: 12044-12049.

Tennant, T. R., Kim, H., Sokoloff, M. and Rinker, S. (2000) The Dunning model. *The Prostate* **43**: 295-302.

Tester, A. M., Sharp, J. A., Dhanesuan, N., Waltham, M. and Thompson, E. W. (2002) Correlation between extent of osteolytic damage and metastatic burden of human breast cancer metastasis in nude mice: real-time PCR quantitation. *Clinical Exp. Metastasis* **19**: 377-383.

Thalmann, G. N., Sikes, R. A., Wu, T. T., Degeorges, A., Chang, S. M., Ozen, M., Pathak, S. and Chung, L. W. (2000) LNCaP progression model of human prostate cancer: androgen-independence and osseous metastasis. *The Prostate* **44**: 91-103.

Urashima, M., Chen, B. P., Chen, S., Pinkus, G. S., Bronson, R. T., Dedera, D. A., Hoshi, Y., Teoh, G., Ogata, A., Treon, S. P., Chauhan, D. and Anderson, K. C. (1997) The development of a model for the homing of multiple myeloma cells to human bone marrow. *Blood* **90**: 754-765.

Vaezy, A. and Budson, D. C. (1978) Phalangeal metastases from bronchogenic carcinoma. *Journal of the American Medical Association* **239**: 226-227.

van der Pluijm, G., Sijmons, B., Vloedgraven, H., Deckers, M., Papapoulos, S. and Lowik, C. (2001) Monitoring metastatic behavior of human tumor cells in mice with species-specific polymerase chain reaction: elevated expression of angiogenesis and bone resorption stimulators by breast cancer in bone metastases. *Journal of Bone and Mineral Research* **16**: 1077-1091.

Varma, V. A. and Austin, G. E. (1990) Morphologic characterization of early prostatic carcinomas in the ACI rat: a light and electron microscopic study. *Experimental Molecular Pathology* **52**: 202-211.

Wang, M. and Stearns, M. E. (1991) Isolation and characterization of PC-3 human prostatic tumor sublines which preferentially metastasize to select organs in S.C.I.D. mice. *Differentiation* **48**: 115-125.

Waters, D. J., Hayden, D. W., Bell, F. W., Klausner, J. S., Qian, J. and Bostwick, D. G. (1997) Prostatic intraepithelial neoplasia in dogs with spontaneous prostate cancer. *The Prostate* **30**: 92-97.

Weber, K. L., Pathak, S., Multani, A. S. and Price, J. E. (2002) Characterization of a renal cell carcinoma cell line derived from a human bone metastasis and establishment of an experimental nude mouse model. *Journal of Urology* **168**: 774-779.

Wetterwald, A., van der, P. G., Que, I., Sijmons, B., Buijs, J., Karperien, M., Lowik, C. W., Gautschi, E., Thalmann, G. N. and Cecchini, M. G. (2002) Optical imaging of cancer metastasis to bone marrow: a mouse model of minimal residual disease. *American Journal of Pathology* **160**: 1143-1153.

Wu, T. T., Sikes, R. A., Cui, Q., Thalmann, G. N., Kao, C., Murphy, C. F., Yang, H., Zhau, H. E., Balian, G. and Chung, L. W. (1998) Establishing human prostate cancer cell xenografts in bone: induction of osteoblastic reaction by prostate-specific antigen-producing tumors in athymic and SCID/bg mice using LNCaP and lineage-derived metastatic sublines. *International Journal Cancer* **77**: 887-894.

Yang, M., Baranov, E., Moossa, A. R., Penman, S. and Hoffman, R. M. (2000) Visualizing gene expression by whole-body fluorescence imaging. *Proceedings of the National Academy of Science U. S. A* **97**: 12278-12282.

Yang, M., Hasegawa, S., Jiang, P., Wang, X., Tan, Y., Chishima, T., Shimada, H., Moossa, A. R. and Hoffman, R. M. (1998) Widespread skeletal metastatic potential of human lung cancer revealed by green fluorescent protein expression. *Cancer Research* **58**: 4217-4221.

Yang, M., Jiang, P., An, Z., Baranov, E., Li, L., Hasegawa, S., Al Tuwaijri, M., Chishima, T., Shimada, H., Moossa, A. R. and Hoffman, R. M. (1999) Genetically fluorescent melanoma bone and organ metastasis models. *Clinical Cancer Research* **5**: 3549-3559.

Yi, B., Williams, P. J., Niewolna, M., Wang, Y. and Yoneda, T. (2002) Tumor-derived platelet-derived growth factor-BB plays a critical role in osteosclerotic bone metastasis in an animal model of human breast cancer. *Cancer Research* **62**: 917-923.

Yoneda, T. (1997) Arterial microvascularization and breast cancer colonization in bone. *Histology and Histopathology* **12**: 1145-1149.

Yoneda, T. (2000) Cellular and molecular basis of preferential metastasis of breast cancer to bone. *Journal of Orthopaedic Science* **5**: 75-81.

Yoneda, T., Michigami, T., Yi, B., Williams, P. J., Niewolna, M. and Hiraga, T. (1999a) Use of bisphosphonates for the treatment of bone metastasis in experimental animal models. *Cancer Treatment Review* **25**: 293-299.

Yoneda, T., Williams, P. J., Myoi, A., Michigami, T. and Mbalaviele, G. (1999b). "Cellular and molecular mechanisms of development of skeletal metastases" In: Body, J-J. (ed.), *Tumor Bone Diseases and Osteoporosis in Cancer Patients*, Marcel Dekker, Inc., pp. 41-69.

Yonou, H., Yokose, T., Kamijo, T., Kanomata, N., Hasebe, T., Nagai, K., Hatano, T., Ogawa, Y. and Ochiai, A. (2001) Establishment of a novel species- and tissue-specific metastasis model of human prostate cancer in humanized non-obese diabetic/severe combined immunodeficient mice engrafted with human adult lung and bone. *Cancer Research* **61**: 2177-2182.

Young, D. M., Fioravanti, J. L., Prieur, D. J. and Ward, J. M. (1976) Hypercalcemic VX-2 carcinoma in rabbits: a clinicopathologic study. *Laboratory Investigations* **35**: 30-46.

Zhang, J., Dai, J., Qi, Y., Lin, D. L., Smith, P., Strayhorn, C., Mizokami, A., Fu, Z., Westman, J. and Keller, E. T. (2001) Osteoprotegerin inhibits prostate cancer-induced osteoclastogenesis and prevents prostate tumor growth in the bone. *Journal of Clinical Investigations* **107**: 1235-1244.

Zhau, H. E., Li, C. L. and Chung, L. W. (2000) Establishment of human prostate carcinoma skeletal metastasis models. *Cancer* **88**: 2995-3001.

Zurcher, C. and Roholl, P. J. M. 1989. "Melanocytic tumors, rat" In: Jones, T. C. (ed.), *Integument and Mammary Glands*, Springer-Verlag, pp. 76-86.

Chapter 4

MIP-1 ALPHA AND MYELOMA BONE DISEASE

G. David Roodman, and Sun Jin Choi
Bone Biology Center of the University of Pittsburgh Medical Center, University of Pittsburgh

INTRODUCTION

Multiple myeloma (MM) is a severely debilitating, incurable, and uniformly fatal neoplastic disease of B cell origin (Barker et al., 1993). Although much effort has been directed at devising effective treatments for these patients, their prognosis and survival have been relatively unchanged over the last 30 years, except for a subgroup of patients undergoing successful autologous or allogeneic stem cell transplantation (Gahrton et al., 2001). The major source of morbidity and possible mortality associated with MM is osteolytic lesions throughout the axial skeleton (Coleman, 1997). Lytic bone lesions occur in over 70-80% of these patients (Anderson, 1999), and are frequently associated with severe bone pain and pathologic fractures. Up to one third of the patients develop hypercalcemia. The bone lesions result from increased osteoclastic bone resorption that occurs adjacent to the myeloma cells and not in areas of normal bone marrow (Anderson et al., 2002). These data suggest that locally acting factors produced by myeloma cells induce extensive bone destruction. Consistent with this hypothesis is the finding that cultures of human myeloma cells in vitro produce several osteoclast activating factors (OAFs), including TNF-α (Garret et al., 1987; Sati et al., 1999), IL-1-β (Lacy et al., 1999; Lust et al., 1999), and IL-6 (Bataille et al., 1995; Epstein et al., 1992; Iwasaki et al., 1999). However, none of these cytokines appears to be clearly responsible for the bone destruction in vivo. The increase in osteoclast (OCL) bone resorption in myeloma is usually associated with a marked impairment in osteoblast function (Alexandrakis et al., 2002). Alkaline phosphatase activity in the serum is decreased or in the normal range, unlike patients with other types of osteolytic bone disease, and radionuclide scans do not show evidence of increased uptake in over 50% of patients with osteolytic lesions, indicating impaired osteoblast responses to the increase in bone resorption.

In this review, we will focus on one of the OAFs implicated in myeloma bone disease, macrophage inflammatory protein-1alpha (MIP-1α).

MIP-1α- A POTENT INDUCER OF OCL FORMATION

In 1992, Kukita et al. reported that recombinant LD78 alpha (MIP-1α) and its variant LD78 beta (MIP-1β) stimulated osteoclast-like cell formation in rat bone marrow cultures in the presence of 1 alpha, 25-dihydroxyvitamin D3 (Kukita et al., 1992). MIP-1α is a member of the small inducible protein family involved in cell growth, wound healing and inflammation. Human macrophage inflammatory protein-1alpha (hMIP-1α) is a member of the chemokine/intercrine family of proteins and is an inhibitor of hematopoietic stem cell proliferation in vitro (Graham et al., 1992). Using a specific monoclonal antibody and in situ hybridization, Kukita et al. have observed significant localization of hMIP-1α in eosinophilic myelocytes in human bone marrow (Kukita et al., 1997). hMIP-1 α mRNA expression was also detected in osteoblasts in the bone-remodeling sites, and osteoclasts were frequently observed in the vicinity of these osteoblasts. hMIP-1α induced osteoclastogenesis on calcified matrices in the absence of any other osteotropic hormones.

Scheven et al. in studies of osteoclast-inducing growth factors (OGF) present in fetal rat calvarial conditioned medium (RCCM) identified macrophage inflammatory protein-1alpha (MIP-1α), a member of the C-C chemokine family, as an essential factor for the induction of osteoclast differentiation in this system (Scheven et al., 1991). Addition of anti-MIP-1α antibody to fetal rat calvarial cultures was accompanied by an increase in the number of macrophage-like cells, suggesting that bone-derived MIP-1α was involved in the direction of preosteoclast formation with an inhibitory action on progenitor cell proliferation (Scheven et al., 1999).

Fuller et al. reported that MIP-1α and IL-8 stimulated osteoclastic motility and increased the osteoclast spread area in a dose-dependent manner. In addition, MIP-1α induced osteoclast orientation in a gradient of the chemokine, and stimulated osteoclast migration. These data suggested that chemokines can promote osteoclast orientation and migration, processes that might be involved in chemotaxis (Fuller et al., 1995).

Votta et al. reported that the chemokines, CKbeta-8, RANTES, and MIP-1α elicited significant chemotactic activity for the tartrate-resistant acid phosphatase (TRAP)-positive subpopulation of mononuclear cells isolated from collagenase digests of human osteoclastoma tissue (osteoclast precursors) but not for either primary osteoblasts derived from human bone explants or the osteoblastic MG-63 cell line (Votta et al., 2000).

These data demonstrated that MIP-1α play an important role in the process of osteoclast recruitment and differentiation, is involved not only in the regulation of hematopoiesis but also in the modulation of bone remodeling and may be a physiologic regulator of bone resorption.

IDENTIFICATION OF MIP-1α AS AN OAF IN PATIENTS WITH MYELOMA

Using a human myeloma cDNA expression library derived from marrow samples from MM patients we identified MIP-1α as a novel OAF produced by myeloma cells (Choi et al., 2000). The human myeloma cDNA library was constructed from bone marrow mononuclear cells from five MM patients who had greater than 60% myeloma cells in their marrow aspirates, had never received any prior chemotherapy or received bisphosphonates prior to collection of their marrow, and had extensive myeloma bone disease.

Our studies demonstrated that elevated levels of MIP-1α mRNA, but not IL-1β, TNFβ, or IL-6 mRNA, were present in freshly isolated bone marrow from MM patients compared to normals (Choi et al., 2000). ELISA results of freshly isolated bone marrow plasma detected elevated concentrations of human MIP-1α (hMIP-1α) (range 75-7784 pg/ml) in 62% (8/13) of patients with active myeloma, in 3/18 (17%) patients with stable myeloma (range 75-190.3), as well as in conditioned media from 4/5 lymphoblastoid cell lines (LCLs) derived from MM patients (Table 1). Mildly increased levels of MIP-1α were only detected in 3/14 (21%) patients with other hematologic diagnoses (range 80.2-118.3; median value of 96 pg/ml) and were not elevated in marrow samples from normals (0/7). Elevated levels of MIP-1α were not detected in the peripheral blood of any MM patients. Furthermore, recombinant hMIP-1α induced OCL formation in human bone marrow cultures (Choi et al., 2000), and importantly, addition of a neutralizing antibody to MIP-1α to human bone marrow cultures treated with freshly isolated marrow plasma from MM patients, blocked the increased OCL formation induced by these marrow plasma samples in 3/5 patients. Anti-MIP-1α had no effect on control levels of OCL formation. Marrow plasma samples from normals did not induce OCL formation. Thus, high levels of MIP-1α are present in marrow samples from MM patients with active disease, but not in marrow from patients with other hematologic disorders or normals, and support an important role for MIP-1α as an OAF in patients with active myeloma. Consistent with our observations is the recent publication by Abe et al., who showed that elevated levels of MIP-1α were present in 15/20 MM patients, and that MIP-1α induced rabbit OCL formation (Abe et al., 2002) and Uneda et al. who showed that the expression levels of MIP-1α produced by myeloma cells is correlated with bone lesions in 16 out of 18 MM patients expressing elevated MIP-1α levels (Uneda et al., 2003).

Table 1. Measurement of MIP-1α levels

Samples	Disease Activity	Elevated MIP-1α
Stage I MM	Inactive	0/2
Stage III MM	Inactive	3/16
Stage III MM	Active	8/13
Others	-	3/14
Normal controls	-	0/7
Cell lines	-	4/5

MIP-1α levels were considered significantly elevated if they were 2 SD above the upper limit of MIP-1α detected in bone marrow plasma from 7 normal individuals; that is, 42.49 + 2 (15.9). MIP-1α levels were measured by ELISA in 2 patients with MM stage I, 16 patients with MM stage III with inactive disease, 13 patients with MM stage III with active disease, 14 patients with non-MM neoplasias, 7 normal controls, and 5 LCLs. The proportion of patients with elevated levels of MIP-1α > 75 pg/mL was significantly higher among patients with MM stage III active disease when compared to all other groups studied (8 of 13 versus 0 of 2, 3 of 16, 3 of 14, 0 of 7, respectively; P < .05). Levels of MIP-1α were highly elevated (>1500 pg/mL) in 4 of 5 LCLs examined. [*]P < .05.

Thus, chemokines in general, and MIP-1α in particular, are attractive candidates for an OAF in MM because: (1) MIP-1α is produced by myeloma cells in vivo and CHO cells expressing MIP-1α can cause osteolytic lesions when injected intracardially in nude mice; (2) Chemokines are only active locally in anatomically restricted sites, but are not active systemically even in high concentrations (Grewal et al., 1997), consistent with MDB being a local rather than a systemic process; (3) Chemokines enhance adhesive interactions between cells or matrix by upregulating integrin effects (Springer, 1994). For example, adhesive interactions between the $\alpha_4\beta_1$ integrin on myeloma cells and the VCAM1 on marrow stromal cells induce

IL-6 secretion by stromal cells and increased expression of Receptor Activator of NF-kappa B Ligand (RANKL), a potent inducer of OCL formation. This enhanced RANKL expression would further increase OCL formation in areas of MM. In addition, we have reported that MIP-1α can enhances the effects of RANKL on OCL formation (Han et al., 2001); (4) MIP-1α is a chemoattractant for OCLs (Fuller et al., 1995) and induces OCL formation in rat marrow cultures (Kukita et al., 1997); (5) MIP-1α enhances the growth of CFU-GM stimulated by GM-CSF but suppresses more primitive hematopoietic precursors (Broxmeyer et al., 1990). CFU-GM are the earliest identifiable OCL precursors; (6) MIP-1α has been implicated in the anemia of myeloma patients (Tsujimoto et al., 1996); and (7) The finding that a chemokine, rather than a known cytokine, may be the OAF in myeloma may explain the inability of previous investigators to identify the cytokine that mediates the bone destruction in myeloma.

EFFECT OF BLOCKING MIP-1α IN AN IN VIVO MODEL OF HUMAN MYELOMA

Alsina et al. developed an in vivo model of human myeloma bone disease, using the human myeloma derived cell line ARH-77 (Alsina et al., 1996), which could engraft in SCID mice and form microscopic osteolytic lesions in the skull and vertebrae (Huang et al., 1993; Tong et al., 1993). The morphology of the ARH-77 cells is plasmoblastic. All ARH-77 transplanted SCID mice, but not control mice, that survived irradiation developed hind limb paralysis 28-35 days after injection of ARH-77 cells and became hypercalcemic (1.35 - 1.46 mmol/L), a mean of 5 days after becoming paraplegic. Lytic bone lesions were detected radiographically in all the hypercalcemic mice examined. No lytic lesions or hypercalcemia developed in the control animals. Bone marrow plasma from ARH-77 mice induced significant bone resorption in the fetal rat long bone resorption assay when compared to controls (percent of total ^{45}Ca released = 35% ± 4 vs. 11% ± 1). Histologic examination of tissues from the ARH-77 mice showed infiltration of myeloma cells in the liver and spleen, and marked infiltration of myeloma cells in vertebrae and long bones, with loss of bony trabeculae and increased OCL numbers. Cultures of bone marrow from ARH-77 bearing mice for early OCL precursors (CFU-GM), revealed a threefold increase in CFU-GM from ARH-77 marrow vs. controls (185 ± 32 vs. 40 ± 3 per 2 X 10^5 cells plated). Human MIP-1α levels were markedly increased in ARH-77 marrow plasma samples (range 20-5000 pg/ml), but were undetectable in control animals. Other bone-resorbing human and murine cytokines such as IL-6, IL-1α or IL-1β, transforming growth factor-alpha (TGFα), lymphotoxin,

PTHrP, HGF, and TNFα were not significantly increased in ARH-77 mouse sera or marrow plasma, compared to control mice, although ARH-77 cells produce IL-6 and lymphotoxin in vitro.

To investigate the roles of MIP-1α in myeloma bone disease in vivo, the human MM-derived cell line ARH-77 was stably transfected with an antisense construct to MIP-1α (AS-ARH) and tested for its capacity to induce MM bone disease in SCID mice. The MIP-1α antisense clone was constructed in the pcDNA3 mammalian expression vector by inserting MIP-1α exon1 cDNA in a reverse orientation. There was no significant difference in the growth characteristics of wild type ARH-77 (WT-ARH), empty vector ARH-77 (EV-ARH), or antisense ARH-77 (AS-ARH) cells. However, MIP-1α levels in media conditioned for 3 days by the cells were significantly different. AS-ARH cells produced approximately 30–50 pg/ml of MIP-1α in the 3-day conditioned media, in contrast to 1,000–1,200 pg/ml of MIP-1α for the WT-ARH cell line or EV-ARH cells. Furthermore, human MIP-1α levels in marrow plasma from AS-ARH mice were markedly decreased compared with controls treated with ARH cells transfected with empty vector (EV-ARH). As shown in Figure 1A, MIP-1α levels were reduced to almost undetectable levels (< 10 pg/ml) in marrow plasma from the vertebrae or femurs of animals transplanted with AS-ARH cells. In contrast, the levels of human MIP-1α, although variable, were markedly elevated in marrow plasma from animals transplanted with either the WT-ARH or the EV-ARH cells. In contrast, the levels of human IgG, which are an indicator of tumor burden, were significantly decreased in the marrow plasma of animals implanted with AS-ARH cells (0.1–1.0 μg/ml) compared with EV-ARH cells or WT-ARH cells (80–120 μg/ml) (Figure 1B). Mice treated with AS-ARH cells lived longer than controls and, unlike the controls, they showed no radiologically identifiable lytic lesions. SCID mice transplanted with AS-ARH cells had a median survival that was longer compared with the mice injected with WT-ARH or EV-ARH cells (AS-ARH, 28 ± 4 days vs. WT-ARH, 20 ± 2 days, or EV-ARH, 23 ± 3 days). These results did not reach statistical significance ($P = 0.06$) because of the large variability in survival of these animals in three independent experiments. However, in all experiments, AS-ARH mice lived longer than EV-ARH or WT-ARH mice. Animals receiving WT- or EV-ARH cells all developed paraplegia before death due to vertebral involvement by myeloma. In contrast, animals receiving AS-ARH cells never developed paraplegia, but died of a wasting disease most likely reflecting extramedullary involvement by their myeloma.

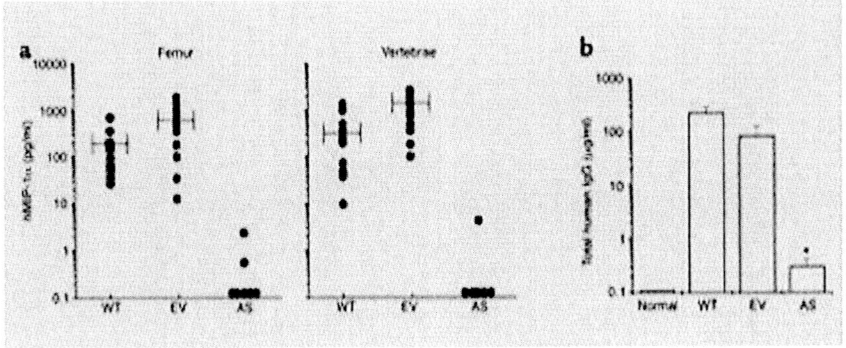

*Figure 1. Expression levels of MIP-1α in vivo. WT-, EV-, and AS-ARH cells were infused intravenously into SCID mice (n=10 per group) and were sacrificed when they became paraplegic. Femurs and vertebrae were then removed and bone marrow plasma obtained by flushing the bones with 1ml of serum-free αMEM. Expression levels of hMIP-1α (a) and human IgG (b) were measured with ELISA kits. KMIP-1α expression in mice implanted with AS-ARH cells was reduced to almost undetectable levels. Human IgG levels, which are indicators of tumor burden, were significantly reduced in AS-ARH mice compared with WT- or EV-ARH mice, but were still detectable (0.1-1 µg/ml). Similar results were seen in three independent experiments (*P<0.0001).*

As shown in Figure 2, animals infused with EV-ARH cells developed lytic bone lesions and increased OCL formation (upper right panel; shown by the red tartrate-resistant acid phosphatase [TRAP] stain). In contrast, animals infused with AS-ARH cells did not demonstrate increased OCL formation or bone resorption (lower right panel). In addition, tumor burden in the bones of animals treated with AS-ARH cells (upper left panel) was markedly decreased compared with animals infused with empty vector-transduced cells (lower left panel). AS-ARH cells could be detected histologically in the bone marrow sections from animals transfected with the antisense construct to MIP-1α, but they were rare. Histomorphometric analysis of the vertebral bodies from these animals demonstrated that OCL numbers per square millimeter of bone and per millimeter of bone surface area were significantly reduced in animals receiving AS-ARH cells compared with EV-ARH cells (Figure. 3). The percentage of tumor per total bone area was also significantly decreased in animals treated with AS-ARH cells compared with animals treated with EV-ARH cells. These data demonstrated that blocking MIP-1α could have a profound effect on bone destruction and tumor growth in multiple myeloma.

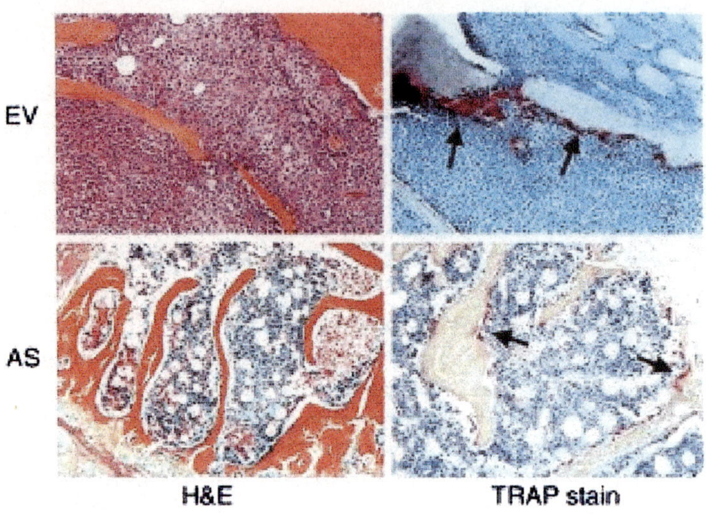

Figure 2. Histology of bone sections from SCID mice implanted with EV- or AS-ARH cells. As shown in the panels stained with hematoxylin and eosin (H and E), mice implanted with AS-ARH cells had significantly reduced tumor burden compared with mice implanted with EV-ARH cells. OCL number was markedly reduced in SCID mice implanted with AS-ARH cells compared with the mice implanted with EV-ARH cells.

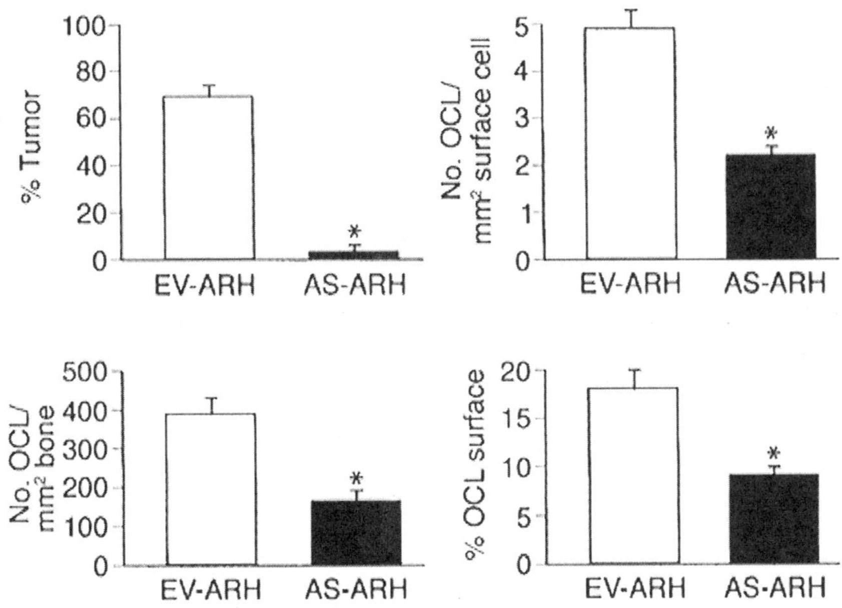

*Figure.3. Histomorphometric analysis of bone sections from SCID mice. Mice treated with AS-ARH cells had markedly reduced tumor burden compared with mice receiving EV-ARH cells. Furthermore, the number of OCLs per square millimeter of surface, the number of OCLs per square millimeter of bone area, and the percentage of active OCL surface were significantly reduced in AS-ARH mice compared with the EV-ARH mice (*P<0.05).*

ROLE OF MIP-1α IN THE ADHESIVE INTERACTIONS OF MYELOMA CELLS WITH MARROW STROMAL IN MYELOMA BONE DISEASE

Adhesive interactions between marrow stromal cells and myeloma cells appear to play a critical role in the bone destructive process ongoing in myeloma as well as to affect tumor cell growth and chemoresistance of myeloma cells to agents such as doxorubicin and melphalan (Cheung et al., 2001). When myeloma cells bind marrow stromal cells, VEGF, IL-6, and RANKL are induced (Vidriales et al., 1996; Gupta et al., 2001). In a murine model of myeloma bone disease, β_1 integrins mediate the adhesive interactions between myeloma cells and marrow stromal cells. Michigami et al have shown that $\alpha_4\beta_1$ integrin plays an important role in inducing a bone-resorbing activity, possibly MIP-1α, when the 5TGM1 murine myeloma cell line binds to the ST2 murine marrow stromal cell line (Michigami et al., 2000). Similarly, Giuliani et al noted that upregulation of RANKL appears to involve in part the integrin $\alpha_4\beta_1$ (Giuliani et al., 2001). Thus, blocking $\alpha_4\beta_1$ binding of myeloma cells to VCAM-1 on stromal cells may decrease the release of bone-resorbing factors by the marrow stromal cells.

Since MIP-1α enhances expression of adhesion molecules on cells (Vaddi et al., 1994; del Pozo et al., 1995), we assessed if blocking MIP-1α expression of myeloma cells result in decreased adherence of myeloma cells to marrow stromal cells using AS-ARH-77 cells as a model. The adherence of AS-ARH cells to ST2 marrow cells was decreased compared with that of EV-ARH cells. We then measured β_1 integrin mRNA levels in EV-ARH and AS-ARH cells. The VLA-4 ($\alpha_4\beta_1$) and VLA-5 ($\alpha_5\beta_1$) integrins have been shown to mediate adherence of myeloma cells to marrow stromal cells (Robledo et al., 1998 ; Michigami et al., 2000). α_4 mRNA expression levels were similar in AS-ARH cells and EV-ARH cells regardless of treatment with a neutralizing antibody to MIP-1α or rhMIP-1α In contrast, the expression of integrin α_5 and β_1 mRNA was decreased and was increased by addition of MIP-1α in AS-ARH cells. Furthermore, treatment of WT-ARH and EV-ARH cells with the anti–MIP-1α antibody decreased $\alpha_5\beta_1$ expression. To confirm that α_5 expression was decreased at the protein level, we analyzed surface expression of β_2 integrin (CD18), β_1 integrin (CD29), and α_5 integrin (CD49e) by immunofluorescence staining and flow cytometry. The results are depicted in Figure 4 demonstrated that a marked decrease in the fluorescence intensity (peak mean channel, or PMC) of β_1 integrin was observed in AS-ARH compared with EV-ARH (from 28–31, to 14 units of fluorescence, respectively) with a concomitant decrease in the percentage of positive cells from 58% to 34%. In contrast to β_1 integrins, no decrease in PMC was observed in surface staining for β_2 integrins between EV-ARH and AS-ARH. Similarly, a decrease in α_5 was also observed in AS-ARH cells compared with EV-ARH cells from 58% positive cells to 22% positive cells, although the overall staining for α_5 was much lower compared with β_1. A concomitant decrease in PMC from 9.3 to 7.1 for α_5 expression by AS-ARH cells was observed, consistent with the observed decrease in the percentage of positive cells (Choi et al., 2001). These data support an important role for MIP-1α in myeloma cell homing, adhesion, and survival, and osteoclastic bone destruction in MM in vivo.

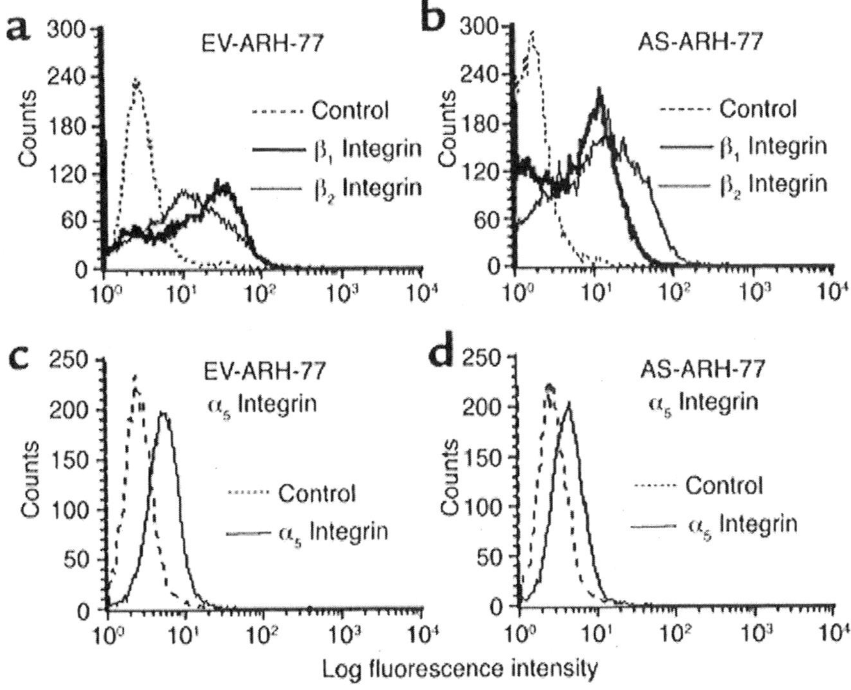

Figure 4. Immunofluorescence staining for CD18, CD29, and CD49e. Staining for EV-ARH cells was compared with AS-ARH cells for a given Ab. For each Ab, cells were also stained with isotype-matched control Ab to correct for background staining. Twenty thousand cells were analyzed for each sample. (a and c) EV-ARH cells. (b and d) AS-ARH cells.

MIP-1α AS A POTENTIAL PROGNOSTIC FACTOR IN MYELOMA

As noted above, elevated levels of MIP-1α in bone marrow plasma samples of MM patients appear to correlate with the activity of their disease (Choi et al., 2000). Therefore, we determined the predictive value of MIP-1α levels present in freshly isolated bone marrow plasma samples in a pilot study of 17 MM patients undergoing peripheral blood stem cell transplantation (PBSCT). Patients were eligible for this study if they had Stage IIIA or IIIB MM and <3 previous infusions of pamidronate. Patients were treated with 6 g/m² of cyclophosphamide and 250 mcg/m²/day of GM-CSF to mobilize their peripheral blood stem cell (PBSC), and received pamidronate (90 or 180 mg IV) before mobilization and on the first day of PBSC collection. After collection of $\geq$ 2 X 10⁶ CD34+ cells/kg, patients were conditioned with melphalan at 200 mg/m² or melphalan/total body irradiation followed by transplantation of CD34+ cells. After engraftment, patients received monthly pamidronate. MIP-1α levels were measured in peripheral blood plasma and bone marrow plasma samples prior to treatment and at 6-month intervals following PBSCT, as well as in daily PBSC collections using standard ELISA assays. Median time from diagnosis to PBSCT was 15 months (range 4-88 months). The disease status of the patients at the time of PBSCT was complete remission: 1 patient; minimal response: 10 patients; partial response: 4 patients; progressive disease: 1 patient. The median percentage of plasma cells in bone marrow aspirates was 14.5% (range 2-86%). Fifteen patients had extensive lytic bone disease. Pretreatment bone marrow plasma levels of MIP-1α ranged from 18-3286 pg/ml (normal < 40 pg/ml). Serial measurements of MIP-1α during PBSC collection did not significantly change over time. Patients with elevated pretreatment levels in bone marrow plasma had elevated MIP-1α levels detected in the PBSC product. Eleven patients were evaluated at a minimum of 1-year after transplantation. Two of two patients with the highest pretreatment MIP-1α levels (1304 and 3286 pg/ml, respectively) relapsed within 6 months of PBSCT. Eight of nine patients with marrow plasma MIP-1α levels <50 pg/ml either prior to transplantation and at follow-up remain in complete remission or had a partial response following PBSCT. One patient relapsed clinically at 1 year after PBSCT. At the 6-month follow-up, his MIP-1α level was elevated (60 pg/ml) and remained so. Pretreatment MIP-1α levels did not correlate with serum β_2 microglobulin levels or % plasma cells in the bone marrow (unpublished data). Recently, Uneda et al. have also reported that high levels of MIP-1α (>100 pg/ml) are associated with a poor prognosis in a series of the MM patients in Japan (Uneda et al., 2003). These data suggest that highly elevated levels of MIP-1α may predict for patients at increased risk for early relapse.

OTHER OSTEOCLAST ACTIVATING FACTORS (OAFS) IN MYELOMA BONE DISEASE

Multiple osteoclastogenic factors in addition to MIP-1α, have been implicated as OAFs that mediate the increased OCL activity in MM patients, including TNFβ, interleukin-1-beta (IL-1β), PTHrP, HGF and IL-6, but none of these factors is present at high levels in the majority of patients or consistently correlate with disease activity (Roodman, 1997). Receptor Activator of NF-kappaB Ligand (RANKL) appears to be a major factor involved in myeloma bone disease in addition to MIP-1α. Receptor activator of NF-kappa B ligand (RANKL) in combination with macrophage colony-stimulating factor (M-CSF) is a potent osteoclastogenic factor in vitro. The relative levels of RANKL and osteoprotegerin (OPG), a decoy receptor for RANKL produced by many different cell types including marrow stromal cells and osteoblasts, determine the level of OCL formation. Giuliani et al have clearly demonstrated that there is an imbalance between OPG and RANKL levels in the bone marrow environment of patients with MM (Giuliani et al., 2001). They examined myeloma cells from 26 patients and 10 myeloma cell lines and demonstrated that myeloma cells failed to express RANKL and produced low amounts of OPG. In coculture systems of human myeloma cells with marrow stromal cells, RANKL expression was upregulated and OPG production strongly downregulated at both the protein and mRNA levels. In addition, Pearse et al have examined marrow biopsy specimens from patients with myeloma and found that RANKL expression was markedly upregulated in bone marrow biopsies from patients with myeloma while OPG was expressed at very low levels compared to normal bone marrow biopsy specimens (Pearse et al., 2001). Taken together, the sets of data suggested that there is a marked imbalance between RANKL expression and OPG levels that favor osteoclastogenesis and OCL activation. In support of these studies is a recent report by Seidel et al from the Nordic Myeloma Group, which showed that OPG levels measured in the serum of patients with MM were significantly lower than those levels in healthy-age and sex-matched controls (Seidel et al., 2001). OPG levels were decreased to a greater extent in myeloma patients with osteolytic disease compared to patients who did not have bone disease. Interestingly, OPG levels did not correlate with clinical stage or survival of the patients. These findings have suggested that OPG may be a reasonable therapeutic agent to treat myeloma bone disease. Several groups have suggested that myeloma cells themselves produce RANKL and directly induce OCL formation, but this has not been a consistent finding. Croucher et al have demonstrated that the murine myeloma cell line, 5T2, expressed RANKL (Croucher et al., 2001). However, Pearse et al. (2001) and Giuliani et al. (2001) failed to demonstrate RANKL expression by human myeloma cells.

In addition to OPG, another antagonist of RANKL is RANK-Fc, a molecule made by fusing the Fc portion of immunoglobulin to a soluble form of the RANK receptor. RANK-Fc has a similar mechanism of action as OPG, but in contrast to OPG, has not been shown to bind TRAIL, a member of the TNF gene family that induces tumor cell apoptosis (Emery et al., 1998). Studies with RANK-Fc in a murine model of humeral hypercalcemia showed that both tumor burden and bone destruction were decreased in these animals when they are treated with RANK-Fc (Oyajobi et al., 2001). Croucher et al have demonstrated that OPG also will inhibit the development of osteolytic bone disease in this model of myeloma (Croucher et al., 2001).

Recently, Yaccoby et al have also examined the potential use of RANK-Fc and bisphosphonates, such as pamidronate or zoledronate, to block bone destruction in the severe combined immunodeficient (SCID)-Hu model of myeloma (Yaccoby et al., 2002). In this model, primary myeloma cells are injected into a human fetal bone rudiment implanted into SCID mice. Both agents decreased bone resorption and tumor burden. Yaccoby et al failed to find any effect on growth of extramedullary myeloma in this model. Taken together, these studies suggest that blocking bone resorption induced by RANKL or MIP-1α may decrease tumor burden as well as bone destruction in patients with myeloma.

SUMMARY

Figure 5 is a proposed model for MIP-1α's effects on myeloma bone disease. MIP-1α is produced by myeloma cells and directly stimulates OCL formation. In addition MIP-1α enhances adhesive interactions between myeloma cells and marrow stromal cells increasing expression of RANKL and IL-6, which further increase bone destruction and tumor burden. The recent evidence from our group and others lead to the conclusion that MIP-1α is an important mediator in the debilitating bone destruction in multiple myeloma. Blocking MIP-1α expression may have profound effects on myeloma cell growth, homing, and bone destruction in this in vivo model of myeloma. These data suggest that antagonists that decrease MIP-1α activity in vivo or blocking MIP-1α signaling by neutralizing its receptor may provide therapeutic alternatives for treating patients with myeloma to decrease both their tumor burden and bone destruction.

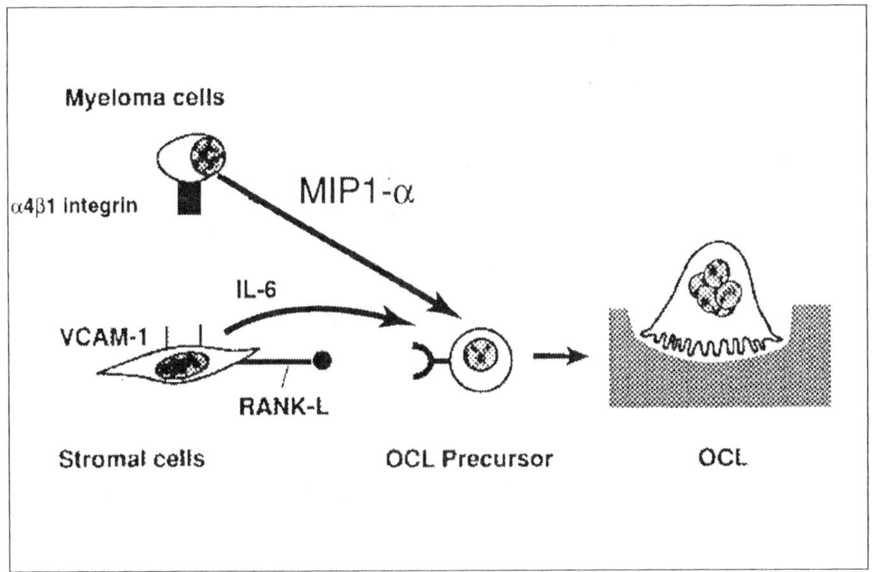

Figure 5. Proposed model for MIP-1α's role in myeloma bone disease. See text for description.

REFERENCES:

Abe, M., Hiura, K., Wilde, J., Moriyama, K., Hashimoto, T., Ozaki, S., Wakatsuki, S., Kosaka, M., Kido, S., Inoue, D. and Matsumoto, T. (2002) Role for macrophage inflammatory protein (MIP)-1alpha and MIP-1beta in the development of osteolytic lesions in multiple myeloma. *Blood* **100**, 2195-2202.

Alexandrakis, M.G., Passam, F.H., Malliaraki, N., Katachanakis, C., Kyriakou, D.S. and Margioris, A.N. (2002) Evaluation of bone disease in multiple myeloma: a correlation between biochemical markers of bone metabolism and other clinical parameters in untreated multiple myeloma patients. *Clin. Chim. Acta.*, **325**, 51-57.

Alsina, M., Boyce, B.F., Devlin, R. Anderson, J.L., Craig, F., Mundy, G.R. and Roodman, G.D. (1996) Development of an in vivo model of human multiple myeloma bone disease. *Blood* **87**, 1495-1501.

Anderson, K. (1999) Advances in the biology of multiple myeloma: therapeutic applications. *Seminars in Oncolgy* **26**, 10–22.

Anderson, K.C., Shaughnessy, J.D. Jr., Barlogie, B., Harousseau, J.L. and Roodman, G.D. (2002) Multiple myeloma. Hematology (Am. Soc. Hematol. Educ. Program.), 214-240

Barker, H.F., Ball, J., Drew, M. and Franklin, I.M. (1993) Multiple myeloma: the biology of malignant plasma cells. *Blood Rev* **7**, 19-23.

Bataille, R., Barlogie, B., Lu, Z.Y., Rossi, J.F., Lavabre-Bertrand, T., Beck, T., Wijdenes, J., Brochier, J. and Klein, B. (1995) Biologic effects of anti-interleukin-6 murine monoclonal antibody in advanced multiple myeloma. *Blood* **86**, 685-691.

Broxmeyer, H.E., Sherry, B., Lu, L., Cooper, S., Oh, K.O., Tekamp-Olson, P., Kwon, B.S. and Cerami, A. (1990) Enhancing and suppressing effects of recombinant murine macrophage inflammatory proteins on colony formation in vitro by bone marrow myeloid progenitor cells. *Blood* **76**, 1110-1116.

Cheung, W.C. and Van Ness, B. (2001) The bone marrow stromal microenvironment influences myeloma therapeutic response in vitro. *Leukemia* **15**, 264-271.

Choi, S.J., Cruz, J.C., Craig, F., Chung, H., Devlin, R.D., Roodman, G.D. and Alsina, M. (2000) Macrophage inflammatory protein 1-alpha is a potential osteoclast stimulatory factor in multiple myeloma. *Blood* **96**, 671-675.

Choi, S.J., Oba, Y., Gazitt, Y., Alsina, M., Cruz, J. anderson, J. and Roodman, G.D. (2001) Antisense inhibition of macrophage inflammatory protein 1-alpha blocks bone destruction in a model of myeloma bone disease. *Journal of Clinical Investigations* **108**, 1833-1841.

Coleman, R.E. (1997) Skeletal complications of malignancy. *Cancer* **80**, 1588-1594.

Croucher, P.I., Shipman, C.M., Lippitt, J., Perry, M., Asosingh, K., Hijzen, A., Brabbs, A.C., van Beek, E.J., Holen, I., Skerry, T.M., Dunstan, C.R., Russell, G.R., Van Camp, B. and Vanderkerken, K. (2001) Osteoprotegerin inhibits the development of osteolytic bone disease in multiple myeloma. *Blood* **98**, 3534–3540.

Damiano, J.S. and Dalton, W.S. (2000) Integrin-mediated drug resistance in multiple myeloma. *Leuk. Lymphoma* **38**, 71-81.

del Pozo, M.A., Sanchez-Mateos, P., Nieto, M. and Sanchez-Madrid, F. (1995) Chemokines regulate cellular polarization and adhesion receptor redistribution during lymphocyte interaction with endothelium and extracellular matrix. Involvement of cAMP signaling pathway. *Journal of Cell Biology* **131**, 495-508.

Emery, J.G., McDonnell, P., Burke, M.B., Deen, K.C., Lyn, S., Silverman, C., Dul, E., Appelbaum, E.R., Eichman, C., DiPrinzio, R., Dodds, R.A., James, I.E., Rosenberg, M., Lee, J.C. and Young, P.R. (1998) Osteoprotegerin is a receptor for the cytotoxic ligand TRAIL. *Journal of Biological Chemistry* **273**, 14363–14367.

Epstein, J. (1992) Myeloma phenotype: Clues to disease origin and manifestation. Hematol Oncol Clin North Am. B Barlogie ed. WB Saunders, **6**, 249-256.

Fuller, K., Owens, J.M. and Chambers, T.J. (1995) Macrophage inflammatory protein-1 alpha and IL-8 stimulate the motility but suppress the resorption of isolated rat osteoclasts. *Journal of Immunology* **154**, 6065-6072.

Gahrton, G., Svensson, H., Cavo, M., Apperly, J., Bacigalupo, A., Bjorkstrand, B., Blade, J., Cornelissen, J., de Laurenzi, A., Facon, T., Ljungman, P., Michallet, M., Niederwieser, D., Powles, R., Reiffers, J., Russell, N.H., Samson, D., Schaefer, U.W., Schattenberg, A., Tura, S., Verdonck, L.F., Vernant, J.P., Willemze, R. and Volin, L. (2001) The European Group for Blood and Marrow Transplantation. Progress in allogenic bone marrow and peripheral blood stem cell transplantation for multiple myeloma: a comparison between transplants performed 1983--93 and 1994--8 at European Group for Blood and Marrow Transplantation centres. *British Journal of Hemaotology* **113**, 209-216.

Garrett, I.R., Durie, B.G.M., Nedwin, G.E., Gillespie, A., Bringman, T., Sabatini, M., Bertolini, D.R. and Mundy, G.R. (1987) Production of the bone resorbing cytokine lymphotoxin by cultured human myeloma cells. *New England Journal of Medicine* **317**, 526-532.

Giuliani, N., Bataille, R., Mancini, C., Lazzaretti, M. and Barille, S. (2001) Myeloma cells induce imbalance in the osteoprotegerin/osteoprotegerin ligand system in the human bone marrow environment. *Blood* **98**, 3527–3533.

Graham, G.J. and Pragnell, I.B. (1992) SCI/MIP-1 alpha: a potent stem cell inhibitor with potential roles in development. *Developmental Biology* **151**, 337-381.

Grewal, I.S., Rutledge, B.J., Fiorillo, J.A., Gu, L., Gladue, R.P., Flavell, R.A. and Rollins, B.J. (1997) Transgenic monocyte chemoattractant protein-1 (MCP-1) in pancreatic islets produces monocyte-rich insulitis without diabetes: Abrogation by a second transgene expressing systemic MCP-1. *Journal of Immunology* **159**, 401-408.

Gupta, D., Treon, S.P., Shima, Y., Hideshima, T., Podar, K., Tai, Y.T., Lin, B., Lentzsch, S., Davies, F.E., Chauhan, D., Schlossman, R.L., Richardson, P., Ralph, P., Wu, L., Payvandi, F., Muller, G., Stirling, D.I. and Anderson, K.C. (2001) Adherence of multiple myeloma cells to bone marrow stromal cells upregulates vascular endothelial growth factor secretion: therapeutic applications. *Leukemia* **15**, 1950-1961.

Han, J.H., Choi, S.J., Kurihara, N., Koide, M., Oba, Y. and Roodman, G.D. (2001) Macrophage inflammatory protein-1alpha is an osteoclastogenic factor in myeloma that is independent of receptor activator of nuclear factor kappaB ligand. *Blood* **97**, 3349-3353.

Huang, Y.W., Richardson, J.A., Tong, A.W., Zhang, B.Q., Stone, M.J. and Vitetta, E.S. (1993) Disseminated growth of a human multiple myeloma cell line in mice with severe combined immunodeficiency disease. *Cancer Research* **53**, 1392-1396.

Iwasaki, T., Hamano, T., Ogata, A. and Kakishita, E. (1999) Clinical significance of interleukin-6 gene expression in the bone marrow of patients with multiple myeloma. *International Journal of Hematology* **70**, 163-168.

Kukita, T., Nakao, J., Hamada, F., Kukita, A., Inai, T., Kurisu, K. and Nomiyama, H. (1992) Recombinant LD78 protein, a member of the small cytokine family, enhances osteoclast differentiation in rat bone marrow culture system. *Bone Miner* **19**, 215-223.

Kukita, T., Nomiyama, H., Ohmoto, Y., Kukita, A., Shuto, T., Hotokebuchi, T., Sugioka, Y., Miura, R. and Iijima, T. (1997) Macrophage inflammatory protein-1 alpha (LD78) expressed in human bone marrow: its role in regulation of hematopoiesis and osteoclast recruitment. *Laboratory Investigations* **76**, 399-406.

Lacy, M.Q., Donovan, K.A., Heimbach, J.K., Ahmann, G.J. and Lust, J.A. (1999) Comparison of interleukin-1 beta expression by in situ hybridization in monoclonal gammopathy of undetermined significance and multiple myeloma. *Blood* **93**, 300-305.

Lust, J.A. and Donovan, K.A. (1999) The role of interleukin-1 beta in the pathogenesis of multiple myeloma. *Hematol. Oncol. Clin. North Am* **13**, 1117-1125.

Michigami, T., Shimizu, N., Williams, P.J., Niewolna, M., Dallas, S.L. and Mundy, G.R. (2000) Cell-cell contact between marrow stromal cells and myeloma cells via VCAM-1 and alpha(4)beta(1)-integrin enhances production of osteoclast-stimulating activity. *Blood* **96**, 1953–1960.

Oyajobi, B.O. anderson, D.M., Traianedes, K., Williams, P.J., Yoneda, T. and Mundy, G.R. (2001) Therapeutic efficacy of a soluble receptor activator of nuclear factor kappaB-IgG Fc fusion protein in suppressing bone resorption and hypercalcemia in a model of humoral hypercalcemia of malignancy. *Cancer Research* **61**, 2572–2578.

Pearse, R.N., Sordillo, E.M., Yaccoby, S., Wong, B.R., Liau, D.F., Colman, N., Michaeli, J., Epstein, J. and Choi, Y. (2001) Multiple myeloma disrupts the TRANCE/ osteoprotegerin cytokine axis to trigger bone destruction and promote tumor progression. *Proceedings of the National Academy of Sciences U S A* **98**, 11581–11586.

Robledo, M.M., Sanz-Rodriguez, F., Hidalgo, A. and Teixido, J. (1998) Differential use of very late antigen-4 and -5 integrins by hematopoietic precursors and myeloma cells to adhere to transforming growth factor-ß$_1$-treated bone marrow stroma. *Journal of Biological Chemistry* **273**, 12056-12060.

Roodman, GD. (1997) Mechanisms of bone lesions in multiple myeloma and lymphoma. *Cancer* **80**, 1557-1563.

Sati, H.I., Greaves, M., Apperley, J.F., Russell, R.G. and Croucher, P.I. (1999) Expression of interleukin-1 beta and tumour necrosis factor-alpha in plasma cells from patients with multiple myeloma. *British Journal of Haematology* **104**, 350-357.

Scheven, B.A., Hamilton, N.J., Duncan, A. and Robins, S.P. (1991) Osteoclast growth factor activity in medium conditioned by fetal rat bones. *Bone Miner* **14**, 221-235.

Scheven, B.A., Milne, J.S., Hunter, I. and Robins, SP. (1999) Macrophage-inflammatory protein-1alpha regulates preosteoclast differentiation in vitro. *Biochemical and Biophysical Research Communications* **254**, 773-778.

Seidel, C., Hjertner, O., Abildgaard, N., Heickendorff, L., Hjorth, M., Westin, J., Nielsen, J.L., Hjorth-Hansen, H., Waage, A., Sundan, A. and Borset, M.; Nordic Myeloma Study Group. (2001) Serum osteoprotegerin levels are reduced in patients with multiple myeloma with lytic bone disease. *Blood* **98**, 2269–2271.

Springer, T. A. (1994) Traffic signals for lymphocyte recirculation and leukocyte emigration: The multistep paradigm. *Cell* **76,** 301-314.

Tong, A.W., Huang, Y.W., Zhang, B.Q., Netto, G., Vitetta, E.S. and Stone, M.J. (1993) Heterotransplantation of human multiple myeloma cell lines in severe combined immunodeficiency (SCID) mice. *Anticancer Research* **13**, 593-597.

Tsujimoto, T., Lisukov, I.A., Huang, N., Mahmoud, M.S. and Kawano, M.M. (1996) Plasma cells induce apoptosis of pre-B cells by interacting with bone marrow stromal cells. *Blood* **87**, 3375-3383.

Uneda, S., Hata, H., Matsuno, F., Harada, N., Mitsuya, Y., Kawano, F. and Mitsuya, H. (2003) Macrophage inflammatory protein-1 alpha is produced by human multiple myeloma (MM) cells and its expression correlates with bone lesions in patients with MM. *British Journal of Haematology* **120**, 53-55.

Vaddi, K. and Newton, R.C. (1994) Regulation of monocyte integrin expression by beta-family chemokines. *Journal of Immunology* **153**, 4721-4732.

Vidriales, M.B. and Anderson, K.C. (1996) Adhesion of multiple myeloma cells to the bone marrow microenvironment: implications for future therapeutic strategies. *Mol. Med. Today*, **2**, 425-431.

Votta, B.J., White, J.R., Dodds, R.A., James, I.E., Connor, J.R., Lee-Rykaczewski, E., Eichman, C.F., Kumar, S., Lark, M.W. and Gowen, M. (2000) CKbeta-8 [CCL23], a novel CC chemokine, is chemotactic for human osteoclast precursors and is expressed in bone tissues. *Journal of Cellular Physiology* **183**, 196-207.

Yaccoby, S., Pearse, R.N., Johnson, CL., Barlogie, B., Choi, Y. and Epstein, J. (2002) Myeloma interacts with the bone marrow microenvironment to induce osteoclastogenesis and is dependent on osteoclast activity. *British Journal of Haematology* **116**, 278–290.

Chapter 5

TYPE I COLLAGEN-MEDIATED CHANGES IN GENE EXPRESSION AND FUNCTION OF PROSTATE CANCER CELLS

Jeffrey Kiefer[1], Angela Alexander, and Mary C. Farach-Carson
Department of Biological Sciences, University of Delaware; [1]Present address: Cancer Drug Development Laboratory, Translational Genomics Research Institute, Gaithersburg, MD

EXTRACELLULAR MATRIX INFLUENCES GENE EXPRESSION

Increasingly it is recognized that the extracellular matrix (ECM) plays a critical role in the normal development and differentiated phenotype of cells and tissues (Lee et al, 1999; Bokel et al, 2002). Engagement of ECM molecules by cells through surface receptors, including integrins, results in the activation of signaling pathways along with specific changes in gene expression. Intracellular signals direct proliferation, survival, migration, invasive potential and differentiation (Giancotti et al, 1999). A well-characterized example of ECM influence over cell phenotype and gene expression is in the control of mammary epithelial cell differentiation by the particular composition of the ECM (Lee et al, 1999; Hansen et al, 2000). Mammary epithelial cells plated onto laminin-1 matrices express proteins associated with milk production, including β-casein, whereas cells plated onto type I collagen do not. Additionally, laminin-1 confers on mammary epithelial cells the capability of being able to respond fully to prolactin-controlled expression of milk proteins. Cells plated onto type I collagen, however, fail to respond (Streuli et al, 1999). Another familiar example of ECM control over cell differentiation and gene expression occurs during osteoblast differentiation. Early studies indicated that contact with type I collagen is required for normal differentiation and eventual matrix secretion and mineralization (Gronowicz et al, 1994; Takeuchi et al, 1997). Subsequent studies showed that type I collagen directs osteoblast differentiation by influencing the activity of a specific transcription factor Cbfa1, also called Runx2, associated with transcriptional activation of a series of genes associated with osteoblast formation (Xiao et al, 1998). The $\alpha_2\beta_1$ integrin serves as the major molecular conduit that mediates type I collagen-dependent osteoblast maturation (Gronowicz et al, 1994; Takeuchi et al, 1997; Xiao et al, 1998). Cbfa1/Runx2 activity, in response to type I collagen binding to the $\alpha_2\beta_1$ integrin, is controlled post-translationally by phosphorylation by MAPK (Xiao et al, 2000). These two examples illustrate the importance of the ECM-directed gene expression for cellular differentiation, and highlight the convergence of intracellular signals that are required for phenotypic and genotypic control.

PROSTATE CANCER BONE METASTASIS AND THE EXTRACELLULAR MATRIX

Bone represents one of the most preferred sites for the metastasis of particular cancer types, especially in the case of breast and prostate cancers (Mundy, 1997). Metastatic cancer cells that have colonized the bone microenvironment have deleterious effects on bone physiology (Sharpe, 1942). Once in bone, cancer cells dramatically alter the normally coupled cycles of bone resorption and formation that occur during normal bone remodeling. For example, in breast cancer, remodeling cycles favor osteoclastic activity producing focal points of osteolysis (Guise et al, 1998). The opposite is often true in prostate cancer, during which the presence of metastatic cells increases osteoblast activity, resulting in an osteoblastic reaction (Mundy, 1997). The actions of metastatic cells in the bone are associated with significant mortality and morbidity. Patients that possess bone metastases often suffer from a number of clinical problems including pathological fracture, bone pain, spinal cord compression and hypercalcemia. Most significantly, metastatic disease in the bone is often refractory to most therapeutic modalities, thus representing a major obstacle in treating patients with advanced disease. Therefore, the development of novel and effective treatments to control the spread and growth of metastatic cancer to bone is an important goal in cancer research.

The seeding of bone by metastatic prostate cells depends on the adhesive interaction between cells and ECM components in the skeletal microenvironment. Site-specific metastasis is thought to involve, in part, adhesion of metastatic cells to endothelial cells of their target tissue (Pauli et al, 1988). Prostate cancer cells adhere to bone marrow derived-endothelial cells to a greater degree than endothelial cells from other tissues (Haq et al, 1992; Lehr et al, 1998). The adhesion between the PC3 prostate cancer cell line and the bone derived endothelial cell can be reduced by blocking antibodies against, galectin-3, vascular cell adhesion molecule (VCAM), CD11a (α_L), CD8 (β_2) and leukocyte functional antigen-1 (LFA-1) (Lehr et al, 1998). RGD blocking peptides used at high concentrations interfere with prostate cell binding to bone endothelial cells (Romanov et al, 1999) suggesting a role for integrins in this process.

The ECM of bone consists of numerous proteins that are able to serve as adhesive substrates for metastatic prostate cells. The organic component of the bone ECM consists primarily (>95%) of type I collagen (Termine, 1996). The remaining non-collagenous component consists of molecules such as BSP, OPN, FN, SPARC, OCN, thrombospondin, and vitronectin. Previous studies show that these non-collagenous proteins either by themselves or in various combinations can promote prostate cancer cell adhesion and growth (Jacob et al, 1999; Koeneman et al, 1999; Thalmann et al, 1999; Lecrone et al, 2000). Additionally, various combinations of non-collagenous protein mixtures mediate attachment of prostate cancer cells in what appears to be an integrin-dependent mechanism (Hullinger et al, 1998; Kiefer, unpublished observations). However, given its abundance in the bone matrix, the role type I collagen may play in prostate cancer bone metastasis has yet to be elucidated. Previous studies demonstrate that type I collagen serves as an adhesive substrate for numerous cancer cells and may influence adhesion and retention of various metastatic cells in skeletal tissue (Klein et al, 1991; Ridley et al, 1993; Kostenuik et al, 1996; Kostenuik et al, 1997). The PC3 prostate cancer cell line rapidly adheres to type I collagen via the $\alpha_2\beta_1$ integrin (Kostenuik et al, 1996). TGF-β was able to increase PC3 cell adhesion to type I collagen, possibly through a mechanism involving up-regulation of collagen-binding integrins (Kostenuik et al, 1997). Type I collagen, therefore, is an attractive candidate molecule capable of influencing homing and adherence of prostate cells to bone. These results illustrate importance of the various ECM molecules in skeletal tissue that influence the behaviour of prostate cancer cells in the skeletal microenivornment.

MICROARRAYS AND CANCER

DNA microarray technology permits the simultaneous monitoring of the expression levels of transcripts encoded by numerous genes under defined experimental conditions. Traditional analysis of gene expression is often tedious and limited with respect to the number of gene transcripts capable of being monitored. Hundreds to thousands of gene transcripts can be analyzed by DNA microarrays. Microarrays are generated by "spotting" oligonucleotides or cDNA molecules onto solid phase supports. Labeled cDNA samples are hybridized to the microarray and the intensity of the hybridized spots are compared and standardized to known controls, allowing for the molecular profiling and comparison between various cell or tissue samples (DeRisi et al, 1999; Khan et al, 1999b; Celis et al, 2000). Microarray technology provides an important tool for elucidating global changes in gene expression associated with specific disease states. For example, microarray analysis of various samples from different tumor stages allows for the generation of a more complete genomic profile associated with the various cancer stages (Dhanasekaran et al, 2001; Sasaki et al, 2002; Dyrskjot et al, 2003; Zhou et al, 2003). Tumor staging has a direct correlation with patient survival and hence is a gauge of patient prognosis. In the near future molecular profiling is likely to allow for the generation of individually tailored therapies (Golub et al, 1999; Alizadeh et al, 2000; Hippo et al, 2001; Watson et al, 2001). Microarray technology also may be used to determine gene expression changes in response to certain experimental manipulations. This approach has been used successfully for profiling expression changes in response to oncogene transfection, viral infection, and cytokine treatments, among others (Der et al, 1998; Zhu et al, 1998; Khan et al, 1999a).

The application of microarray technology to prostate cancer, particularly to the area of bone metastasis, and related areas of research are quickly expanding our knowledge of the molecular development and progression of metastatic disease. One area of investigation that has been amenable to microarray analysis is in the profiling of gene expression changes in response to androgen deprivation (Bubendorf et al, 1999a; Amler et al, 2000; Vaarala et al, 2000; Nelson et al, 2002). Early stages of prostate cancer growth are dependent on the presence of androgens, however, during disease progression this androgen-dependence is lost. Pilot microarray studies profiling gene expression changes accompanying transitions to androgen-independence have utilized androgen responsive prostate cancer cell lines. Results of these studies show that gene products associated with cellular proliferation are up-regulated in androgen-independent cell lines (Bubendorf et al, 1999a; Amler et al, 2000; Vaarala et al, 2000; Nelson et al, 2002). Profiling studies between normal and cancerous prostate tissue also have been performed and have revealed novel changes in certain gene products between these two types of tissue (Bubendorf et al, 1999b; Elek et al, 2000;

Xu et al, 2000; Dhanasekaran et al, 2001; Brooks, 2002; Rhodes et al, 2002). These changes may represent new tumor markers or new targets for therapeutic intervention. Another area of microarray analysis in prostate cancer is in the monitoring of gene expression changes in response to ECM components. Calaluce et. al., monitored gene transcript expression in prostate cancer cell lines in response to the addition of laminin-5. Results from the microarray analysis revealed potential target gene products that may influence the initial stages of prostate tumor development (Calaluce et al, 2001).

Recently published results from our laboratory (Kiefer et al, 2001) suggest that type I collagen, influences the proliferative capacity of bone-derived PC3 prostate cancer cells. We wished to follow up these studies with a cDNA microarray strategy designed to characterize changes in gene transcript expression occurring in PC3 cells plated on type I collagen rather than on standard tissue culture plastic. The microarray results, some of which are reported in this chapter, reveal changes in the expression of gene products associated with cellular signaling, cell metabolism, regulation of gene transcription and protein translation. The changes in gene transcript expression profile are indicative of cells that are proliferating, consistent with the earlier functional studies (Kiefer et al, 2001), and further support the significant role that type I collagen may play in prostate cancer cell gene expression in the bone microenvironment.

OVERVIEW OF METHODS USED IN THIS STUDY

Cell Culture and RNA Isolation. Serum starved (24 hr) PC3 cells were harvested with 0.5 mM EDTA/1X PBS and collected by centrifugation and washed twice with 1X PBS. Cells were seeded onto either uncoated tissue culture wells or tissue culture wells coated with rat-tail type I collagen. Total RNA was harvested with the RNeasy® Total RNA System (QIAGEN Inc.-USA, Valencia, CA) according to manufacturer's instructions. Purified total RNA was treated with DNAse I (Ambion, Austin, TX.) to remove genomic DNA contamination. DNAse I was removed according to manufacturer's instructions and RNA stored at -80° C

cDNA Labeling, Hybridization, and Scanning of Microarray. The microarray analyses were performed using a sequence validated human prostate tissue cDNA array (Human Prostate-Specific GeneFilters® Microarray, Release I, GF221, Invitrogen Corporation, Carlsbad, CA). This particular array consisted of an estimated 5,000 genes or ESTs spotted onto a nylon filter. Each spot on the membrane contains approximately 0.5 ng of insert DNA from an I.M.A.G.E. cDNA clone containing the 3' end of a gene. The array was probed with cDNA from PC3 cells grown in serum free media on either tissue culture plastic or type I collagen for 24 hr. Equal amounts of total RNA (10 μg) from cells grown on plastic and type I collagen were used for generation of cDNA probes. Probe labeling was carried out using the GeneFilters® Probe Labeling and Purification Kit (Invitrogen) according to manufacturer's instructions. Briefly, total RNA was subjected to oligo-dT primed reverse transcription in the presence of ^{33}P-dCTP for 2 hr at 42°C. Probe was gel purified with manufacturer supplied spin columns. Purified probe was denatured for 5 min in a boiling water bath. The denatured probe was added directly to hybridization solution and placed with a pre-hybridized blot in a roller bottle. Hybridization was performed at 42°C for 18 hr. Hybridized membranes were washed twice in low stringency wash solution (2X SSC, 1.0% (w/v) SDS) and once in high stringency wash solution (0.5X SSC, 1.0% (w/v) SDS) at 55°C. Membranes were exposed to PhosphorImager plates for 96 hr. The PhosphorImager screens were scanned on the Molecular Dynamics Storm Imager® at 50 μM resolution. Scanned images were analyzed with Pathways® 3.0 software (Invitrogen). Image normalization was accomplished by global nomalization all membrane spots. Pair wise analysis of plastic vs. collagen I RNA preparation was conducted on normalized images. Gene transcript expression changes were marked at an arbitrarily established cutoff intensity ratio of 2.0. The membrane was hybridized with cDNA from two independent experiments to insure reproducible and consistent gene transcript expression profiles between experiments.

EST Analysis. Because information is constantly being added to national databases, we devised a strategy for identifying ESTs of unknown function whose expression changed significantly as a result of growth on type I collagen. The standard BLAST program of the NCBI (http://www.ncbi.nlm.nih.gov/Tools/index.html) was used to scan regions of nucleotide or translated protein sequence associated with genes listed as ESTs. In cases where the entire nucleotide sequence failed to detect a known homologue, regions representing shorter (25-30 nucleotides) sequences were submitted independently. Sequences also were translated in Six-Frame (http://searchlauncher.bcm.tmc.edu/seq-util/Options/sixframe.html) and the best (fewest stop codons) translated sequence was analyzed by BLAST against Swiss-Prot Protein Knowledgebase (http://ca.expasy.org/sprot/).

RESULTS OF CDNA MICROARRAY ANALYSIS

Our cDNA microarray strategy revealed numerous changes in the gene transcript expression profile of the PC3 prostate cancer cell line plated on a type I collagen matrix rather than standard tissue culture plastic. A representative scanned microarray phosphorimage is shown in figure 1. Normalization of membrane data was performed using all data points. The measured intensities of the array elements are represented in figure 2 as a simple bivariate scatter plot. As shown, this plot compares spot intensity distribution between the cells plated on type I collagen (Y axis) and the cells plated on tissue culture plastic (X axis). Data points above the arbitrarily set slope line represents gene transcripts whose intensity is increased in the type I collagen samples.

A comparison of the gene product expression profiles of PC3 cells plated on type I collagen relative to tissue culture plastic revealed that 78 known gene products were increased 2-fold or more. A decrease in 38 gene transcripts and expressed sequence tags (ESTs) were observed, however the expression was below the arbitrary control point normalization levels set by the software and were excluded from further analysis.

Grouping of the increased gene transcripts into four clusters based on function identified four functional classes of gene products. The four gene clusters included molecules associated with ECM and cytoskeleton function (cluster 1), components of cellular signaling pathways (cluster 2), modulators of metabolic activity (cluster 3), and products involved in gene transcription, DNA synthesis and repair, and protein translation (cluster 4). These four clusters are shown in tables 1-4. In addition, 27 ESTs and gene transcripts of unknown function according to the manufacturer were found to change significantly on type I collagen. Our EST analysis method allowed us to tentatively identify or classify about 25% of these ESTs, some of which fell into a known cluster and were added to the tables. The overall profile of gene transcript expression changes is consistent with a phenotype of cells in a highly proliferative state when plated onto collagen. Each of the various clusters is discussed below and a more detailed analysis of particular components and their significance to prostate cancer bone metastasis is presented.

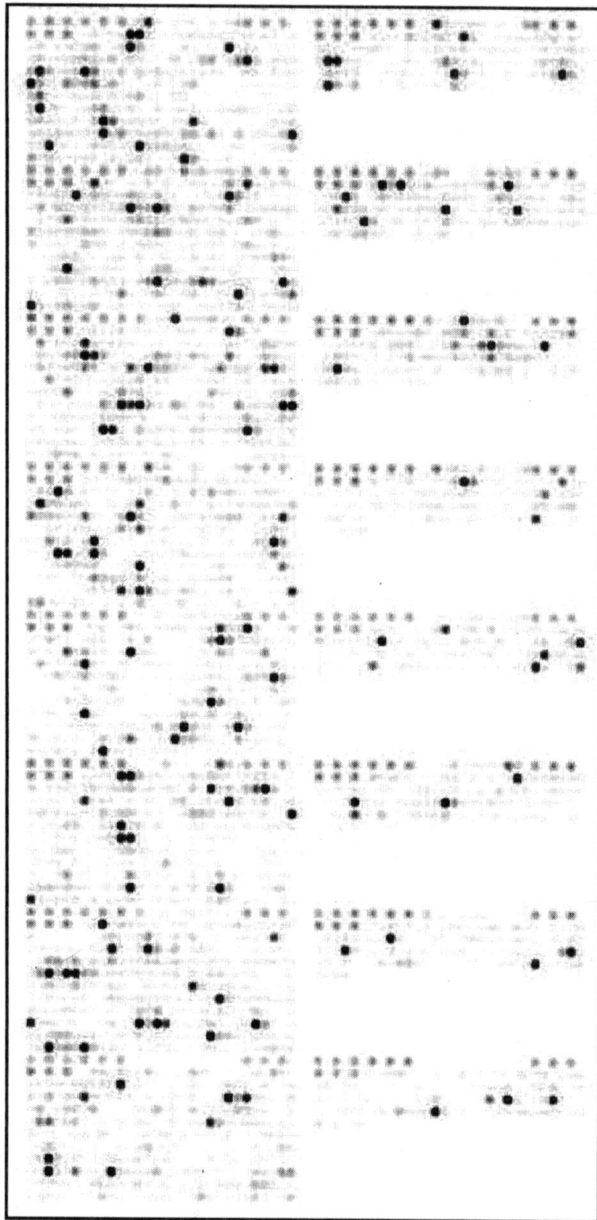

Figure 1. Scanned Phosphorimage of cDNA Microarray. cDNA derived from RNA extracted from PC3 cells plated on type I collagen for 24 hr in serum free medium was hybridized to the Human Prostate-Specific GeneFilter Microarray, Release I, GF221.

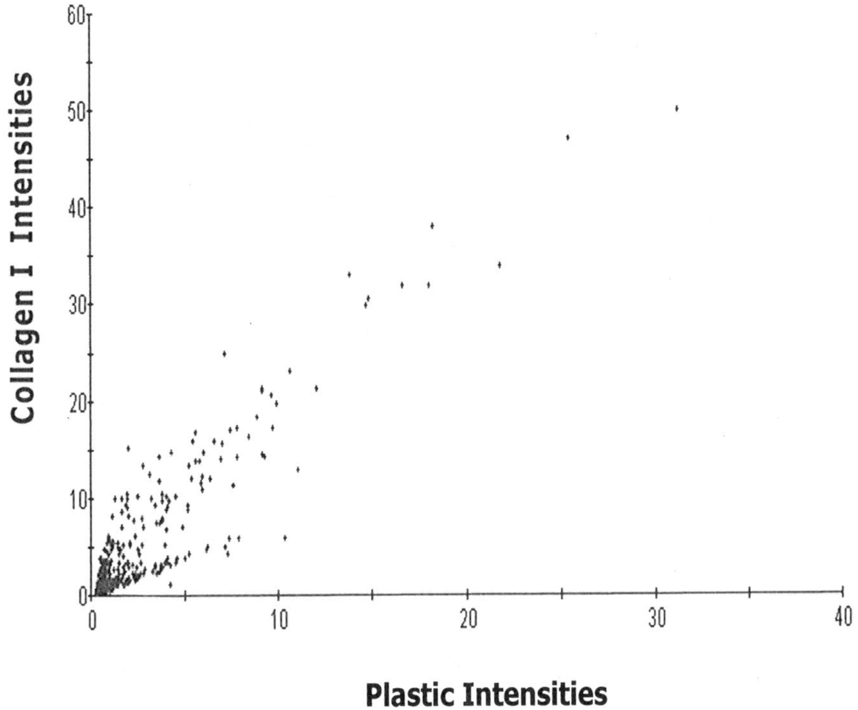

Figure 2. Global Intensity Distribution of Microarray Data. Sample data point intensities of the type I collagen treated cDNA (Y axis) are graphed against the sample data point intensities of the plastic samples (X axis). Points above the arbitrarily drawn slope line represent increases in gene expression reflected in individual data points.

Cluster 1: ECM and Cytoskeleton Function

The ECM and cytoskeleton cluster 1 contained 18 gene transcripts with expression ratios ranging from 2.3 to 3.9 (Table 1). This cluster contains genes such as tubulin (2.5-fold increase), amyloid beta precursor binding protein 2 (3.8-fold) and collagen type XVII alpha 1 (3.3), which are important in the control of cellular structure and integrity. Additionally, cellular adhesion modulators, CD44 (3.2) and ezrin (2.7), are increased within this cluster. Together, these various components participate in aspects of cell adhesion and structure that are important in many aspects of cell behavior.

Table 1. Cluster 1: Extracellular Matrix and Cytoskeletal RElated Gene Transcripts

Gene	Function	Ratio	Gene Bank Number
Adaptor-Related Protein Complex 1 Gamma 1 Subunit	Clathrin Coated Pit Formation	3.05	Y12226
Adaptor-Related Protein Complex 3 Delta 1 Subunit	Clathrin Coated Pit Formation	3.99	NM_003938
Amyloid Beta Precursor Binding Protein 2	Basolateral Sorting	3.81	NM_006380
Ataxin 2 Related Protein	Unknown	2.59	NM_007245
Caldesmon 1	Regulates Actomycin	2.6	NM_004342
Calponin 3	Unknown	2.33	NM_001839
CD44	Cell Adhesion Receptor	3.23	BC004372
Collagen, Type XVII, Alpha 1	Hemidesmosome Assembly	3.29	NM_000494
Ezrin	Adhesion, Migration, Signal Transduction	2.69	X51521
Kinesin Family Member 5B	Intracellular Organelle Movement	2.49	NM_004521
Major Histocompatibility Complex Class 1, A	Lymphocyte Immune Co-Receptor	3.89	M24095
Major Histocompatibility Complex Class II, DQ Beta	Lymphocyte Immune Co-Receptor	3.43	M81141
Matrix Gla Protein	Calcification	3.5	M55270
Neurexin III	Neural Cell Adhesion	2.87	NM_004796
Syntaxin 5A	Vesicle Docking	2.28	U26648
Transforming Growth Factor Beta-induced, 68kD	ECM Molecule Found in the Eye	2.92	M77349
Tubulin, Beta Polypepticle	Cytoskeletal Scaffolding	2.477	NM_001069

Cluster 2: Cell Signaling Modulators

This cluster contains molecules involved in the various aspects of cell signaling (Table 2). An increase in 18 gene transcripts was observed with expression ratios of 2.2 to 8.8. Additionally, five identified ESTs were added to this cluster. Potential growth factors, such as granulin (2.5), and growth factor receptors, such as, colony stimulating factor 2 receptor alpha (CSF2RA) (3.1) and jagged-2 (3.5) exhibit an increase in response to type I collagen attachment. The gene transcripts for signaling modulators, such as enigma (2.6) and serum/glucocorticoid kinase (3.3), also exhibit an increase in expression. Of note, one particular interesting gene product that functions in cell cycle progression, the CDC28 protein kinase 1, which shows an increase of 2.8 fold in expression, was identified. Finally, several molecules known to be regulated by calcium and cAMP were identified which is of interest given our previously published findings that ECM from bone matrix is associated with calcium influx into PC-3 cells (Lecrone et al, 2000). The list of gene products within this category represent exciting potential molecules that participate in the increase of cell proliferation observed in PC3 cells plated on type I collagen, and because many of them are enzymes or regulators of enzyme-controlled signaling pathways, they also represent exciting potential therapeutic targets.

Table 2. Cluster 2: Cell Signaling Modulatory Transcripts

Gene	Function	Ratio	Gene Bank Number
BRCA1 Associated Protein I (BAP1)	Modulates BRCA-1 Signaling	3.39	AF045581
Colony Stimulating Factor 2 Receptor, Low-Affinity Alpha Subunit	GM-CSF Receptor	3.12	NM_006140
CDC28 Protein Kinase I	Cell Cycle Progression	2.77	X54941
Calcineurin Binding Protein 1	Inhibits Calcineurin Function	2.24	NM_012295
Enigma (LIM Domain Protein)	Signal Transduction Adaptor Protein duction	2.55	NM_005451
Granulin	Cysteine-Rich Growth Factor (Oncogenic Activity)	2.48	M75165
Guanine Nucleotide Binding Protein Alpha Inhibiting Activity Polypeptide 3 (GNA13)	G-Protein Inhibition	5.46	NM_006496

(Table 2 continued on next page)

(Table 2 continued)

Guanine Nucleotide Binding Protein-Like I (GNL1)	Unknown	3.22	NM_005275
Jagged-2	Notch Receptor Ligand	3.51	AF003521
Papillary Renal Cell Carcinoma (Translocation-Associated)	Oncogenic Transcription Factor	3.37	X97124
Phosphoserine Phosphatase-Like	Unknown	6.55	NM_003832
Pim-1 Oncogene	Serine/Threonine Kinase	4.17	M16750
Rho GTPase Activating Protein (CDC42)	cdc42 GTPase	2.81	NM 004308
similar to cAMP-binding guanine exchange factor IV	GEF	6.5	W15542
similar to type III adenylyl cyclase	Adenylyl cyclase activity	2.0	**AA400482**
Serum/Glucocorticoid Regulated Kinase	Serine/Threonine Kinase	3.32	NM_005627
Solute Carrier Family 7 Cationic Amino Acid Transporter y+ System	Amino Acid Transport	2.9	M80244
Solute Carrier Family 9 (Sodium/Hydrogen Exchanger) Isoform 3	Interaction with ERM Proteins	2.67	AF036241
TGFBI-Induced Anti-Apoptotic Factor 1	Inhibits TNF Apoptosis	8.79	NM_004740
Thyroid Hormone Receptor Interactor 12 (TRIP 12)	Interaction with Thyroid Hormone Receptor	2.76	Q14669

Cluster 3: Cellular Metabolism and Energy Generation

A wide array of gene products which function in cellular metabolism and energy generation, and whose expression was increased in type I collagen samples compared to plastic controls (Table 3) are represented in this cluster. The levels of these 24 gene products are associated with various aspects of cellular metabolic activity, including reactive oxygen regulated pathways. It is well accepted that an increase in metabolic function occurs in cells that are actively proliferating. This is of particular importance since PC3 cell grown on type I collagen demonstrate increased proliferation over cells plated on plastic (Kiefer et al, 2001). Gene products such as cytochrome C oxidase subunit VIIc (5.0), NADH dehydrogenase 1 beta subcomplex 10 (2.9), and lactate dehydrogenase A (2.6) are intimately involved in various pathways associated with energy generation. Additionally, two gene products, glutathione-s-transferase omega and superoxide dismutase 2, that function in controlling the accumulation of deleterious side products generated during high rates of energy production are increased 3.1 and 2.9-fold, respectively, in this cluster. The total outcome of the activities of the gene products in this cluster likely plays an important role in supporting prostate cancer cell proliferation.

Table 3. Cluster 3: Cellular Metabolism and Energy Generation Transcripts

Gene	Function	Ratio	Gene Bank Number
3-Oxoacid CoA Transferase	Ketone Metabolism	2.64	U62961
Alpha-2-Plasmin Inhibitor	Plasmin Inhibitor	5.27	D00174
Apolipoprotein E	Cell Surface Endocytosis	2.5	M12529
Cytochrome c Oxiclase Subunit VIIc	Mitochondrial Respiration	5.02	NM_001867
D-dopachrome Tautomerase	Tautomerase Activity	3.38	U84143
Endoplasmic Reticulum Lumenal Protein	Protein Secretion	3.16	X94910
Galactosylceramidase (Krabbe Disease)	Lysosoma Galactosylceramide of Catabolism	4.08	L23116
GCN5 (Amino-Acid Synthesis Yeast Homolog)	Amino Acid Transcription Control	4.39	S82447
Glucosamine-6-Phosphate Deaminase	Glucosamine Catabolism	3	AF048826
Glucose Phosphate Isomerase	lycolytic Enzyme	4.38	NM_000175
Glucosidase I	N-Linked Protein Glycosylation	5.87	NM_006302
Glutathione Peroxidase 3 (Plasma)	Reduction of Reactive Oxygen Species	3.39	X58295
Glutathione-S-Transferase like Glutathione Transferase Omega	Glutathione- Dependent Detoxification Reactions	3.12	AF212303

(Table 3 continued on next page)

(Table 3 continued)

Heat Shock 40kD Protein 1	Molecular Chaperone	3.18	D49547
Lactate Dehydrogenase A	Pyruvate Reduction to Lactate	2.56	NM_005566
Low Density Lipoprotein Related Peptide 1	Cell Surface Endocytosis	2.7	X13916
Metallothionein 1G	Metal Transfer	2.36	NM_005951
NADH Dehydrogenase (Ubiquinone) 1 Beta Subcomplex 10 (22kD)	Mitochondrial Respiration	2.93	XM_007919
Proteasome (prosome,macropain) Subunit, Alpha Type 1	Subunit of 20S Proteosome	3.94	NM_002786
Proteosome (Prosome, Macropain) Inhibitor Subunit 1 (P131)	Inhibitor of 20S Proteosome	6.25	D88378
Superoxide Dismutase 2	ROS Scavenger	2.93	X65965
Surfeit 1	Association with Cytochrome c Oxidase	3.54	Z35093
Ubiquinol-Cytochrome c Reductase Rieske Iron-Sulfur Polypeptide	Mitochondrilal Respiration	5.51	NM_006003
Ubiquitin-Conjugating Enzyme E21	Ubiquitin-Mediated Protein Digestion	3.07	U45328

Cluster 4: Transcription, DNA Synthesis, Repair, and Protein Translation

The gene products in this category exert control over gene expression and protein translation. This cluster contains 17 gene transcripts that were increased in PC-3 plated on type I collagen (Table 4). The two gene products, poly (a) polymerase and polymerase (RNA) II polypeptide J play pivotal roles in the gene transcription and were increased 3.1 and 2.8-fold, respectively. The glutamyl-prolyl-tRNA synthetase and phenylalanine-tRNA synthetase gene products function in the charging of amino acids for use in translation. Therefore, genes such as these would be important in the facilitating the overall changes in gene expression mediated by binding to type I collagen.

Table 4. Cluster 4: Transcription, DNA Synthesis, Repair and Protein Translation Transcripts

Gene	Function	Ratio	Number
Apex Nuclease Multifunctional DNA Repair Enzyme	DNA Repair and Editing	8.76	D90373
Bromodomain Adjacent to Zinc Finger Domain 2A	Unknown	5.67	W88615
cAMP Responsive Element Binding Protein 3	cAMP Responsive Transcription Factor	3.26	AF211848
DEAD/H Box Binding Protein 1	Inhibits Stat Activity	2.4	U78524
Eukaryotic Translation Initiation Factor 4B	mRNA Binding to Ribosome	5.89	X55733
Glutamyl-Prolyl- tRNA Synthetase	Charge Glutamic Acid and Proline to tRNA	5.54	NM_00446
Heterogeneous Nuclear Ribonucleoprotein U (Scaffold Attachment Factor)	Pre-RNA Processing	3.51	AF068846
LPS-Induced TNF-alpha Factor (Pig7)	TNF alpha Transcription	8.19	U77396
MORF-Related Gene X	Unknown	3.18	XM_010125
Phenylalanine-tRNA Sythetase-Like	Charge Phenylalanine to tRNA	3.33	NM_004461
Poly (a) Polymerase	Synthesis of Poly A Tails	3.11	X76770
Polymerase (RNA) II (DNA Directed) Polypeptide J	Component of RNA Polymerase II	2.76	NM_006234
Pre-RNA Splicing Factor PrP16	Pre-RNA Splicing	3.05	AF038392
Primase, Polypeptide 2A (58kD)	Synthesis of Primers for DNA Synthesis	3.15	NM_000947
Ribophorin	Ribosome Binding	2.35	Y00281
Ribosomal Protein S5	Ribosomal Subunit Membe	2.24	U14970
RNA Helicase-Related Protein	RNA Processing And Ribosome Binding	2.07	AF083255
similar to SH3 domain binding protein SNP70	Pre-mRNA processing	4.6	AA454654

GENE PRODUCT VALIDATION

To confirm the validity of the gene expression changes observed on the microarray, Northern blot analyses were performed for select genes. Two interesting and novel genes, enigma and CDC28, were selected for our initial analysis and verification. The enigma gene product was chosen because of its unique function in modulating growth factor signaling pathways. By Northern blot analysis, approximately a two-fold induction in enigma message was observed in the type I collagen sample compared to the plastic control sample (data not shown). Additionally, because of its critical role in cell cycle progression, CDC28 transcript levels were also confirmed by Northern blot analysis. Although to a lesser extent than enigma, CDC28 message increased approximately 1.4 fold on collagen type I compared to plastic (data not shown). Additional studies are aimed at validating the changes in expression of the other gene products and in elucidating the pathways in which they are likely to function during cancer progression in the context of tissue ECM.

ARRAY ANALYSIS IN THE CONTEXT OF CANCER CELL INTERACTIONS WITH ECM

It is clear that various ECM components play critical roles in cancer development and progression (Tlsty, 1998; Park et al, 2000). Among ECM molecules, type I collagen provides a proliferative signal to the PC-3 prostate cancer cell line (Kiefer et al, 2001). Given the fact that type I collagen is the major organic constituent of skeletal tissue, these results have important implications for prostate cancer bone metastasis. The microarray analysis comparing the gene expression changes in PC3 cells plated on type I collagen to cells plated on tissue culture plastic reveals a profile indicative of actively proliferating cells. The pattern changes seen in the four gene clusters suggest that significant gene expression changes occur during prostate cancer bone metastasis and in growth in a collagen I rich tissue including bone marrow stroma or bone. Such findings have implications for other types of cancer as well, particularly those that grow in bone marrow or tend to invade bone during disease progression. The demonstration that collagen receptors such as $\alpha_2\beta_1$, and perhaps $\alpha_3\beta_1$, are likely mediators of these genotypic changes (Kiefer et al, 2001) identifies new molecular targets for growth intervention during cancer therapy.

Cluster analysis revealed specific categories of gene transcripts that are up-regulated in PC-3 cells plated on type I collagen relative to plastic. The activity of the various gene products in these clusters likely plays a role in prostate cancer bone metastasis. One cluster of special note is the metabolism cluster 3 of gene products. Previous studies have demonstrated that an increase in energy metabolism sustains increased rates of cellular proliferation (Newsholme et al, 1985; Newsholme et al, 1991; Mazurek et al, 1998; Newell et al, 1999). The increase in these gene transcripts in this cluster correlates with the increased rates of proliferation observed in PC3 cells plated on type I collagen. A cluster of genes (Table 4) associated with the control of gene transcription and translation was also found to be up-regulated. These gene products are important drivers of gene expression changes initiated by binding to type I collagen. It is interesting to note the increased expression of gene transcripts associated with the control of protein translation such as glutamyl-prolyl-tRNA synthetase and phenylalanine-tRNA synthetase, that possess a 5'-TOP sequence. As previously mentioned, 5'-TOP containing gene transcripts are rapidly translated in response to various mitogenic signaling pathways (Thomas et al, 1997). The up-regulation of these gene products in this system may further potentiate changes in translation that sustain increased rates of proliferation.

SPECIFIC GENES

Enigma

Enigma is a member of a family of proteins characterized by the presence of two protein-protein interaction motifs, the PDZ and LIM domain (Gill, 1995). PDZ domains, so named for the three proteins that they were first recognized (postsynaptic density-95, discs large, and zo1 tight junction protein), are protein interaction motifs that characterize proteins involved in scaffolding large protein-protein structures involved in cell-cell adhesion and signaling complexes. LIM domains, also named for three proteins that they were first discovered in (lin-11, isl-1, and mec-1), are cysteine-rich protein interaction domains involved in mediating interactions among signaling molecules and transcription factors (Gill, 1995; Ranganathan et al, 1997). The PDZ domain in enigma mediates interactions with actin filaments. Enigma contains three LIM motifs (Gill, 1995). These motifs couple enigma to a variety of signaling molecules including, c-Ret receptor tyrosine kinase, insulin receptor, and protein kinase β-1. c-Ret mitogenic signaling requires the interaction of the second LIM domain (Durick et al, 1996). Ret expression has been detected in prostate cancer specimens and may play a role in signaling for prostate cancer cell growth (Dawson et al, 1998). Recently, overexpression of Enigma has been demonstrated, by microarray analysis, in prostate cancer specimens (Dhanasekaran et al, 2001). Further study is needed to systematically determine what role enigma may play in transducing type I collagen-mediated growth signals and its role in prostate cancer.

CD44 and ezrin

CD44 and ezrin are two proteins that interact to during the process of cell adhesion and have been implicated in tumor progression and metastasis (Rudzki et al, 1997; Vaheri et al, 1997). CD44 is a large transmembrane adhesion receptor for hyaluronate and osteopontin. CD44 functions in cell migration, homotypic cell adhesion, and lymphocyte activation. CD44 is alternatively spliced with different splice variants controlling different cellular functions (Ponta et al, 1998). A large amount of literature exists implicating CD44 in the invasion and metastatic spread of numerous cancer types, including prostate cancer (Stevens et al, 1996; Rudzki et al, 1997; Herrlich et al, 1998). The short cytoplasmic tail of CD44 associates with the members of the ERM (ezrin-moesin-radixin) family of proteins (Vaheri et al, 1997). ERM proteins concentrate in actin-enriched areas and function as membrane cytoskeleton linkers. ERMs are thought to play a role in cell adhesion, migration, and in the modulation of adhesion signal transduction pathways (Vaheri et al, 1997). One member of this family, ezrin, has been associated with cancer metastasis (Jiang et al, 1996; Vaheri et al, 1997; Akisawa et al, 1999). This microarray screen revealed the up-regulation of CD44 and ezrin in PC3 cells plated on type I collagen. This is an interesting finding that possibly suggests that adhesion to type I collagen might facilitate metastatic behavior in PC3 cells by altering the expression of components involved in adhesion pathways. An interesting scenario may exist whereby type I collagen signals for the up-regulation of CD44 and ezrin, which may then bind to osteopontin in the bone matrix thereby facilitating the growth and survival of prostate cells in bone.

CSFR2A and Granulin

Prostate cancer progression is often driven by paracrine and autocrine derived growth factors (Cussenot, 1997). Two interesting gene products that function in growth factor signaling were up-regulated in PC3 cells plated on type I collagen. The first was CSFR2A. This is one part of the granulocyte-macrophage colony stimulating factor (GM-CSF) growth factor receptor. Previous work indicated PC-3 cell lines produce GM-CSF and proliferate in response to it (Lang et al, 1994). The up-regulation of the receptor for GM-CSF by type I collagen may offer a possible explanation for the proliferative effect observed. It is also tempting to speculate that up-regulation of the CSFR2A in response to the collagenous microenvironment in bone may facilitate the survival and growth of metastatic prostate cells. The second gene associated with growth factor signaling that was up-regulated was granulin. Granulin is one of a family of small growth modulatory proteins associated with epithelial and hematopoietic tissue (Bateman et al, 1998). The overexpression of granulin correlates with increased growth and confers anchorage-independent growth in epithelial cells in culture (He, 1999). The overexpression of granulin is detected in glial tumors (Zanocco-Marani et al, 1999; Markert et al, 2001). No published studies exist investigating granulin expression or function in prostate cancer; however, the aforementioned studies indicate that granulin might be involved in prostate cancer progression.

CDC28 Protein Kinase 1

Previous work demonstrated the importance of the expression of cell cycle related gene changes in PC3 plated on type I collagen (Kiefer et al, 2001). The CDC28 protein kinase 1 product is another gene product that functions in the regulation of cell cycle. This particular protein is important in controlling the ubiquitin-mediated destruction of the $p27^{kip}$ cyclin-dependent kinase inhibitor (Ganoth et al, 2001). $p27^{kip}$ prevents progression from the G1 to S phase of the cell cycle. CDC28 protein kinase 1 promotes the degradation of $p27^{kip}$ leading to the progression through the cell cycle (Ganoth et al, 2001).

SUMMARY

In this study, cDNA microarrays were used to characterize gene expression changes elicited in prostate cancer cells by plating them on type I collagen. The results clearly reveal changes in the expression of genes associated with cellular signaling, cellular metabolism, gene transcription and gene translation which are indicative of cells that are actively proliferating. Together these results suggest that these changes in the gene expression profiles mediated by type I collagen may influence the proliferative capacity of prostate cancer cells in the bone microenvironment and facilitate development of prostate cancer bone metastases. Additionally, the microarray approach provides an invaluable tool to determine and track changes in gene expression in numerous disease states including prostate cancer. This technology is certain to facilitate discovery of new therapeutic gene targets.

ACKNOWLEDGMENTS

The authors thank Dr. Robert Sikes and Dr. Carlton Cooper for reading the chapter prior to its submission.

REFERENCES

Akisawa, N., Nishimori, I., Iwamura T., Onishi, S. and Hollingsworth, M.A. (1999) High levels of ezrin expressed by human pancreatic adenocarcinoma cell lines with high metastatic potential. *Biochemical and Biophysical Research Communications*, **258**, 395-400.

Alizadeh, A.A., Eisen, M.B., Davis, R.E., Ma, C., Lossos, I.S., Rosenwald, A., Boldrick, J.C., Sabet, H., Tran, T., Yu, X., Powell, J.I., Yang, L., Marti, G.E., Moore, T., Hudson, J., Jr., Lu, L., Lewis, D.B., Tibshirani, R., Sherlock, G., Chan, W.C., Greiner, T.C., Weisenburger, D.D., Armitage, J.O., Warnke, R., Staudt, L.M. et al. (2000) Distinct types of diffuse large B-cell lymphoma identified by gene expression profiling. *Nature* **403**, 503-11.

Amler, L.C., Agus, D.B., LeDuc, C., Sapinoso, M.L., Fox, W.D., Kern, S., Lee, D., Wang, V., Leysens, M., Higgins, B., Martin, J., Gerald, W., Dracopoli, N., Cordon-Cardo, C., Scher, H.I. and Hampton, G.M. (2000) Dysregulated expression of androgen-responsive and nonresponsive genes in the androgen-independent prostate cancer xenograft model CWR22-R1. *Cancer Research* **60**, 6134-41.

Bateman, A. and Bennett, H.P. (1998) Granulins: the structure and function of an emerging family of growth factors. *Journal of Endocrinology* **158**, 145-51.

Bokel, C. and Brown, N.H. (2002) Integrins in development: moving on, responding to, and sticking to the extracellular matrix. *Dev Cell* **3**, 311-21.

Brooks, J.D. (2002) Microarray analysis in prostate cancer research. *Current Opinions in Urology*, **12**, 395-9.

Bubendorf, L., Kolmer, M., Kononen, J., Koivisto, P., Mousses, S., Chen, Y., Mahlamaki, E., Schraml, P., Moch, H., Willi, N., Elkahloun, A.G., Pretlow, T.G., Gasser, T.C., Mihatsch, M.J., Sauter, G. and Kallioniemi, O.P. (1999a) Hormone therapy failure in human prostate cancer: analysis by complementary DNA and tissue microarrays. *Journal of the National Cancer Institute* **91**, 1758-64.

Bubendorf, L., Kononen, J., Koivisto, P., Schraml, P., Moch, H., Gasser, T.C., Willi, N., Mihatsch, M.J., Sauter, G. and Kallioniemi, O.P. (1999b) Survey of gene amplifications during prostate cancer progression by high-throughout fluorescence in situ hybridization on tissue microarrays. *Cancer Research* **59**, 803-6.

Calaluce, R., Kunkel, M.W., Watts, G.S., Schmelz, M., Hao, J., Barrera, J., Gleason-Guzman, M., Isett, R., Fitchmun, M., Bowden, G.T., Cress, A.E., Futscher, B.W. and Nagle, R.B.

(2001) Laminin-5-mediated gene expression in human prostate carcinoma cells. *Molecular Carcinoma* **30**, 119-29.

Celis, J.E., Kruhoffer, M., Gromova, I., Frederiksen, C., Ostergaard, M., Thykjaer, T., Gromov, P., Yu, J., Palsdottir, H., Magnusson, N. and Orntoft, T.F. (2000) Gene expression profiling: monitoring transcription and translation products using DNA microarrays and proteomics. FEBS Lett, **480**, 2-16.

Cussenot, O. (1997) Growth factors and prostatic tumors. Ann Endocrinology **58**, 370-80.

Dawson, D.M., Lawrence, E.G., MacLennan, G.T., Amini, S.B., Kung, H.J., Robinson, D., Resnick, M.I., Kursh, E.D., Pretlow, T.P. and Pretlow, T.G. (1998) Altered expression of RET proto-oncogene product in prostatic intraepithelial neoplasia and prostate cancer. *Journal of the National Cancer Institute* **90**, 519-23.

Der, S.D., Zhou, A., Williams, B.R. and Silverman, R.H. (1998) Identification of genes differentially regulated by interferon alpha, beta, or gamma using oligonucleotide arrays. *Proceedings of the National Academy of Sciences U S A* **95**, 15623-8.

DeRisi, J.L. and Iyer, V.R. (1999) Genomics and array technology. *Current Opinions in Oncology* **11**, 76-9.

Dhanasekaran, S.M., Barrette, T.R., Ghosh, D., Shah, R., Varambally, S., Kurachi, K., Pienta, K.J., Rubin, M.A. and Chinnaiyan, A.M. (2001) Delineation of prognostic biomarkers in prostate cancer. *Nature* **412**, 822-6.

Durick, K., Wu, R.Y., Gill, G.N. and Taylor, S.S. (1996) Mitogenic signaling by Ret/ptc2 requires association with enigma via a LIM domain. *Journal of Biological Chemistry* **271**, 12691-4.

Dyrskjot, L., Thykjaer, T., Kruhoffer, M., Jensen, J.L., Marcussen, N., Hamilton-Dutoit, S., Wolf, H. and TF, O.R. (2003) Identifying distinct classes of bladder carcinoma using microarrays. *Nat Genet* **33**, 90-6.

Elek, J., Park, K.H. and Narayanan, R. (2000) Microarray-based expression profiling in prostate tumors. *In Vivo* **14**, 173-82.

Ganoth, D., Bornstein, G., Ko, T.K., Larsen, B., Tyers, M., Pagano, M. and Hershko, A. (2001) The cell-cycle regulatory protein Cks1 is required for SCF(Skp2)- mediated ubiquitinylation of p27. *Nat Cell Biol* **3**, 321-4.

Giancotti, F.G. and Ruoslahti, E. (1999) Integrin signaling. *Science*, **285**, 1028-32.

Gill, G.N. (1995) The enigma of LIM domains. *Structure* **3**, 1285-1289.

Golub, T.R., Slonim, D.K., Tamayo, P., Huard, C., Gaasenbeek, M., Mesirov, J.P., Coller, H., Loh, M.L., Downing, J.R., Caligiuri, M.A., Bloomfield, C.D. and Lander, E.S. (1999) Molecular classification of cancer: class discovery and class prediction by gene expression monitoring. *Science* **286**, 531-7.

Gronowicz, G.A. and Derome, M.E. (1994) Synthetic peptide containing Arg-Gly-Asp inhibits bone formation and resorption in a mineralizing organ culture system of fetal rat parietal bones. *Journal of Bone and Mineral Research* **9**, 193-201.

Guise T.A. and Mundy G.R. (1998) Cancer and bone. *Endocrinology Review* **19**, 18-54.

Hansen, R.K. and Bissell, M.J. (2000) Tissue architecture and breast cancer: the role of extracellular matrix and steroid hormones. *Endocr Relat Cancer* **7**, 95-113.

Haq, M., Goltzman, D., Tremblay, G. and Brodt, P. (1992) Rat prostate adenocarcinoma cells disseminate to bone and adhere preferentially to bone marrow-derived endothelial cells. *Cancer Research* **52**, 4613-9.

He, Z.a.B.A. (1999) Progranulin gene expression regulates epithelial cell growth and promotes tumor growth in vivo. *Cancer Research* **59**, 3222-3229.

Herrlich, P., Sleeman, J., Wainwright, D., Konig, H., Sherman, L., Hilberg, F. and Ponta, H. (1998) How tumor cells make use of CD44. *Cell Adhes Commun* **6**, 141-7.

Hippo, Y., Yashiro, M., Ishii, M., Taniguchi, H., Tsutsumi, S., Hirakawa, K., Kodama, T. and Aburatani, H. (2001) Differential gene expression profiles of scirrhous gastric cancer cells with high metastatic potential to peritoneum or lymph nodes. *Cancer Research* **61**, 889-95.

Hullinger, T.G., McCauley, L.K., DeJoode, M.L. and Somerman, M.J. (1998) Effect of bone proteins on human prostate cancer cell lines in vitro. *The Prostate* **36**, 14-22.

Jacob, K., Webber, M., Benayahu, D. and Kleinman, H.K. (1999) Osteonectin promotes prostate cancer cell migration and invasion: a possible mechanism for metastasis to bone. *Cancer Research* **59**, 4453-7.

Jiang, W.G. and Hiscox, S. (1996) Cytokine regulation of ezrin expression in the human colon cancer cell line HT29. *Anticancer Research* **16**, 861-5.

Khan, J., Bittner, M.L., Saal, L.H., Teichmann, U., Azorsa, D.O., Gooden, G.C., Pavan, W.J., Trent, J.M. and Meltzer, P.S. (1999a) cDNA microarrays detect activation of a myogenic transcription program by the PAX3-FKHR fusion oncogene. *Proceedings of the National Academy of Sciences U S A* **96**, 13264-9.

Khan, J., Saal, L.H., Bittner, M.L., Chen, Y., Trent, J.M. and Meltzer, P.S. (1999b) Expression profiling in cancer using cDNA microarrays. *Electrophoresis* **20**, 223-9.

Kiefer, J.A. and Farach-Carson, M.C. (2001) Type I collagen-mediated proliferation of PC3 prostate carcinoma cell line: implications for enhanced growth in the bone microenvironment. *Matrix Bioliogy* **20**, 429-37.

Klein, C.E., Dressel, D., Steinmayer, T., Mauch, C., Eckes, B., Krieg, T., Bankert, R.B. and Weber, L. (1991) Integrin alpha 2 beta 1 is upregulated in fibroblasts and highly aggressive melanoma cells in three-dimensional collagen lattices and mediates the reorganization of collagen I fibrils. *Journal of Cellular Biology* **115**, 1427-36.

Koeneman, K.S., Yeung, F. and Chung, L.W. (1999) Osteomimetic properties of prostate cancer cells: a hypothesis supporting the predilection of prostate cancer metastasis and growth in the bone environment. *The Prostate*, **39**, 246-61.

Kostenuik, P.J., Sanchez-Sweatman, O., Orr, F.W. and Singh, G. (1996) Bone cell matrix promotes the adhesion of human prostatic carcinoma cells via the alpha 2 beta 1 integrin. *Clinical Experimental Metastasis* **14**, 19-26.

Kostenuik, P.J., Singh, G. and Orr, F.W. (1997) Transforming growth factor beta upregulates the integrin-mediated adhesion of human prostatic carcinoma cells to type I collagen. *Clinical Experimental Metastasis* **15**, 41-52.

Lang, S.H., Miller, W.R., Duncan, W. and Habib, F.K. (1994) Production and response of human prostate cancer cell lines to granulocyte macrophage-colony stimulating factor. *International Journal of Cancer* **59**, 235-41.

Lecrone, V., Li, W., Devoll, R.E., Logothetis, C. and Farach-Carson, M.C. (2000) Calcium signals in prostate cancer cells: specific activation by bone- matrix proteins. *Cell Calcium*, **27**, 35-42.

Lee, Y.J. and Streuli, C.H. (1999) Extracellular matrix selectively modulates the response of mammary epithelial cells to different soluble signaling ligands. *Journal of Biological Chemistry* **274**, 22401-8.

Lehr, J.E. and Pienta, K.J. (1998) Preferential adhesion of prostate cancer cells to a human bone marrow endothelial cell line *Journal of the National Cancer Institute* **90**, 118-23.

Markert, J.M., Fuller, C.M., Gillespie, G.Y., Bubien, J.K., McLean, L.A., Hong, R.L., Lee, K., Gullans, S.R., Mapstone, T.B. and Benos, D.J. (2001) Differential gene expression profiling in human brain tumors. *Physiol Genomics* **5**, 21-33.

Mazurek, S., Grimm, H., Wilker, S., Leib, S. and Eigenbrodt, E. (1998) Metabolic characteristics of different malignant cancer cell lines. *Anticancer Research* **18**, 3275-82.

Mundy, G.R. (1997) Mechanisms of bone metastasis. *Cancer* **80**, 1546-56.

Nelson, P.S., Clegg, N., Arnold, H., Ferguson, C., Bonham, M., White, J., Hood, L. and Lin B. (2002) The program of androgen-responsive genes in neoplastic prostate epithelium. *Proceedings of the National Academy of Sciences U S A*, **99**, 11890-5.

Newell, M.K., Harper, M.E., Fortner, K., Desbarats, J., Russo, A. and Huber, S.A. (1999) Does the oxidative/glycolytic ratio determine proliferation or death in immune recognition? *Ann N Y Acad Sci* **887**, 77-82.

Newsholme, E.A. and Board, M. (1991) Application of metabolic-control logic to fuel utilization and its significance in tumor cells. *Adv Enzyme Regul* **31**, 225-46.

Newsholme, E.A., Crabtree, B. and Ardawi, M.S. (1985) The role of high rates of glycolysis and glutamine utilization in rapidly dividing cells. *Biosci Rep* **5**, 393-400.

Park, C.C., Bissell, M.J. and Barcellos-Hoff, M.H. (2000) The influence of the microenvironment on the malignant phenotype. *Mol Med Today* **6**, 324-9.

Pauli, B.U. and Lee, C.L. (1988) Organ preference of metastasis. The role of organ-specifically modulated endothelial cells. *Laboratory Investigations* **58**, 379-87.

Ponta, H., Wainwright, D. and Herrlich, P. (1998) The CD44 protein family. *International Journal Biochemistry and Cell Biology* **30**, 299-305.

Ranganathan, R. and Ross, E.M. (1997) PDZ domain proteins: scaffolds for signaling complexes. *Current Biology* **7**, R770-3.

Rhodes, D.R., Barrette, T.R., Rubin, M.A., Ghosh, D. and Chinnaiyan, A.M. (2002) Meta-analysis of microarrays: interstudy validation of gene expression profiles reveals pathway dysregulation in prostate cancer. *Cancer Research* **62**, 4427-33.

Ridley, R.C., Xiao, H., Hata, H., Woodliff, J., Epstein, J. and Sanderson R.D. (1993) Expression of syndecan regulates human myeloma plasma cell adhesion to type I collagen. *Blood* **81**, 767-74.

Romanov, V.I. and Goligorsky, M.S. (1999) RGD-recognizing integrins mediate interactions of human prostate carcinoma cells with endothelial cells in vitro. *Prostate*, **39**, 108-18.

Rudzki, Z. and Jothy, S. (1997) CD44 and the adhesion of neoplastic cells. *Molecular Pathology* **50**, 57-71.

Sasaki, H., Ide, N., Fukai, I., Kiriyama, M., Yamakawa, Y. and Fujii, Y. (2002) Gene expression analysis of human thymoma correlates with tumor stage. *International Journal of Cancer* **101**, 342-7.

Sharpe, W.a.M.J. (1942) Reaction of bone to metastsis from carcinoma of the breast and prostate. *Arch Pathol* **17**, 312-325.

Stevens, J.W., Palechek, P.L., Griebling, T.L., Midura, R.J., Rokhlin, O.W. and Cohen, M.B. (1996) Expression of CD44 isoforms in human prostate tumor cell lines *Prostate*, **28**, 153-61.

Streuli, C.H. and Gilmore, A.P. (1999) Adhesion-mediated signaling in the regulation of mammary epithelial cell survival. *Journal of Mammary Gland Biol Neoplasia* **4**, 183-91.

Takeuchi, Y., Suzawa, M., Kikuchi, T., Nishida, E., Fujita, T. and Matsumoto, T. (1997) Differentiation and transforming growth factor-beta receptor down- regulation by collagen-alpha2beta1 integrin interaction is mediated by focal adhesion kinase and its downstream signals in murine osteoblastic cells. *Journal of Biological Chemistry* **272**, 29309-16.

Termine, J.D.a.R., P. G (1996) "Bone Matrix Proteins and the Mineralization Process" In *Prime on the Metabolic Bone Diseases and Disorders of Mineral Metabolism* (ed. M. J. Favus). Philadelphia: Lippincott-Raven.

Thalmann, G.N., Sikes, R.A., Devoll, R.E., Kiefer, J.A., Markwalder, R., Klima, I., Farach-Carson, C.M., Studer, U.E. and Chung, L.W. (1999) Osteopontin: possible role in prostate cancer progression. *Clinical Cancer Research* **5**, 2271-7.

Thomas, G., Hall, M.N. (1997) TOR signalling and control of cell growth. *Current Opinions in Cell Biology* **9**, 782-7.

Tlsty, T.D. (1998) Cell-adhesion-dependent influences on genomic instability and carcinogenesis. *Current Opinions in Cell Biology* **10**, 647-53.

Vaarala, M.H., Porvari, K., Kyllonen, A. and Vihko, P. (2000) Differentially expressed genes in two LNCaP prostate cancer cell lines reflecting changes during prostate cancer progression. *Laboratory Investigations* **80**, 1259-68.

Vaheri, A., Carpen, O., Heiska, L., Helander, T.S., Jaaskelainen, J., Majander-Nordenswan, P., Sainio, M., Timonen, T. and Turunen, O. (1997) The ezrin protein family: membrane-cytoskeleton interactions and disease associations. *Current Opinions in Cell Biology* **9**, 659-66.

Watson, M.A., Perry, A., Budhjara, V., Hicks, C., Shannon, W.D. and Rich, K.M. (2001) Gene expression profiling with oligonucleotide microarrays distinguishes World Health Organization grade of oligodendrogliomas. *Cancer Research* **61**, 1825-9.

Xiao, G., Jiang, D., Thomas, P., Benson, M.D., Guan, K., Karsenty, G. and Franceschi R.T. (2000) MAPK pathways activate and phosphorylate the osteoblast-specific transcription factor, Cbfa1. *Journal of Biological Chemistry* **275**, 4453-9.

Xiao, G., Wang, D., Benson, M.D., Karsenty, G. and Franceschi, R.T. (1998) Role of the alpha2-integrin in osteoblast-specific gene expression and activation of the Osf2 transcription factor. *Journal of Biological Chemistry* **273**, 32988-94.

Xu, J., Stolk, J.A., Zhang, X., Silva, S.J., Houghton, R.L., Matsumura, M., Vedvick, T.S., Leslie, K.B., Badaro, R. and Reed, S.G. (2000) Identification of differentially expressed genes in human prostate cancer using subtraction and microarray. *Cancer Research* **60**, 1677-82.

Zanocco-Marani, T., Bateman, A., Romano, G., Valentinis, B., He, Z.H. and Baserga, R. (1999) Biological activities and signaling pathways of the granulin/epithelin precursor. Cancer Research **59**, 5331-40.

Zhou, J., Zhao, L.Q., Xiong, M.M., Wang, X.Q., Yang, G.R., Qiu, Z.L., Wu, M. and Liu, Z.H. (2003) Gene expression profiles at different stages of human esophageal squamous cell carcinoma. *World Journal of Gastroenterology* **9**, 9-15.

Zhu, H., Cong, J.P., Mamtora, G., Gingeras, T. and Shenk, T. (1998) Cellular gene expression altered by human cytomegalovirus: global monitoring with oligonucleotide arrays. *Proceedings of the National Academy of Sciences U S A*, **95**, 14470-5.

Chapter 6

PTHRP AND SKELETAL METATASIS

Laurie K. McCauley[1,2] and Abraham Schneider[1]
[1]*University of Michigan Department of Periodontics/Prevention/Teriatrics, School of Dentistry;* [2]*University of Michigan, Department of Pathology, Medical School*

INTRODUCTION

Skeletal metastasis is a common event in many advanced-stage cancer patients, with half of the common primary tumors eventually metastasizing to bone (Rubens, 2000). In most cases, it is the metastasis rather than the primary tumor that is responsible for the cancer-associated mortality (Chambers et al., 2002). Certain solid tumors such as cancer of the prostate, breast, and lung preferentially metastasize to bone (Rubens, 2000; Mundy, 2002). All of these tumors have been found to produce parathyroid hormone-related protein (PTHrP) (Keller et al., 2001; Martin and Moseley, 2000; Käkönen and Mundy, 2003). The levels of PTHrP produced by tumors in the bone marrow are dramatically higher than what is normally produced by cells resident in bone and bone marrow thus setting up a scenario where the bone is exposed to supraphysiologic levels of this highly bone active cytokine. The precise levels of PTHrP in the bone marrow microenvironment in metastatic lesions and among various tumors are as yet unknown. Most studies have focused on circulating levels of PTHrP that are readily measurable but do not necessarily reflect the levels in the metastatic environment, and on the production of PTHrP by various tumor cell lines *in vitro* that may be very different than what the tumor produced *in situ*. Once in the bone marrow microenvironment, PTHrP is localized to its key target tissue, which is bone. For most tumors, PTHrP may be the most 'bone-active' cytokine produced in this lesion and hence understanding the actions of PTHrP are critical to the pathophysiology of bony metastases.

than normal growth plates (Jobert et al., 1998). Jansen's metaphyseal chondrodysplasia is also a PTH-1 receptor mutation where a constitutively active receptor leads to dwarfism due to a delay in maturation of chondrocytes (Schipani et al., 1995). Both these human conditions manifest their skeletal impact during development and less is known regarding alteration of PTHrP signaling after growth is complete and in the site of skeletal metastasis. Interestingly, the response to PTHrP in the bone microenvironment of the metastatic lesion may recapitulate some aspects of development and hence it is important to be familiar with effects of PTHrP on the mature and developing skeleton. Metastatic tumor induced alterations in bone remodeling can be grouped into the following categories: 1) lytic, 2) blastic, or 3) mixed lytic and blastic lesions. In actuality it is likely that all lesions are mixed lytic and blastic ones, but that either the resorptive or formative activity predominates and as a result the overall presentation is that of either more or less bone than in the non-cancerous state (Mundy, 2002). PTHrP has both anabolic and catabolic actions in bone and hence may participate in the development of all types of lesions; although the most definitive role that PTHrP has been found to have is in the resorptive aspects of metastatic bony lesions (Guise et al., 1994; Mundy, 2002).

PTHrP, like PTH is responsible for inducing bone resorption based on its interaction with the PTH-1 receptor on osteoblasts exerting this action indirectly as it is not well accepted that PTH acts directly on osteoclasts. Through this interaction, PTHrP induces the expression of factors such as receptor activator of NFκB ligand (RANKL) that increase osteoclast development and subsequently lead to a loss of bone. At the same time, PTH and PTHrP stimulate bone formation, which although known for a long time, has just recently reached the point where PTH is being utilized for its potential to treat conditions such as osteoporosis where bone volume is critically reduced. In fact, recent reports suggest that PTH may be the best anabolic agent to treat osteoporosis currently available. Results of the first multicenter clinical trial with its use were reported last year and data indicated a 65% reduction in vertebral fracture in patients administered PTH over 2 years (Neer et al., 2001). Why is this important when considering cancer metastasis to bone? There are many similarities between the systemic response to PTH or its homologous counterpart PTH-related peptide (PTHrP), and PTHrP has also been under investigation for its anabolic potential (Horwitz et al., 2003). Observations such as these, and data of the production of PTHrP by many carcinomas with a variety of osseous responses dictate the need to more closely evaluate the role of PTHrP in the skeletal response to metastatic tumors. Most reports indicate that anabolic actions of PTH or PTHrP appear to depend on an intermittent dosing regime, although other modes of administration including a more sustained release formulation, continuous infusion, local gene therapy, an animal model with constitutively active receptors and a model of blocked desensitization of the PTH-1R may challenge dependence on an intermittent regime (Kostenuik et al., 2001; Fang et al., 1996; Chen et al., 2002; Calvi et al., 2001; Zhou et al., 2001; Spurney et al., 2002). The condition of humoral hypercalcemia of malignancy that is attributed to high PTHrP levels results in alterations in the normal osteoblast-osteoclast coupling that typically result in a reduction in osteoblastic activity; however, it is unclear whether a pulsatile secretion of PTHrP by a tumor of neuroendocrine origin may have opposite effects (Stewart, 2002). Furthermore, increased osteoblastic activity is found at an early stage of humoral hypercalcemia of malignancy suggesting a temporal or dose dependent response of PTHrP on osteoblasts (Yamato et al., 1995). There is much as yet unclear regarding anabolic actions of PTH or PTHrP, but it is well accepted that high continuous PTH or PTHrP leads to a catabolic response. In contrast, it appears that either high dose intermittent or low dose continuous PTH or PTHrP may lead to an anabolic response. Interestingly, intermittent administration of PTH also leads to dose dependent bone proliferative lesions including osteosarcoma, focal osteoblast hyperplasia, osteoma, and osteoblastoma in rats (Vahle et al., 2002). Furthermore, there was an increased incidence in soft tissue metastases in these rats treated with PTH for 2 years. This underscores the importance of determining the impact of tumor-derived PTHrP on bone in the microenvironment of the metastatic lesion.

PTHrP protein structure and peptide fragments

There are three PTHrP mRNA products that result from alternative splicing and result in three protein products of differing lengths, 139, 141, and 173 amino acids (Philbrick, 2001) (Figure 2). Normal prostate epithelium has been found to have all three transcripts (Cramer et al., 1996), but recently, PC-3 cells were found to only have one major transcript (Tovar Sepulveda and Falzon, 2002a). Further post-translational modifications of these PTHrP gene products have been found to include amino terminal peptides, midregion peptides and carboxy-terminal peptides. A prominent cleavage site at the arginine residue at position 37 generates a biologically active PTHrP 1-36 peptide. A midregion PTHrP 38-111 has been found in circulation with shorter peptides having carboxy termini at residues 94, 95, and 101 also identified (Philbrick, 2001). Interestingly, a midregion peptide containing amino acids 38-94 was found to inhibit growth and invasion of human breast cancer suggesting this midregion may play a role in pathologic growth and differentiation (Luparello et al., 2001). A nuclear targeting sequence in PTHrP has also been under intensive investigation and most recently has been localized to amino acids 66-94 or 88-106 with direct interaction with importin β resulting in translocation into the nucleus (Cingolani et al., 2002). Carboxy terminal fragments of PTHrP have also been found in circulation in renal disorders and in the urine of normal individuals. Carboxy terminal fragments of PTHrP containing residues 107-139 have been suggested to inhibit osteoclastic activity in vitro (Fenton et al., 1991). Unfortunately, although these fragments have been found, their precise role has not been determined. An interesting finding regarding the ability of PSA to cleave PTHrP was reported in 1996 (Cramer et al., 1996). These *in vitro* data indicated that PTHrP 1-141 was specifically cleaved by PSA with a preferred cleavage site at amino acid 23 rendering its ability to stimulate cAMP completely abolished. Unfortunately, little has been done to follow up on this phenomenon and it is virtually unknown whether this occurs *in vivo*.

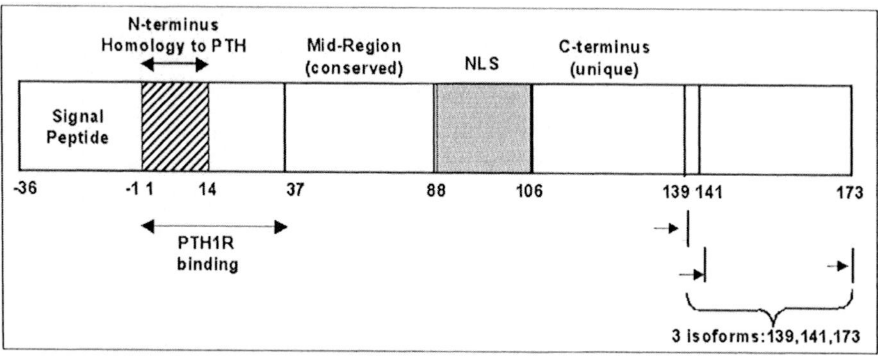

Figure 2. Structural features of PTHrP. PTHrP is a single gene product with three splice variants producing peptides of 139, 141, or 173 amino acids in length. The first 13 amino acids of PTHrP have 70% homology with PTH but it is in the region extending to amino acids 35 that binding to the shared PTH-1 receptor occurs. The mid-region of PTHrP is relatively conserved across species whereas the C-terminus is more divergent. The region of amino acids 88-106 contains a nuclear localization sequence that is responsible for translocation of PTHrP to the nucleus.

PTHrP and apoptosis

That PTHrP may be protective against apoptosis is intriguing and well substantiated based on reports of its activity in chondrocytes and recent reports of PTH's anti-apoptotic activity in bone (Jilka et al., 1999). PTHrP has been reported to have anti-apoptotic effects in chondrocytes and in prostate carcinoma epithelial cells attributed to its nuclear localization sequence. In *in vitro* culture systems, PTHrP production was associated with a protection from apoptosis whereas deletion of the nuclear localization sequence (amino acids 87-107) resulted in apoptosis levels that reversed to control values (Dougherty et al., 1999; Henderson et al., 1995). It is still unclear what the mechanisms for this apoptosis inhibition are and whether it is dependent on the PTH-1 receptor. One potential candidate is the protective oncogene *bcl-2*, that has been shown to be upregulated by PTHrP (Amling et al., 1997). In osteoblasts, PTH has been shown to be anti-apoptotic and one explanation for the promising anabolic actions of PTH (Jilka et al., 1999). In the bone multicellular unit (BMU), 65% of the osteoblasts that originally assembled at the remodeling site die (Manolagas, 2000). The remaining cells are either converted to lining cells or entombed in the bone as osteocytes. The frequency of osteoblast apoptosis is such that its alteration could have a significant impact on the number of osteoblasts capable of forming bone. PTH increases the life span of mature osteoblasts *in vivo* by reducing their apoptosis nearly 10-fold (Jilka et al., 1999). One can speculate that tumor-derived PTHrP would have similar effects due to its signaling through the same receptor, but these studies have not been reported. More recent data indicates that PTH and PTHrP are anti-apoptotic in less differentiated osteoblasts but are pro-apoptotic in more differentiated osteoblasts (Chen et al., 2002). These findings suggest that PTH and PTHrP may promote more cells to become active matrix producing osteoblasts by inhibiting their apoptosis. Once they have achieved their matrix production their clearance may be facilitated by the pro-apoptotic effects.

PTHrP signaling

Signaling through the PTH-1 receptor has been intensively investigated and although the immediate second messengers are known, the transcriptional mediators responsible for regulation of downstream genes are still unclear. It is well known that PTH and PTHrP interact with the PTH-1 receptor and activate protein kinase A (PKA) and protein kinase C (PKC) pathways. The activation of phospholipase C and PKC has recently been shown to oppose the dominant effects of cAMP-dependent signaling (Guo et al., 2002). The PKA pathway has received more attention since it is directly involved in the biologic activities of PTH and PTHrP and their anabolic actions (Ouyang et al., 2000). PKA has been implicated in the phosphorylation of the cyclic AMP response element binding protein (CREB) at serine 133 (Pearman et al., 1996). Particularly relevant, CREB has been found in several cell systems to be anti-apoptotic (Wilson et al., 1996; Riccio et al., 1999; Bonni et al., 1999). To our knowledge, this has not been explored in cells of the osteoblast lineage, but one recent paper indicates that protection from apoptosis is associated with cAMP activation

(Machwate et al., 1998). The phosphorylated CREB binds to the cyclic AMP response element (CRE) in the promoter region of the c-*fos* proto-oncogene and transcriptionally activates its expression.

The Fos protein forms a heterodimer with members of the Jun family to form the AP-1 transcription factor that binds to the promoter region of various target genes (Curran and Franza, 1988). Work including both *in vitro* and *in vivo* studies has suggested that c-*fos* is a key mediator of PTH and PTHrP actions in development. Interestingly, recent studies indicate that c-*fos* acts as a sensor for the signal duration of growth factors that alter proliferation and differentiation of cells (Murphy et al., 2002). *In vivo* data demonstrate that c-*fos* is critical for anabolic actions of PTH (Demiralp et al., 2002). This intriguing new information make it tempting to speculate that the Fos protein may be a master switch of anabolic and catabolic actions of PTH and PTHrP. That c-*fos* encodes a factor implicated in osteosarcomas and that PTHrP increases c-*fos* expression, a link between tumor-derived PTHrP, c-*fos* and skeletal response seems likely.

Traditionally, PTH and PTHrP have been associated with signaling via the PKA or PKC pathway. Recently, evidence is building for a role of the MAPK pathway in actions of PTH and PTHrP in bone and cartilage. Various cell model systems are turning up with evidence of crosstalk between cAMP and MAPK signaling (Stork and Schmitt, 2002; Belcheva and Coscia, 2002). This crosstalk may occur via cAMP activation of Epac, Rap1 and B-Raf (Enserink et al., 2002). It is virtually unknown whether signaling via this pathway contributes positively, negatively or at all in the actions of PTHrP in the metastatic lesion.

PTHRP AND BREAST CANCER

PTHrP is a central mediator of osteolytic bone metastasis associated with breast cancer

Several lines of evidence support PTHrP as one of the key mediators responsible for the osteolytic bone response associated with advanced breast cancer metastasis to the skeleton (Käkönen and Mundy, 2003). PTHrP expression is markedly increased in human breast carcinoma metastatic to the skeleton compared to the primary site or non-osseous metastases (Southby et al., 1990; Powell et al., 1991; Bundred et al., 1992; Vargas et al., 1992; Liapis et al., 1993; Henderson et al., 2001). PTHrP-positive tumor cells have been detected in 92% of bone metastases (Powell et al., 1991), approximately 70% of primary breast tumors (Southby et al., 1990; Bundred et al., 1992; Vargas et al., 1992; Liapis et al., 1993; Henderson et al., 2001) but only 17% of soft tissue metastases (Powell et al., 1991). Furthermore, expression of the PTH-1 receptor is present in breast carcinomas and reportedly higher in bone metastases than primary breast carcinomas (Hoey et al., 2003). These observations have prompted insightful investigation about the role of PTHrP in osteolytic metastasis associated with breast cancer.

Established breast carcinoma cell lines as well as the use of stable genetic modifications with activating or inactivating mutations have facilitated *in vitro* and *in vivo* studies to elucidate the impact of PTHrP in the development and progression of breast carcinoma-related metastatic bone disease. These studies clearly suggest that once tumor cells disseminate to the skeleton, the bone microenvironment exhibits unique properties to enhance tumor-derived PTHrP production in the metastatic lesion, leading to the development of local bone destruction. *In vivo* experimental studies supporting the role of breast carcinoma PTHrP in osteolytic bone metastasis have been reported based on the use of the intracardiac inoculation model, where tumor cells are directly injected into the vascular system (Nakai et al., 1992; Guise et al., 1996; Guise et al., 2002). This model has been instrumental in supporting the association between PTHrP with metastatic end points that occur following tumor cell entry into the blood circulation.

In recent years special attention has been devoted to dissect the cellular and molecular mechanisms of PTHrP-mediated osteolysis associated with breast carcinoma. As a bone-resorbing cytokine, PTHrP stimulates osteoclastic activity by modulating the production of osteoblast-derived activating and inhibitory osteoclastogenic factors that belong to the tumor necrosis factor (TNF) receptor family (Lee and Lorenzo, 1999). Regulation of RANKL and osteoprotegerin (OPG), is pivotal for the proper maturation and activity of osteoclasts in the bone marrow microenvironment (Lacey et al., 1998; Yasuda et al., 1998). The formation of multinucleated osteoclasts occurs when RANKL binds to its cognate receptor RANK, a membrane-bound TNF-related receptor identified in osteoclast precursors. OPG inhibits RANKL/RANK interaction by acting as a secreted decoy receptor for RANKL to prevent the binding to RANK and to ultimately limit osteoclast formation and bone resorption (Anderson et al., 1997; Simonet et al., 1997; Yasuda et al., 1998). Osteoclast-mediated bone destruction associated with breast carcinoma bone metastasis is in part due to the action of tumor-produced PTHrP on RANKL and OPG expression by osteoblasts (Thomas et al., 1999). Osteoblastic RANKL and OPG mRNA expression levels were increased and decreased, respectively, in cocultures with the PTHrP-negative breast carcinoma cell line MCF-7 experimentally induced to overexpress PTHrP. On the contrary, no changes in RANKL and OPG mRNA levels were observed in cocultures with parental MCF-7 cells. When osteoclast precursors were included in the cocultures, multinucleated osteoclasts developed without the supplementation of any osteoclastogenic factors. Cocultures with parental or empty vector-transfected MCF-7 cells, in contrast, required exogenous factors to induce osteoclastogenesis. Furthermore, bone metastases established by the intracardiac inoculation of MCF-7 cells overexpressing PTHrP, significantly resulted in more osteolytic lesions together with elevated serum PTHrP and calcium levels compared to mice inoculated with parental or empty vector controls. These results clearly implicate PTHrP as a critical tumor-derived factor responsible for stimulating osteoblast-mediated osteoclast development and activation.

Bone resorption as a consequence of osteoclast activation results in the release of bone matrix cytokines and growth factors into the bone marrow microenvironment (Hauschka et al., 1986). Among these factors, transforming growth factor β (TGF-β) is an important regulator of breast carcinoma-derived PTHrP production. Studies using MDA-MB-231 cells expressing mutant TGF-β receptors have provided evidence of the central role of TGF-β in stimulating tumor-derived PTHrP secretion (Yin et al., 1999). Enhanced PTHrP production and more osteolytic lesions and tumor burden with decreased animal survival were observed when breast cancer cells overexpressing constitutively active TGF-β type I receptors were used *in vitro* and in an animal model of bone metastasis, respectively. Blockade of these effects was obtained by utilizing MDA-MB-231 cells transfected with dominant negative TGF-β II receptors. Further, PTHrP overexpressing cells transfected with dominant negative TGF-β II receptors resulted in constitutive production of PTHrP *in vitro* together with increased osteolytic lesions and tumor growth in vivo. Recent molecular studies suggest that TGF-β effects on PTHrP production are mediated via the Smad as well as the p38 mitogen-activated protein (MAP) kinase signaling pathways (Kakonen et al., 2002). Taken together, these findings indicate that once breast cancer cells colonize the bone microenvironment, they secrete PTHrP and regulate the production of osteoblastic cell-derived RANKL and OPG resulting in osteoclastic bone resorption. Bone matrix-derived TGFβ, released in active form into the bone microenvironment following osteolysis, stimulates PTHrP production by tumor cells via TGF-β receptors which relay its downstream signals through the Smad and MAP kinase pathways. This results in the establishment of a detrimental vicious cycle involving bi-directional interactions between tumor cells and the bone microenvironment.

Contributing to this cycle may also be the extracellular calcium that is released from the bone and provides a feedback mechanism for increased PTHrP production reported to occur in breast carcinoma cells with calcium-sensing receptors (Sanders et al., 2003). Overall, these studies have improved our understanding of the unique and complex interactions between the bone microenvironment and tumor cell-derived PTHrP to support both local osteolysis and tumor growth in the bone metastatic lesions. In particular, they are paving the way to develop and implement novel therapeutics aimed at preventing and controlling this devastating complication of malignancy.

PTHrP secretion by breast carcinoma as a predictor of bone metastasis

The implications of breast carcinoma-derived PTHrP as a central mediator of osteoclast activation in the metastatic bone lesion are well substantiated; however, it still remains unclear if primary tumor-produced PTHrP serves as a good prognostic indicator for the potential to metastasize to the skeleton. Some clinical studies have reported that PTHrP expression by tumor cells correlates with the onset of bone metastasis (Bundred et al., 1992; Bouizar et al., 1993). However, a recent prospective clinical study in 367 women with invasive breast cancer found that PTHrP-positive breast carcinoma is associated with increased patient survival and reduced incidence of bone metastasis as compared to PTHrP-negative breast cancer (Henderson et al., 2001). Moreover, in some patients whose primary tumors were negative for PTHrP production, their bone metastases demonstrated PTHrP-positive lesions. These results suggest that PTHrP might be a downregulator of the primary tumor invasive phenotype. However, once breast carcinoma disseminates to bone, the local microenvironment contributes to the development of metastatic lesions by enhancing PTHrP tumor production as demonstrated by other studies (Guise et al., 1996). These findings are in agreement with recent studies utilizing murine orthotopic breast carcinoma models that suggest that primary tumor-produced PTHrP is not sufficient to induce skeletal metastasis (Lelekakis et al., 1999; Wysolmerski et al., 2002). Therefore, PTHrP production by breast carcinoma in the bone metastatic lesion in response to local bone-derived factors appears to be more significant to the development of bone metastases than PTHrP produced at the primary tumor site.

PTHrP regulates breast cancer cell growth via autocrine, paracrine and intracrine actions

PTHrP is known to modulate cell behavior by affecting tumor cell proliferation, differentiation and survival. PTHrP expression and production is significantly increased in highly tumorigenic human mammary epithelial cell lines (Cataisson et al., 2000). Recently, PTHrP overexpressed in MCF-7 cells has been associated with increased tumor cell proliferation apparently mediated via an intracrine mechanism since overexpressed PTHrP targeted to the perinuclear region (Falzon and Du, 2000). PTHrP stimulation of tumor cell proliferation occurred through regulatory effects on the cell cycle and anti-apoptotic actions mediated by the Bcl-2 pro- and anti-apoptotic protein family in response to serum starvation (Tovar Sepulveda and Falzon, 2002b). Interestingly, similar cells treated with exogenous PTHrP, which mediates its effects by binding to the PTH/PTHrP receptor, exhibited decreased cell growth. Thus, these studies indicate that PTHrP exerts opposing mitogenic actions *in vitro* that depend on whether they are mediated through autocrine/paracrine or intracrine signaling pathways.

PTHRP AND PROSTATE CANCER

Metastatic bone disease associated with advanced prostate carcinoma is one of the leading causes of morbidity and mortality in men. Accumulating data in recent years have identified prostate-derived PTHrP as one of the contributing factors for the pathogenesis and progression of prostate cancer (Deftos, 2000). Many features of PTHrP make it an attractive candidate for influencing prostate carcinoma growth. PTHrP is produced by normal prostate epithelial cells, from which prostate carcinoma arises, and PTHrP is found in the seminal fluid (Iwamura et al., 1994a; Deftos, 2000). PTHrP has been immunohistochemically identified in prostate cancer tissue in patients with clinically localized disease (Iwamura et al., 1993), is found in higher levels in prostate intraepithelial neoplasia than in normal prostate epithelium, is found in higher levels in prostate carcinoma than in benign prostatic hyperplasia (Iwamura et al., 1995; Asadi et al., 1996), and is found in metastatic lesions in bone (Dougherty et al., 1999).

These initial findings suggested that PTHrP might play important roles in the regulation of normal prostatic function, promotion of neoplastic transformation and development of bone metastasis. PTHrP isoforms (1-139), (1-141) and (1-173) are differentially expressed in normal prostate compared to prostate cancer. Whereas all three isoforms are present in normal and malignant tissue, only PTHrP (1-139) is markedly increased in prostatic adenocarcinoma (Wu et al., 1998). Interestingly, PSA, a serine protease that is used as a screening marker of prostate cancer, cleaves PTHrP (1-141) at the amino-terminus and inactivates PTHrP bioactivity (Cramer et al., 1996). However, it is not known whether this proteolytic processing is relevant to PTHrP actions *in vivo*. Vitamin D_3 and androgens have also been reported to negatively regulate the expression of PTHrP in prostate cancer cells (Tovar Sepulveda and Falzon, 2002a). Animal models of prostate carcinoma metastasis utilize PTHrP as a marker of a bone active protein produced by cancer cells (Corey et al., 2002). The impact of PTHrP on angiogenesis relative to tumor progression has also been the focus of recent investigation where PTHrP was found to inhibit angiogenesis in a PKA-dependent manner (Bakre et al., 2002).

PTHrP regulates prostate cancer cell growth and survival

Recent evidence indicates that PTHrP positively regulates the growth of prostate tumors. Experimental evidence demonstrates that growth rates and size of tumors derived from PTHrP-overexpressing prostate cancer cells are significantly enhanced when compared to tumors generated from cells producing lower levels of PTHrP (Dougherty et al., 1999). These findings indicate that PTHrP is bioavailable during tumor formation *in vivo*. *In vitro*, PTHrP appears to mediate prostate cancer cell growth via autocrine, paracrine and intracrine actions (Iwamura et al., 1994b; Dougherty et al., 1999; Tovar Sepulveda and Falzon, 2002b). PTHrP targeted to the nucleus appears to promote a growth advantage by protecting tumor cells from apoptotic stimuli (Dougherty et al., 1999). This observation suggests that intracrine PTHrP activity may be critical to stimulate primary prostate tumor growth and perhaps the development and progression of bone metastasis. Interestingly, prostate carcinoma cells, have been reported to have functional calcium-sensing receptors that respond to elevated extracellular calcium with a prevention of apoptosis (Lin et al., 1998). These findings along with the findings of extracellular calcium increasing PTHrP secretion from breast carcinoma cells suggest a cyclic response may result. Calcium released from the bone via the osteolytic action of PTHrP may feedback to increase PTHrP and the PTHrP-mediated prevention of apoptosis may positively regulate tumor growth (Sanders et al., 2003).

PTHrP in the development and progression of prostate cancer bone metastases

PTHrP immunoreactivity in clinical and experimental bone metastases associated with prostate cancer suggests that PTHrP may contribute to the development of these lesions, which are frequently osteoblastic in nature (Dougherty et al., 1999; Iddon et al., 2000; Bryden et al., 2002; Corey et al., 2002). Recently, more detailed morphological and *in vivo* studies have revealed that prostate cancer-related bone metastases also contain an osteolytic component at some point in their progression (Rabbani et al., 1999; Mundy, 2002). Using a rodent model of intracardiac injection, PTHrP-overexpressing MatLyLu rat prostate cancer cells resulted in more osteolytic lesions in lumbar vertebrae than control animals (Rabbani et al., 1999). However, other studies utilizing a similar experimental model found no evidence to support a role for PTHrP in promoting skeletal metastasis (Blomme et al., 1999). As a potent regulator of bone remodeling, PTHrP is likely to promote both increases in osteoblast and osteoclast activity in the metastatic lesion (Stewart, 2002). However, more comprehensive studies are needed to validate this hypothesis.

OTHER CANCERS AND PTHRP

PTHrP has been reported to be produced by virtually every cancer identified but its localization in sites of skeletal metastasis has not been as extensive, likely due to the access to such tissues for analysis. In addition to breast and prostate where much of the work has been performed, other tumors that metastasize to bone and produce PTHrP include: lung (Iwaniec et al., 2002), ovarian cancer (Kitazawa et al., 1997), and gastric cancer (Ito et al., 1997). In a subpopulation of patients with lung carcinoma, high serum PTHrP levels (<150 pmol/L) were reported to be a predictor of bone metastasis and decreased survival (Iwaniec et al., 2002). However, in another study of 690 patients with lung carcinoma including 207 squamous cell carcinomas, 75 small cell carcinomas and 29 large cell carcinomas, there was no relationship between serum PTHrP levels of patients with or without bone metastasis (Takai et al., 1996). Seventeen patients had tumor-induced hypercalcemia and 15 of these had elevated PTHrP levels. However, in an experimental model of lung carcinoma metastasis, antibodies to PTHrP reduced the incidence of bone metastases and tumor volume, suggesting that PTHrP promotes skeletal metastasis in this model system (Iguchi et al., 1996). In another lung cancer model system, the formation of bone metastases was directly correlated with the expression of PTHrP in 8 different cell lines (Miki et al., 2000). Discrepancies between experimental models and the human condition with varied results supporting or not supporting the role of PTHrP as a significant contributor in the ability of tumors to metastasize makes it difficult to resolve this issue and further studies are clearly necessary.

PTHrP is likely the most potent regulator of bone turnover present in the bone microenvironment when cancers metastasizes to bone. Relative to the other bone active growth factors produced by tumors, PTHrP has a profound impact on skeletal development when its presence or activity is altered. Understanding its effects on bone in the metastatic environment is critical to better address the consequences of tumor metastasis. Unfortunately, there are no studies that accurately compare the levels of PTHrP from metastatic sites of different tumors so it has been impossible to attribute findings from various tumors to the correlative impact on the bone in the metastatic lesion.

THERAPEUTIC APPROACHES TO CONTROL PTHRP ACTIVITY

The central role of tumor-derived PTHrP in the development and progression of bone metastases provides clear evidence to target PTHrP by pharmacological means to prevent and control the skeletal morbidity associated with malignancy. This rationale has led investigators to actively search for novel drugs capable of blocking PTHrP activity. Experimental studies in immunocompromised mice have demonstrated positive results with the use of neutralizing monoclonal antibodies directed against PTHrP (1-34), which caused a significant reduction in local osteolytic disease and tumor burden in metastatic breast cancer (Guise et al., 1996; Käkönen and Mundy, 2003). Neutralizing antibodies to PTHrP also have been utilized to reduce serum calcium levels associated with humoral hypercalcemia of malignancy (HHM) in experimental animals (Guise et al., 1993; Kukreja et al., 1988). Currently, this therapeutic approach is under clinical investigation to be considered as part of the medical management of osteolytic bone metastases in humans (Mundy, 2002). Recent developments in the search for PTHrP inhibitory drugs have also identified small-molecule compounds that inhibit PTHrP production *in vitro* and in experimental models of osteolytic bone metastasis and HHM in mice (Gallwitz et al., 2002). Anticancer agents such as the guanine nucleotide analogs 6-thioguanine and 6-thioguanosine effectively diminished PTHrP production in both breast and lung cancer cell lines as well as reduced bone destruction and hypercalcemia in mice. The reduced PTHrP production appears to be associated with mechanisms that specifically inhibit PTHrP promoter activity, thus, affecting its transcriptional activity and limiting its expression. In addition, vitamin D_3 analogues have been found to inhibit PTHrP production in prostate cancer cells *in vitro* (Tovar Sepulveda and Falzon, 2002a). Taken together, these promising data indicate that drugs that specifically target and inhibit tumor-derived PTHrP in both metastatic bone disease and HHM may serve in the future as therapeutic adjuvants to either prevent the occurrence or delay the devastating consequences of the skeletal complications of malignancy.

Table 1. Tumor-derived PTHrP Actions in Bone Metastasis

Biologic activity	In vitro	In vivo	References
Tumor growth		Stimulatory	(Dougherty et al., 1999; Wysolmerski et al., 2002)
Mitogenesis	No effect		(Dougherty et al., 1999)
	Stimulatory		(Iwamura et al., 1994b; Cataisson et al., 2000; Falzon and Du, 2000)
Cell survival	Stimulatory		(Dougherty et al., 1999; Tovar Sepulveda and Falzon, 2002b)
Dissemination to bone		Stimulatory	(Bundred et al., 1992; Bouizar et al., 1993; Guise et al., 1996; Thomas et al., 1999; Yin et al., 1999; Rabbani et al., 1999; Käkönen and Mundy, 2003; Gallwitz et al., 2002; Guise et al., 2002; Iguchi et al., 1996; Miki et al., 2000)
		Inhibitory or no effect	(Henderson et al., 2001; Lelekakis et al., 1999; Bendre et al., 2002; Takai et al., 1996)
Alterations of bone remodeling in the metastatic site		Increased osteoclastic activity	(Guise et al., 1996; Thomas et al., 1999; Rabbani et al., 1999; Yin et al., 1999; Käkönen et al., 2002; Gallwitz et al., 2002; Guise et al., 2002)

REFERENCES

Amizuka, N., Henderson, J.E., White, J.H., Karaplis, A.C., Goltzman, D., Sasaki, T. and Ozawa, H. (2000) Recent studies on the biological action of parathyroid hormone (PTH)-related peptide (PTHrP) and PTH/PTHrP receptor in cartilage and bone. *Histology and Histopathology* **15**, 957-970.

Amling, M., Neff, L., Tanaka, S., Inoue, D., Kuida, K., Weir, E., Philbrick, W., Broadus, A.E. and Baron, R. (1997) Bcl-2 lies downstream of PTHrP in a signaling pathway that is required for normal skeletal development. *Journal of Cellular Biology* **136**, 205-213.

Anderson, D.M., Maraskovsky, E., Billingsley, W.L., Dougall, W.C., Tometsko, M.E., Roux, E.R., Teepe, M.C., DuBose, R.F., Cosman, D. and Galibert, L. (1997) A homologue of the TNF receptor and its ligand enhance T-cell growth and dendritic-cell function. *Nature* **390**, 175-179.

Asadi, F., Farraj, M., Sharifi, R., Malkouti, S., Antar, S. and Kukreja, S. (1996). Enhanced expression of parathyroid hormone-related protein in prostate cancer as compared with benign prostatic hyperplasia. *Human Pathology* **27**,1319-1323.

Bakre, M.M., Zhu, Y., Yin, H., Burton, D.W., Terkeltaub, R., Deftos, L.J. and Varner, J.A. (2002). Parathyroid hormone-related peptide is a naturally occuring protein kinase A-dependent angiogenesis inhibitor. *Nature Medicine* **8**, 995-1003.

Belcheva, M.M. and Coscia, C.J. (2002) Diversity of G Protein-coupled receptor signaling pathways to ERK/MAP kinase. *Neurosignals* **11**, 34-44.

Bendre, M.S., Gaddy-Kurten, D., Mon-Foote, T., Akel, N.S., Skinner, R.A., Nicholas, R.W. and Suva, L. (2002) Expression of Interleukin 8 and not parathyroid hormone-related protein by human breast cancer cells correlates with bone metastasis in vivo. *Cancer Research* **62**, 5571-5579.

Blomme, E.A.G., Dougherty, K.M., Pienta, K.J., Capen, C.C., Rosol, T.J. and McCauley, L.K. (1999) Skeletal metastasis of prostate adenocarcinoma in rats: Morphometric analysis and role of parathyroid hormone-related protein. *The Prostate* **39**, 187-197.

Bonni, A., Brunet, A., West, A.E., Datta, S.R., Takasu, M.A. and Greenberg, M.E. (1999) Cell survival promoted by the Ras-MAPK signaling pathway by transcription-dependent and -independent mechanisms. *Science* **286**, 1358-1362.

Bouizar, Z., Spyratos, F., Deytieux, S., de Vernejoul, M. and Jullienne, A. (1993) Polymerase chain reaction analysis of parathyroid hormone-related protein gene expression in breast cancer patients and occurrence of bone metastasis. *Cancer Research* **53**, 5076-5078.

Bryden, A.A., Islam, S., Freemont, A.J., Shanks, J.H., George, N.J. and Clarke, N.W. (2002) Parathyroid hormone-related peptide: expression in prostate cancer bone metastasis. *Prostate Cancer and Prostatic Diseases* **5**, 59-62.

Bundred, N.J., Walker, R.A., Ratcliffe, W.A., Warwick, J., Morrison, J.M. and Ratcliffe, J.G. (1992) Parathyroid hormone related protein and skeletal morbidity in breast cancer. *European Journal of Cancer* **28**, 690-692.

Calvi, L.M., Sims, N.A., Hunzelman, J.L., Knight, M.C., Giovannetti, A., Saxton, J.M., Kronenberg, H.M., Baron, R. and Schipani, E. (2001) Activated parathyroid hormone/parathyroid hormone-related protein receptor in osteoblastic cells differentially affects cortical and trabecular bone. *Journal of Clinical Investigation* **107**, 277-286.

Cataisson, C., Lieberherr, M., Cros, M., Gauville, C., Graulet, A.M., Cotton, J., Calvo, F., Vernejoul, M., Foley, J.J. and Bouizar, Z. (2000) Parathyroid hormone-related peptide stimulates proliferation of highly tumorigenic human SV 40-immortalized breast epithelial cells. *Journal of Bone and Mineral Research* **15**, 2129-2139.

Chambers, A.F., Groom, A.C. and MacDonald, I.C. (2002) Dissemination and growth of cancer cells in metastatic sites. *Nature Reviews: Cancer* **2**, 563-572.

Chen, H., Demiralp, B., Schneider, A., Koh, A.J., Silve, C., Wang, C.Y. and McCauley, L.K. (2002) Parathyroid Hormone and Parathyroid Hormone Related Protein Exert Both Pro- and Anti-apoptotic Effects in Mesenchymal Cells. *Journal of Biological Chemistry* **277**, 19374-19381.

Chen, H., Frankenberg, L., Goldstein, S.A. and McCauley, L.K. (2002) The combination of local and systemic PTH enhances fracture healing. *Clin Orthop Relat Res* (in press).

Cingolani, G., Bednenko, J., Gillespie, M.T. and Gerace, L. (2002) Molecular basis for the recognition of a nonclassical nuclear localization signal by importin β. *Molecular Cell* **10**, 1345-1353.

Corey, E., Quinn, J.E., Bladou, F., Brown, L.G., Roudier, M.P., Brown, J.M., Buhler, K.R. and Vessella, R.L. (2002) Establishment and characterization of osseous prostate cancer models: intra-tibial injection of human prostate cancer cells. *Prostate* **52**, 20-23 (Abstract).

Cramer, S.D., Chen, Z. and Peehl, D.M. (1996) Prostate specific antigen cleaves parathyroid hormone-related protein in the PTH-like domain: Inactivation of PTHrP-stimulated cAMP accumulation in mouse osteoblasts. *Journal of Urology* **156**, 526-531.

Curran, T. and Franza., B.R. (1998) Fos and Jun: the AP-1 connection. Cell **55**,:395-397.

Deftos, L.J. (2000) Prostate carcinoma: production of bioactive factors. *Cancer* **88** (12 Suppl), 3002-3008.

Demiralp, B., Chen, H., Koh-Paige, A.J., Keller, E.T. and McCauley, L.K. (2002) Anabolic effects of parathyroid hormone during endochondral bone growth are dependent on c-fos. *Endocrinology* **143**, 4038-4047.

Dougherty, K.M., Blomme, E.A.G., Koh, A.J., Henderson, J.E., Pienta, K.J., Rosol, T.J. and McCauley, L.K. (1999) Parathyroid hormone related protein (PTHrP) as a growth regulator of prostate carcinoma. *Cancer Research* **59**, 6015-6022.

Enserink, J.M., Christensen, A.E., deRooij, D., vanTriest, M., Schwede, F., Genieser, H.G., Doskeland, S.O., Blank, J.L. and Bos, J.L. (2002) A novel Epac-specific cAMP analogue demonstrates independent regulation of Rap1 and ERK. Nature Cell Biology Published on-line:28 October, 2002.

Falzon, M. and Du, P. (2000) Enhanced growth of MCF-7 breast cancer cells overexpressing parathyroid hormone-related peptide. *Endocrinology* **141**, 1882-1892.

Fang, J., Zhu, Y.Y., Smiley, E., Bonadio, J., Rouleau, J.P., Goldstein, S.A., McCauley, L.K., Davidson, B.L. and Roessler, B.L. (1996) Stimulation of new bone formation by direct transfer of osteogenic plasmid genes. *Proceedings of the National Academy of Sciences of the United States of America* **93**, 5753-5758.

Fenton, A.J., Kemp, B.E., Kent, G.N., Moseley, J.M., Zheng, M.H., Rowe, D.J., Britto, J.M., Martin, T.J. and Nicholson, G.C. (1991) A carboxyl-terminal peptide from the parathyroid hormone-related protein inhibits bone resorption by osteoclasts. *Endocrinology* **129**, 1762-1768.

Gallwitz, W.E., Guise, T.A. and Mundy, G.R. (2002) Guanosine nucleotides inhibit different syndromes of PTHrP excess caused by human cancers in vivo. *Journal of Clinical Investigations* **110**, 1559-1572.

Guise, T.A., Taylor, S.D., Yoneda, T., Sasaki, A., Wright, K., Boyce, B.F., Chirgwin, J.M. and Mundy, G.R. (1994) Parathyroid hormone-related protein (PTHrP) expression by breast cancer cells enhance osteolytic bone metastases in vivo. *Journal of Bone and Mineral Research* **9**, S128

Guise, T.A., Yin, J.J., Taylor, D., Kumagai, Y., Dallas, M., Boyce, B.F., Yoneda, T. and Mundy, G.R. (1996) Evidence for a causal role of parathyroid hormone-related protein in the pathogenesis of human breast cancer-mediated osteolysis. *Journal of Clinical Investigations* **98**, 1544-1549.

Guise, T.A., Yin, J.J., Thomas, R.J., Dallas, M., Cui, Y. and Gillespie, M.T. (2002) Parathyroid hormone-related protein (PTHrP)-(1-139) isoform is efficiently secreted in vitro and enhances breast cancer metastasis to bone in vivo. *Bone* **30**, 670-676. (Abstract)

Guise, T.A., Yoneda, T., Yates, A.J.P. and Mundy, G.R. (1993) The combined effect of tumor-produced parathyroid hormone-related peptide and transforming growth factor-α enhance hypercalcemia in vivo and bone resorption in vitro. *Journal of Clinical Endocrinology Metabolism* **77**, 40-45.

Guo, J., Chung, U., Kondo, H., Bringhurst, F.R. and Kronenberg, H. (2002) The PTH/PTHrP Receptor Can Delay Chondrocyte Hypertrophy In Vivo without Activating Phospholipase C. *Developmental Cell* **3**, 183-194.

Hauschka, P.V., Mavrakos, A.E., Iafrati, M.D., Doleman, S.E. and Klagsbrun, M. (1986) Growth factors in bone matrix. Isolation of multiple types by affinity chromatography on heparin-sepharose. *Journal of Biological Chemistry* **261**, 12665-12674.

Henderson, J.E., Amizuka, N., Warshawsky, H., Biasotto, D., Lanske, B.M., Goltzman, D. and Karaplis, A.C. (1995) Nucleolar localization of parathyroid hormone-related peptide enhances survival of chondrocytes under conditions that promote apoptotic cell death. *Molecular and Cellular Biology* **15**, 4064-4075.

Henderson, M.A., Danks, J.A., Moseley, J.M., Slavin, J.L., Harris, T.L., McKinlay, M.R., Hopper, J.L. and Martin, T.J. (2001) Parathyroid hormone-related protein production by breast cancers, improved survival, and reduced bone metastases. *Journal of the National Cancer Institute* **93**, 234-237.

Hoey, R.P., Sanderson, C., Iddon, J., Brady, G., Bundred, N.J. and Anderson, N.G. (2003) The parathyroid hormone-related protein receptor is expressed in breast cancer bone metastases and promotes autocrine proliferation in breast carcinoma cells. *British Journal of Cancer* **88**, 567-573.

Horwitz, M.J., Tedesco, M.B., Gundberg, C., Garcia-Ocana, A. and Stewart, A.F. (2003) Short-term, high dose parathyroid hormone-related protein as a skeletal anabolic agent for the treatment of postmenopausal osteoporosis. *Journal of Clinical Endocrinology Metabolism* **88**, 569-575.

Iddon, J., Bundred, N.J., Hoyland, J., Downey, S.E., Baird, P., Salter, D., McMahon, R. and Freemont, A.J. (2000) Expression of parathyroid hormone-related protein and its receptor in bone metastases from prostate cancer. *Journal of Pathology* **191**, 170-174.

Iguchi, H., Tanaka, S., Ozawa, Y., Kashiwakuma, T., Kimura, T., Hiraga, T., Ozawa, H. and Kono, A. (1996) An experimental model of bone metastasis by human lung cancer cells: the role of parathyroid hormone-related protein in bone metastasis. *Cancer Research* **56**, 4040-4043.

Ito, M., Nakashima, M., Alipov, G.K., Matasuzaka, S., Ohtsuru, A., Yano, H., Yamashita, S. and Sekine, I. (1997) Gastric cancer associated with overexpression of parathyroid hormone-related peptide (PTHrP) and PTH/PTHrP receptor in relation to tumor progression. *Journal of Gastroenterology* **32**, 396-400.

Iwamura, M., Abrahamsson, P.A., Foss, K.A., Wu, G., Cockett, A.T.K. and Deftos, L.J. (1994b). Parathyroid hormone-related protein:a potential autocrine growth regulator in human prostate cancer lines. *Urology* **43**, 675-679.

Iwamura, M., Abrahamsson, P.A., Schoen, S., Cockett, A.T.K. and Deftos, L.J. (1994a) Immunoreactive parathyroid hormone-related protein is present in human seminal plasma and is of prostate origin. *Journal of Andrology* **15**, 410-414.

Iwamura, M., di Sant 'Agnese, P.A., Wu, G., Benning, C.M., Cockett, A.T., Deftos, L.J. and Abrahamsson, P.A. (1993) Immunohistochemical localization of parathyroid hormone related protein in human prostate cancer. *Cancer Research* **53**, 1724-1726.

Iwamura, M., Gershagen, S., Lapets, O., Moynes, R., Abrahamsson, P., Cockett, A.T.K., Deftos, L.J. and di Sant'agnese, P.A. (1995) Immunohistochemical localization of parathyroid hormone-related protein in prostatic intraepithelial neoplasia. *Human Pathology* **26**, 797-801.

Iwaniec, U.T., Mosekilde, L., Mitova-Caneva, N.G., Thomsen, J.S. and Wronski, T.J. (2002) Sequential treatment with basic fibroblast growth factor and PTH is more efficacious than treatment with PTH alone for increasing vertebral bone mass and strength in osteopenic ovariectomized rats. *Endocrinology* **143**, 2515-2526.

Jilka, R.L., Weinstein, R.S., Bellido, T., Roberson, P., Parfitt, A.M. and Manolagas, S.C. (1999). Increased bone formation by prevention of osteoblast apoptosis with parathyroid hormone. *Journal of Clinical Investigation* **104**, 439-446.

Jobert, A.S., Zhang, P., Couvineau, A., Bonaventure, J., Roume, J., Le Merrer, M. and Silve, C. (1998) Absence of functional receptors for parathyroid hormone and parathyroid hormone-related peptide in Blomstrand chondrodysplasia. *Journal of Clinical Investigation* **102**, 34-40.

Käkönen, S.M. and Mundy, G.R. (2003) Mechanisms of osteolytic bone metastases in breast carcinoma. *Cancer* **97**(3 Suppl), 834-839.

Käkönen, S.M., Selander, K.S., Chirgwin, J.M., Yin, J.J., Burns, S., Rankin, W.A., Grubbs, B.G., Dallas, M., Cui, Y. and Guise, T.A. (2002). Transforming gowth factor-β stimulates parathyroid hormone-related protein and osteolytic metastases via Smad and mitogen-activated protein kinases signaling pathways. *Journal of Biology Chemistry* **277**, 24571-24578.

Keller, E.T., Zhang, J., Cooper, C.W., Smith, P.C., McCauley, L.K., Pienta, K.J. and Taichman, R.T. (2001) Prostate carcinoma skeletal metastases: cross-talk between tumor and bone. *Cancer Metastasis Reviews* **20**, 333-349.

Kitazawa, R., Kitazawa, S., Matui, T. and Maeda, S. (1997) In situ detection of parathyroid hormone-related protein in ovarian clear cell carcinoma. *Human Pathology* **28**, 379-382.

Kostenuik, P.J., Morony, S., Warmington, K.S., Porkess, M.V., Geng, Z., Boone, T., Delaney, J. and Lacey, D.L. (2001) Twice-weekly injection of a sustained-duration PTH construct increases cortical and trabecular bone density in adult mice. *Journal of Bone and Mineral Research* **16**, S221 (Abstract).

Kukreja, S.C., Shevrin, D.H., Wimbiscus, S.A., Ebeling, P.R., Danks, J.A., Rodda, C.P., Wood, W.I. and Martin, T.J. (1988) Antibodies to parathyroid hormone-related protein lower serum calcium in athymic mouse models. *Journal of Clinical Investigation* **82**, 1798-1802.

Lacey, D.L., Timms, E., Tan, H.-L., Kelley, M.J., Dunstan, C.R., Burgess, T., Elliott, R., Colombero, A., Elliott, G., Scully, S., Hsu, H., Sullivan, J., Hawkins, N., Davy, E., Capparelli, C., Eli, A., Qian, Y.-X., Kaufman, S., Sarosi, I., Shalhoub, V., Senaldi, G., Guo, J., Delaney, J. and Boyle, W.J. (1998) Osteoprotegerin ligand is a cytokine that regulates osteoclast differentiation and activation. *Cell* **93**, 165-176.

Lanske, B., Amling, M., Neff, L., Guiducci, J., Baron, R. and Kronenberg, H. (1999) Ablation of the PTHrP gene or the PTH/PTHrP receptor gene leads to distinct abnormalities in bone development. *Journal of Clinical Investigation* **104**, 399-407.

Lee, S.K. and Lorenzo, J.A. (1999) Parathyroid hormone stimulates TRANCE and inhibits osteoprotegerin messenger ribonucleic acid expression in murine bone marrow cultures: correlation with osteoclast-like cell formation. *Endocrinology* **140**, 3553-3561.

Lelekakis, M., Moseley, J.M., Artin, T.J., Ards, D., Williams, E., Ho, P., Lowe, D., Javni, J., Miller, F.R., Slavin, J. and Anderson, R.L. (1999) A novel orthotopic model of breast cancer metastasis to bone. *Clinical Experimental Metastasis* **17**, 163-170.

Liapis, H., Crouch, E.C., Grosso, L.E., Kitazawa, S. and Wick, M.R. (1993) Expression of parathyroid like protein in normal, proliferative and neoplastic human breast tissues. *American Journal of Pathology* **143**, 1169-1178.

Lin, K.I., Chattopadhyay, N., Bai, M., Alvarez, R., Dang, C.V., Baraban, J.M., Brown, E.M. and Ratan, R.R. (1998) Elevated extracellular calcium can prevent apoptosis via the calcium-sensing receptor. *Biochem Biophys Res Commun* **249**, 325-331.

Luparello, C., Romanotto, R., Tipa, A., Sirchia, R., Olmo, N., De Silanes, I.L., Turnay, J., Lizarbe, M.A. and Stewart, A.F. (2001) Midregion parathyroid hormone-related protein inhibits growth and invasion in vitro and tumorigenesis in vivo of human breast cancer cells. *Journal of Bone and Mineral Research* **16**, 2173-2181.

Machwate, M., Rodan, S.B., Rodan, G.A. and Harada, S.I. (1998) Sphingosine kinase mediates cyclic AMP suppression of apoptosis in rat periosteal cells. *Molecular Pharmacology* **54**, 70-77.

Manolagas, S.C. (2000) Birth and death of bone cells: Basic regulatory mechanisms and implications for the pathogenesis and treatment of osteoporosis. Endocr Rev **21**, 115-137.

Martin, T.J. and Moseley, J.M. (2000) Mechanisms in the skeletal complications of breast cancer. *Endocrine Related Cancer* **7**, 271-284.

Miki, T., Yano, S., Hanibuchi, M. and Sone, S. (2000) Bone metastasis model with multiorgan dissemination of human small-cell lung cancer (SBC-5) cells in natural killer cell-depleted SCID mice. *Oncology Research* **12**, 209-217.

Mundy, G.R. (2002) Metastasis to bone: Causes, consequences and therapeutic opportunities. *Nature Reviews: Cancer* **2**, 584-593.

Murphy, L.O., Smith, S., Chen, R.H., Fingar, D.C. and Blenis, J. (2002) Molecular interpretation of ERK signal duration by immediate early gene products." *Nature Cell Biology* **4**, 556-564.

Nakai, M., Mundy, G.R., Williams, P.J., Boyce, B. and Yoneda, T. (1992) A synthetic antagonist to laminin inhibits the formation of osteolytic metastases by human melanoma cells in nude mice. *Cancer Research* **52**, 5395-5399.

Neer, R.M., Arnaud, C.D., Zanchetta, J.R., Prince, R., Gaich, G.A., Reginster, J.Y., Hodsman, A.B., Eriksen, E.F., Ish-Shalom, S., Genant, H., Wang, O. and Mitlak, B.H. (2001) Effect of parathyroid hormone (1-34) on fractures and bone mineral density in postmenopausal women with osteoporosis. *New England Journal of Medicine* **10**, 1434-1441.

Ouyang, H., Franceschi, R.T., McCauley, L.K., Wang, D. and Somerman, M.J. (2000) Parathyroid hormone-related protein downregulates bone sialoprotein gene expression in cementoblasts: role of the protein kinase A pathway. *Endocrinology* **141**, 4671-4680.

Pearman, A.T., Chou, W.Y., Bergman, K.D., Pulumati, M.R. and Partridge, N.C. (1996) Parathyroid hormone induces c-fos promoter activity in osteoblastic cells through phosphorylated cAMP response element (CRE)-binding protein binding to the major CRE. *Journal of Biological Chemistry* **271**, 25715-25721.

Philbrick, W. (2001) Parathyroid hormone-related protein:Gene structure, biosynthesis, metabolism, and regulation. In: The parathyroids. Edited by Bilezikian, J.P., R. Marcus, and M.A. Levine. San Diego: Academic Press, p.31.

Powell, G.J., Southby, J., Danks, J.A., Stillwell, R.G., Hayman, J.A., Henderson, M.A., Bennett, R.C. and Martin, T.J. (1991) Localization of parathyroid hormone-related protein in breast cancer metastasis: increased incidence in bone compared with other sites. *Cancer Research* **51**, 3059-3061.

Rabbani, S.A., Gladu, J., Harakidas, P., Jamison, B. and Goltzman, D. (1999) Over-production of parathyroid hormone-related peptide results in increased osteolytic skeletal metastasis by cancer cells in vivo." *International Journal of Cancer* **80**, 257-264.

Riccio, A., Ahn, S., Davenport, C.M., Blendy, J.A. and Ginty, D.D. (1999) Mediation by a CREB family transcription factor of NGF-dependent survival of sympathetic neurons. *Science* **286**, 2358-2361.

Rosol, T.J. and Capen, C.C. (1992) Biology of Disease: Mechanisms of cancer-induced hypercalcemia. *Laboratory Investigations* **67**, 680-702.

Rubens, R.D. (2000) Clinical aspects of bone metastases. In: Tumor bone diseases and osteoporosis in cancer patients. Edited by Body, J.J. Brussels: Marcel Dekker, Inc., p.85.

Sanders, J.L., Chattopadhyay, N., Kifor, O., Yamaguchi, T., Butters, R.R. and Brown, E.M. (2003) Extracellular calcium-sensing receptor expression and its potential role in regulating parathyroid hormone-related peptide secretion in human breast cancer cell lines. *Endocrinology* **141**, 4357-4364.

Schipani, E., Kruse, K. and Jueppner, H. (1995) A constitutively active mutant PTH/PTHrP receptor in Jansen-type metaphyseal chondrodysplasia. *Science* **268**, 98-100.

Simonet, W.S., Lacey, D.L., Dunstan, C., Kelly, M., Chang, M.S., Nguyen, H.Q., Wooden, S., Bennett, L., Boone, T., Shimamoto, G., DeRose, M., Elliott, R., Colombero, A., Tan, H.L., Trail, G., Sullivan, J., Davey, E., Bucay, N., Renshaw-Gegg, L., Hughes, T.M., Hill, D., Pattison, W., Campbell, P., Boyle, W.J. and et.al. (1997) Osteoprotegerin: a novel secreted protein involved in the regulation of bone density. *Cell* **89**, 159-161.

Southby, J., Kissin, M.W., Danks, J.A., Hayman, J.A., Moseley, J.M., Henderson, M.A., Bennett, R.C. and Martin, T.J. (1990) Immunohistochemical localization of parathyroid hormone-related protein in human breast cancer. *Cancer Research* **50**, 7710-7716.

Spurney, R.F., Flannery, P.J., Garner, S.C., Athirakul, K., Liu, S., Guilak, F. and Quarles, L.D. (2002) Anabolic effects of a G protein-coupled receptor kinase inhibitor expressed in osteoblasts. *Journal of Clinical Investigation* **109**, 1361-1371.

Stewart, A.F. (2002) Hyperparathyroidism, humoral hypercalcemia of malignancy, and the anabolic actions of parathyroid hormone and parathyroid hormone-related protein on the skeleton. *Journal of Bone and Mineral Research* **17**, 753-757.

Stork, P.J.S. and Schmitt, J.M. (2002) Crosstalk between cAMP and MAP kinase signaling in the regulation of cell proliferation. *Trends in Cell Biology* **12**, 258-266.

Strewler, G.J. (2000) Mechanisms of disease: The physiology of parathyroid hormone-related protein. *New England Journal of Medicine* **342**, 177-185.

Takai, E., Yano, T., Igushi, H., Fukuyama, Y., Yokoyama, H., Asoh, H. and Ichinose, Y. (1996) Tumor-induced hypercalcemia and parathyroid hormone-related protein in lung carcinoma. *Cancer* **78**, 1384-1387.

Thomas, R.J., Guise, T.A., Yin, J.J., Elliot, J., Horwood, N.J., Martin, T.J. and Gillespie, M.T. (1999) Breast cancer cells interact with osteoblasts to support osteoclast formation. *Endocrinology* **140**, 4451-4458.

Tovar Sepulveda, V.A. and Falzon, M.. (2002b) Parathyroid hormone-related protein enhances PC-3 prostate cancer cell growth via both autocrine/paracrine and intracrine pathways. *Regulatory Peptides* **105**, 109-120.

Tovar Sepulveda, V.A. and Falzon, M. (2002a) Regulation of PTH-related protein gene expression by vitamin D in PC-3 prostate cancer cells. *Molecular Cellular Biology* **190**, 115-124.

Vahle, J.L., Sato, M., Long, M., Long, G.G., Young, J.K., Francis, P.C., Engelhardt, J.A., Westmore, M.S., Ma, L.Y. and Nold, J.B. (2002) Skeletal changes in rats given daily subcutaneous injections of recombinant human parathyroid hormone (1-34) for 2 years and relevance to human safety. *Toxicologic Pathology* **30**, 312-321.

Vargas, S.J., Gillespie, M.T., Powell, G.J., Southby, J., Danks, J.A., Moseley, J.M. and Martin, T.J. (1992) Localization of parathyroid hormone-related protein mRNA expression in breast cancer and metastatic lesions by in situ hybridization. *Journal of Bone and Mineral Research* **7**, 971-979.

Wilson, B.E., Mochon, E. and Boxer, L.M. (1996) Induction of bcl-2 expression by phosphorylated CREB proteins during B-cell activation and rescue from apoptosis. *Molecular and Cellular Biology* **16**, 5546-5556.

Wu, G., Iwamura, M., di Sant'agnese, A., Deftos, L.J., Cockett, A.T. and Gershagen, S. (1998) Characterization of the cell-specific expression of parathyroid hormone-related protein in normal and neoplastic prostate tissue. *Urology* **51**(5A suppl), 110-120.

Wysolmerski, J.J., Dann, P.R., Zelazny, E., Dunbar, M.E., Insogna, K.L., Guise, T.A. and Perkins, A.S. (2002) Overexpression of parathyroid hormone-related protein causes hypercalcemia but not bone metastases in a murine model of mammary tumorigenesis. *Journal of Bone and Mineral Research* **17**, 1164-1170. (Abstract)

Yamato, H., Nagai, Y., Inoue, D., Ohnishi, Y., Ueyama, Y., Ohno, H., Matsumoto, T., Ogata, E. and Ikeda, K. (1995) Association between histomorphometry and biochemical markers of bone turnover in a longitudinal rat model of parathyroid hormone-related peptide (PTHrP)-mediated tumor osteolysis. *Journal of Bone and Mineral Research* **10**, 36-45.

Yasuda, H., Shima, N., Nakagawa, N., Mochizuki, S.I., Yano, K., Fujise, N., Sato, Y., Goto, M., Yamaguchi, K., Kuriyama, M., Kanno, T., Murakami, A., Tsuda, E., Morinaga, T. and Higashio, K. (1998) Identity of osteoclastogenesis inhibitory factor (OCIF) and osteoprotegerin (OPG): a mechanism by which OPG/OCIF inhibits osteoclastogenesis in vitro. *Endocrinology* **139**, 1329-1337.

Yasuda, H., Shima, N., Nakagawa, N., Yamaguchi, K., Kinoshaki, M., Mochizuki, S., Tomoyasu, A., Yano, K., Goto, M., Murakami, A., Tsuda, E., Morinaga, T., Higashio, K., Udagawa, N., Takahashi, N. and Suda, T. (1998) Osteoclast differentiation factor is a ligand for osteoprotegerin/osteoclastogenesis-inhibitory factor and is identical to TRANCE/RANKL. *Proc Natl Acad Sci U S A* **95**, 3602

Yin, J.J., Selander, K., Chirgwin, J.M., Dallas, M., Grubbs, B.G., Wieser, R., Massague, J., Mundy, G.R. and Guise, T.A. (1999) TGF-beta signaling blockade inhibits PTHrP secretion by breast cancer cells and bone metastases development. *Journal of Clinical Investigation* **103**, 197-206.

Zhou, H., Shen, V., Dempster, D. and Lindsay, R. (2001). Continuous parathyroid hormone and estrogen administration increases vertebral cancellous bone volume and cortical width in the estrogen-deficient rat. *Journal of Bone and Mineral Research* **16**, 1300-1307.

Chapter 7

OPG, RANKL, AND RANK IN CANCER METASTASIS: EXPRESSION AND REGULATION

Julie M. Brown[1], Jian Zhang[2], and Evan T. Keller[2]
[1]*Oncology Research Centre, UNSW Department of Clinical Medicine, Prince of Wales Hospital, Randwick, NSW2031, Australia;* [2]*Unit for Laboratory Animal Medicine and Department of Pathology, University of Michigan, Ann Arbor, MI 48109 USA*

INTRODUCTION

In normal adult human bone, the skeleton is renewed on a continuous basis in a dynamic, highly regulated process known as the bone remodeling sequence. The synthesis of new bone by osteoblasts is consequent to the critical primary step of excavation of old bone (resorption or osteolysis) by large multinucleated osteoclasts. These processes are tightly coupled such that, in normal bone homeostasis, the formative and resorptive phases are balanced [reviewed in (Mundy, 1999)].

In pathological processes, this equilibrium is compromised. In metabolic bone disease such as osteoporosis, and in some cancers that metastasize to bone, including most breast cancers and multiple myeloma, there is a net increase in bone resorption [reviewed in (Coleman, 1997)]. Prostate cancer (CaP) is atypical of osteotropic cancers in that CaP bone metastases are distinctively osteoblastic or mixed (Coleman, 1997), although concomitant increases in bone resorption have been described in several studies (Revilla *et al*, 1998; Brown *et al*, 2001a; Jung *et al*, 2001) [and as reviewed in (Yoneda, 1998; Goltzman, 2001)]. The manipulation by cancer cells of the bone remodeling pathway, directly or indirectly, results in a dramatic weakening of bone structure that produces fractures, compressions and pain, and can result in hypercalcemia (Coleman, 1997). These complications are of profound concern to clinicians, particularly since treatment options at this pathological stage are limited in their effectiveness. An understanding of the basic processes at work in normal circumstances may therefore help us to elucidate the mechanisms through which tumor cells disrupt bone homeostasis and may reveal novel therapeutic approaches.

THE OPG, RANKL AND RANK AXIS

Osteoclasts are the primary determinants of bone resorption. The increased activity of osteoclasts causes many pathophysiological conditions of bone, such as osteoporosis, Paget's disease, and the osteolytic components of bone lesions from cancer metastases. The interaction between mesenchymally-derived osteoblasts or bone marrow stromal cells and mononucleate hematopoietic osteoclast precursors results in the formation of actively resorbing osteoclasts (Takahashi *et al*, 1988; Roodman, 1999). Until the discovery of osteoprotegerin (OPG), receptor activator of NFκB ligand (RANKL) and receptor activator of NFκB (RANK), the molecular mediators of bone resorption, studies on osteoclastogenesis demanded the presence of osteoblasts or bone marrow stromal cells (Rodan Martin, 1981; Takahashi *et al*, 1988) [reviewed in (Roodman, 1996)]. This was further supported by studies in Cbfa1 gene-deficient mice, in which the reduction in mature osteoblasts is accompanied by a marked decrease in the numbers of osteoclasts (Komori *et al*, 1997) and a diminished ability of calvarial cells from these mice to support osteoclastogenesis *in vitro* (Gao *et al*, 1998).

The major negative regulator of bone resorption, osteoprotegerin (OPG), was identified by two independent groups through screening of a fetal rat intestinal cDNA library (Simonet *et al*, 1997) and through purification from the tissue culture supernatant of human fibroblasts (Tsuda *et al*, 1997). Its familial identity was revealed by sequencing of its amino terminus, whereupon it was determined to be a member of the tumor necrosis factor (TNF) receptor superfamily. Several features, including a hydrophobic leader sequence and the absence of a hydrophobic transmembrane-spanning region, suggested that OPG could be secreted (Simonet *et al*, 1997). Four transcripts ranging in size from 2.4kb to 6.5kb have been detected in a range of fetal and adult tissues (Simonet *et al*, 1997; Morinaga *et al*, 1998; Yasuda *et al*, 1998a): of these, it is the major 2.4kb transcript that is known to encode the full-length 401 amino acid peptide that contains 4 N-terminal domains, which permit anti-resorptive activity *in vitro* and *in vivo* (Yasuda *et al*, 1998a) [reviewed in (Hofbauer Heufelder, 2001)]. Transgenic mice with hepatic overexpression of OPG exhibited increased bone mineral density and decreased numbers of osteoclasts, indicative of an osteopetrotic phenotype (Simonet *et al*, 1997), whereas the bones of *opg*$^{-/-}$ mice had thin cortices, with reductions in trabecular bone volume, and decreased bone mineral density, strength and rigidity, suggestive of osteoporosis (Mizuno *et al*, 1998). The osteoprotective function of OPG was confirmed in two studies: administration of exogenous OPG to rats for two weeks increased bone volume and bone mineral density (Yasuda *et al*, 1998a); and, a single subcutaneous dose of human OPG at 3mg/kg was able to reduce the levels of urine deoxypyridinolines, a bone resorption systemic marker, by 80% within 5 days in postmenopausal women (Bekker *et al*, 2001).

The ligand for OPG was discovered using cross-linking studies, where OPG bound to a cell membrane-bound 40kD protein on murine ST2 cells that had been treated with calcitriol (Yasuda *et al*, 1998a). This was supported by generation of a cDNA library from ST2 cells that had been treated with calcitriol and dexamethasone, which produced a clone that could stimulate osteoclastogenesis and whose activity was abrogated upon addition of exogenous OPG (Yasuda *et al*, 1998b). This pro-resorptive factor was identified as RANKL, a member of the TNF superfamily. Three isoforms of RANKL have since been identified: a truncated intracellular form, and mature functional membrane-bound and soluble forms (Ikeda *et al*, 2001), the latter of which can be expressed as a separate entity or produced through cleavage of the membrane-bound isoform by TNF-alpha converting enzyme-like proteases or related metalloprotease-disintegrins (Lum *et al*, 1999). RANKL was first identified in the immune system, where it has a pivotal role in T cell proliferation and acts a survival factor for mature T cells (Anderson *et al*, 1997) and dendritic cells (Wong *et al*, 1997). In the skeleton, RANKL is the master inducer of bone resorption, where it stimulates osteoclast formation (Matsuzaki *et al*, 1998), activation (Fuller *et al*, 1998; Burgess *et al*, 1999; Udagawa *et al*, 1999), adherence (O'Brien *et al*, 2000) and survival (Lacey *et al*, 2000) by ligation with RANK, which is expressed on osteoclast precursors (Nakagawa *et al*, 1998; Hsu *et al*, 1999; Udagawa *et al*, 1999; Li *et al*, 2000).

The binding of RANKL with RANK initiates and maintains the osteoclastogenic cascade: an intracellular signaling cascade involving TNF receptor-associated factors [reviewed in (Wong *et al*, 1999a) and (Lee Kim, 2003)] transduces nuclear factor-κB (Wong *et al*, 1998), mitogen-activated protein kinases (Mizukami *et al*, 2002), c-jun N-terminal kinase (Lee *et al*, 2000), extracellular signal-related kinase (ERK), and phosphatidylinositol 3-

kinase (P13K) pathways (Wong *et al*, 1999b; Arron *et al*, 2001). This results in the fusion of osteoclast precursors (Matsuzaki *et al*, 1998; Yasuda *et al*, 1998b), their maturation and activation (Fuller *et al*, 1998; Burgess *et al*, 1999), and their survival (Fuller *et al*, 1998; Lacey *et al*, 1998; Yasuda *et al*, 1998b). The necessity of this interaction for the generation of functional osteoclasts and for bone resorption was indicated by the osteopetrotic phenotypes demonstrated in *rankl*$^{-/-}$ and *rank*$^{-/-}$ transgenic mice (Kong *et al*, 1999), where an absence of osteoclasts was noted, and by the inability of hematopoietic cells from *rank*$^{-/-}$ mice to differentiate into osteoclasts *ex vivo* (Dougall *et al*, 1999). Furthermore, administration of soluble RANKL to mice resulted in hypercalcemia, thinned bones and larger osteoclasts (Lacey *et al*, 1998).

Osteoblasts and bone marrow stromal cells express RANKL and can therefore mediate the extent of osteoclastogenesis and of consequent bone resorption. These cells also express OPG, suggesting the possibility that these cells can control the relative availability of both factors. Many studies have been published describing the interaction between OPG and RANKL, whereby OPG binds to RANKL and hinders its ligation to RANK [reviewed in (Horowitz *et al*, 2001)]. Through this interference, OPG acts as a decoy receptor for RANKL and as a negative regulator of bone resorption by inhibiting osteoclastogenesis (Simonet *et al*, 1997; Lacey *et al*, 1998; Yasuda *et al*, 1998a; Yasuda *et al*, 1998b). These data collectively suggest that the relative abundancies of OPG and RANKL regulate bone resorption: a net increase in OPG results in osteopetrosis whereas a net increase in RANKL causes excessive bone resorption and osteoporosis.

OPG, RANKL AND RANK EXPRESSION

The establishment of tumor cells in bone, and their subsequent growth as metastases, is thought to be dependent upon a primary osteolytic event (Roland, 1958; Nielsen *et al*, 1991). It was therefore postulated that cancer cells in bone might aberrantly express OPG, RANKL and/ or RANK, or modulate the expression of these molecules by bone-derived cells, which could provide a mechanism through which abnormal osteolysis might occur. As shown in Table 1, several studies have recently determined the expression of OPG, RANKL and RANK by tumor cells and by other non-malignant local cells in bone. OPG, RANKL and RANK expression by cells in other tumors that also metastasize to bone, such as lung and renal cancer, have not yet been documented, but it is likely that the expression of at least one of these proteins is altered in the metastasis of these cancers to bone.

Table 1. Expression of OPG, RANKL and RANK in cancer specimens. IHC: immunohistochemistry. ICC: immunocytochemistry. FC: flow cytometry. RT-PCR: reverse-transcription polymerase chain reaction. IF: immunofluorescnece. ISH: in situ hybridization. FISH: fluorescent ISH.

Tumor	Specimen	Cells	Factor	Method	Reference
Multiple myeloma	Bone marrow sample	Reticular stromal cells	RANKL+	IHC (n=15)	(Roux *et al,* 2002a)
		Erythroblasts	RANK+		
		Bone marrow plasma cells	RANKL+ (10/10)	IF	(Sezer *et al,* 2002a)
		Multiple myeloma cells	RANKL+ (6/6)	ICC, FC	(Sezer *et al,* 2002b)
		Multiple myeloma cells	RANKL-, OPG+ (3/21)	RT-PCR (n=21), IHC	(Giuliani *et al*, 2001)
		Stromal cells	RANKL+	(n=15)	
		Osteoblasts	OPG+		
		Stromal cells	RANKL+	ISH, IHC	(Pearse *et al*, 2001)
		T cells		(n=14)	
		Megakaryo-cytes	OPG decreased	IHC	
		Stromal cells			
		Vessels			
Breast cancer	Primary	Homogenized samples	RANKL-; OPG+; RANK+ (12/12)	RT-PCR + Southern	(Thomas *et al*, 1999)
	Bone mets	Breast cancer cells	RANKL+	IHC (4/4),	(Huang *et al*, 2002)
		Osteoblasts		ISH	
		Fibroblasts			
Adult T cell leukemia + hyper-calcemia	Bone marrow sample	ATL cells	RANKL+ (7/8), OPG+ (3/8)	RT-PCR	(Nosaka *et al*, 2002)

(Table 1 continued on next page)

(Table 1 continued)

Prostate cancer	Primary	Prostate cancer cells	RANKL+ (9/11); OPG+ (2/10)	IHC	(Brown *et al*, 2001b)
	Non-osseous mets	CaP cells in lymphoid mets	RANKL+ (3/4); OPG+ (2/4)		
		CaP cells in appendix met	RANKL- (1/1);		
		CaP cells in liver mets	OPG- (1/1) RANKL- (3/3);		
		CaP cells in bone mets	OPG- (3/3)		
	Bone mets		RANKL+ (9/9); OPG+ (8/9)		
	Bone mets	Prostate cancer cells Osteoblasts Fibroblasts	RANKL+	IHC (2/2), ISH	(Huang *et al*, 2002)
Lung cancer	Bone mets	Lung cancer cells Osteoblasts Fibroblasts	RANKL+	IHC (6/6), ISH	(Huang *et al*, 2002)
Follicular thyroid cancer	Bone mets	Thyroid cancer cells	RANKL+	IHC (4/4), ISH	(Huang *et al*, 2002)
Osteo-clastoma	Primary	Stromal cells Giant cells	RANKL+, OPG+ RANKL+, OPG+, RANK+	RT-PCR (n=8)	(Atkins *et al*, 2000)
		Giant cells Stromal (tumor) cells Macrophage-like cells	OPG+, RANK+ RANKL+ OPG+, OPG+, RANK+	FISH (n=5)	(Huang *et al*, 2000)
Hodgkin's disease	Lymph node biopsy	Homogenized	RANKL+ (4/4), OPG+ (4/4), RANK- (4/4W) (7/7, IHC)	Western blot (all) + IHC (RANK)	(Fiumara *et al*, 2001)
Plasma cell leukemia	Bone marrow or peripheral blood sample	Homogenized	RANKL-, OPG+ (1/5)	RT-PCR	(Giuliani *et al*, 2001)

The expression of OPG, RANKL and RANK has also been determined in a range of primary cells *in vitro*, and in cell lines that are commonly used to model cancers (see Table 2). Several of the cell lines stimulated osteoclastogenesis in the absence of stromal cells, which was blocked by addition of exogenous OPG, suggesting that the expressed RANKL was functional (Atkins *et al*, 2001; Zhang *et al*, 2001; Nosaka *et al*, 2002; Yonou *et al*, 2003). These data imply a direct mechanism for the action of cancer cells on osteoclasts, and therefore on bone resorption, without the requirement of a stromal intermediate. However, others have found that the role of the osteoclast in the development of a metastatic lesion is variable depending on the prostate cancer cell phenotype and tumor-induced osteolysis may not be required for osteoblastic metastases (Lee *et al*, 2003).

Table 2. Expression of OPG, RANKL and RANK in cell lines. PMSCs: primary murine stromal cells. MBMCs: bone marrow cells.

Cell	Factor	Method	Reference
Primary murine osteoblasts	RANKL+, OPG+	RT-PCR + Northern blot	(Thomas *et al*, 1999)
	RANKL decreases, OPG increases post-confluence	RT-PCR	(Thomas *et al*, 2001)
PMSCs	RANKL-	RT-PCR	(Pearse *et al*, 2001)
MBMCs	RANKL-, OPG+	RT-PCR	(Michigami *et al*, 2001)
Prostate cancer cell lines			
LNCaP	RANKL+, OPG+	RT-PCR, Western	(Zhang *et al*, 2001),
		(RANKL)	(Penno *et al*, 2002)
LNCaP-C4-2B	RANKL+, OPG+	RT-PCR (OPG)	(Lin *et al*, 2001)
PC-3	OPG+	RT-PCR, ELISA	(Penno *et al*, 2002), (Lee *et al*, 2003)
DU 145	OPG+		(Holen *et al*, 2002)
LAPC-9	OPG+, RANKL-	RT-PCR	(Lee *et al*, 2003)
Breast cancer cell lines			
MDA-MB-231	RANKL-, OPG+, RANK+	RT-PCR + Northern blot	(Thomas *et al*, 1999)
MCF-7	RANKL-, OPG+, RANK+		
T47D	RANKL-, OPG+, RANK+		
Hodgkin's disease cell lines			
KM-H2	RANKL+, OPG+, RANK-	Western blot	(Fiumara *et al*, 2001)
HDLM-2	RANKL+, OPG+, RANK+		
L-428	RANKL+, OPG+, RANK+		
HD-MYZ	RANKL+, OPG+, RANK-		

(Table 2 continued on next page)

(Table 2 continued)
Myeloma cell lines

XG-1	RANKL-, OPG-	RT-PCR	(Giuliani *et al*, 2001)
XG-6	RANKL-, OPG-		
MDN	RANKL-, OPG-		
HMCL U266	RANKL-, OPG-		
HMCL LP-1	RANKL-, OPG-		
OPM-2	RANKL-, OPG-		
JJN-3	RANKL-, OPG-		
ARP-1+ PMSCs or MG-63 cells	PMSCs: RANKL+ MG-63: OPG+	RT-PCR (RANKL), Northern blot (OPG)	(Pearse *et al*, 2001)
ARH-77 + PMSCs or MG-63 cells	PMSCs: RANKL+ MG-63: OPG-		
U266 + PMSCs or MG-63 cells	PMSCs: RANKL+ MG-63: OPG+		
H929 + PMSCs or MG-63 cells	PMSCs: RANKL+ MG-63: OPG+		
RPMI 8226 + PMSCs or MG-63 cells	PMSCs: RANKL+ MG-63: OPG-		
Other hematopoietic and leukemic cell lines			
DHL-1	RANKL-, OPG+, RANK+/-	Western blot	(Fiumara *et al*, 2001)
HL-60	RANKL-, OPG+, RANK-		
Jurkat	RANKL-, OPG+, RANK+/-		
SUP-M2	RANKL+, OPG+, RANK-		
8226	RANKL+, OPG+, RANK+		
Osteosarcoma cell lines			
MG-63	OPG+ (strong)	Northern blot	(Pearse *et al*, 2001)
Neuroblastoma cell line			
NB-19	RANKL-, OPG-	RT-PCR	(Michigami *et al*, 2001)
NB-19 + MBMCs	RANKL+, OPG+		

Since OPG is soluble, it was suggested that measurement of serum OPG levels might be useful as a marker of metastatic bone disease. Thus far, it has been determined that serum OPG levels are decreased in multiple myeloma (Giuliani *et al*, 2001; Seidel *et al*, 2001; Lipton *et al*, 2002) and sarcoma (Lipton *et al*, 2002) but are increased in prostate cancer (Brown *et al*, 2001a; Jung *et al*, 2001), pancreatic and colorectal cancers, and Hodgkin's and non-Hodgkin's disease (Lipton *et al*, 2002). Studies on the utility of RANKL as a marker of bone metastatic disease have not yet been published. However, in a preliminary investigation, we found that soluble RANKL production is increased in the bone-metastatic LNCaP-C4-2B prostate cancer subline when compared with parental LNCaP cells (unpublished data). Furthermore, prostate cancer patients with bone metastases have elevated levels of soluble RANKL in serum when compared with patients without bone metastases (unpublished data).

The altered expression of RANKL and/or OPG and/or RANK is evident in many cancers that metastasize to bone, such as prostate cancer (Brown *et al*, 2001b), breast cancer (Thomas *et al*, 1999; Bhatia *et al*, 2002; Roux *et al*, 2002b) and multiple myeloma (Pearse *et al*, 2001; Seidel *et al*, 2001) [reviewed in (Tricot, 2000)]. This suggests that these molecules may be involved in the localized destruction of bone that is mediated by these cancers.

REGULATION OF OPG, RANKL AND RANK EXPRESSION

Bone resorption can be affected by therapeutic treatments, such as glucocorticoid therapy, and by osteotropic factors, including growth factors and cytokines. Many studies have been published on the examination of how such factors modulate the expression of OPG, RANKL and RANK, although this work has been performed predominantly with bone-derived cells.

Steroid hormones

Exposure of murine stromal-like cells to calcitriol alone or in combination with dexamethasone inhibited the expression of OPG and stimulated that of RANKL at the mRNA level (Horwood *et al*, 1998; Nagai Sato, 1999; Huang *et al*, 2000;) and at the protein level (Nakashima *et al*, 2000). In mouse calvarial cultures, treatment with calcitriol or dexamethasone decreased OPG protein levels (O'Brien *et al*, 2001). In primary murine osteoblasts, calcitriol stimulated the expression of RANKL mRNA (Horwood *et al*, 1998; Quinn *et al*, 2001; Thomas *et al*, 2001), whereas the expression of OPG mRNA varied from study to study: vitamin D had no effect in one investigation (Thomas *et al*, 2001), but decreased OPG mRNA levels in others (Horwood *et al*, 1998; Murakami *et al*, 1998). Dexamethasone had a biphasic effect where a short exposure inhibited OPG mRNA expression but a longer exposure produced an increase over basal levels (Murakami *et al*, 1998).

The effects of vitamin D were tested in human osteoblastic cells: in hFOBs and hMS cells, calcitriol stimulated OPG mRNA levels, whereas these were unaffected in primary osteoblasts (Hofbauer *et al*, 1998). The glucocorticoids dexamethasone and cortisol inhibited OPG mRNA expression in primary osteoblasts (Vidal *et al*, 1998a; Viereck *et al*, 2002): dexamethasone also inhibited OPG protein secretion in bone marrow stromal cells (Brändström *et al*, 2001) and cortisol decreased OPG mRNA in MG-63 osteosarcoma cells (Vidal *et al*, 1998a). Estrogen stimulated OPG mRNA production in primary osteoblasts as well as in immortalized osteoblasts transfected with a wild-type estrogen receptor, in the latter of which OPG protein expression was also increased (Hofbauer *et al*, 1999a).

Growth factors

Members of the transforming growth factor (TGFβ) superfamily typically stimulate osteoblastogenesis, but can also affect bone resorption. TGFβ$_1$ increased OPG mRNA and/ or decreased RANKL mRNA in human osteosarcoma cells (Pearse *et al*, 2001) and in murine osteoblastic cells (Horwood *et al*, 1998; Quinn *et al*, 2001; Thirunavukkarasu *et al*, 2001) and stimulated RANK mRNA and protein levels in murine hematopoietic cells in the presence or absence of colony-stimulating factor-1 (Kaneda *et al*, 2000; Yan *et al*, 2001). The effects on OPG mRNA and protein levels are likely to be mediated through the Cbfa1 and Smad-binding sites located within the proximal promoter region of the OPG gene (Thirunavukkarasu *et al*, 2001). Bone morphogenetic proteins (BMPs) are also members of the TGFβ superfamily and stimulate OPG expression (Hofbauer *et al*, 1998), likely through the Hoxc-8 sites in the OPG promoter (Wan *et al*, 2001).

Fibroblastic growth factor (FGF)-2 stimulated osteoclastogenesis in a mouse spleen-osteoblastic co-culture system: this was due to the stimulation of RANKL (Chikazu *et al*, 2001) and inhibition of OPG mRNA levels in the primary mouse osteoblasts (Nakagawa *et al*, 1999a), which was supported by inhibition of OPG secretion. However, FGF-2 suppressed the induction of osteoclasts by calcitriol through inhibiting its stimulation of RANKL expression (Nakagawa *et al*, 1999b).

Treatment with prostaglandins inhibits OPG mRNA levels in human bone marrow stromal cells (BMSCs) (Brändström *et al*, 1998) and in primary mouse osteoblasts (Murakami *et al*, 1998) and decreases protein secretion in human BMSCs (Brändström *et al*, 2001) and in calvarial cultures (O'Brien *et al*, 2001).

Parathyroid hormone (PTH) and PTH-related protein (PTHrP) are known to stimulate bone resorption and can cause hypercalcemia. Studies show that PTH stimulates RANKL and/ or decreases OPG expression in rodent bone marrow cultures, neonatal calvariae and in osteoblastic cells (Horwood *et al*, 1998; Murakami *et al*, 1998; Lee Lorenzo, 1999; Onyia *et al*, 2000; O'Brien *et al*, 2001; Halladay *et al*, 2002).

Cytokines

The interleukin (IL) family has been shown to affect bone turnover by acting directly on bone-derived cells or by stimulating T cells: for example, IL-1 stimulates expression of RANKL mRNA in T cells (Weitzmann *et al*, 2000). Most published studies to date have focused on the effects of IL-1α and β. IL-1α stimulates OPG protein secretion in human bone marrow stromal cells (Brändström *et al*, 2001), primary human osteoblasts (Vidal *et al*, 1998b) and osteosarcoma cells (Vidal *et al*, 1998b), whereas OPG mRNA is decreased in primary mouse osteoblasts (Murakami *et al*, 1998). IL-1β stimulates RANKL mRNA in pre-osteoblasts (Hofbauer *et al*, 1999b; Giuliani *et al*, 2001), marrow stromal cells and osteosarcoma cells (Hofbauer *et al*, 1999b), and increases OPG mRNA expression in osteosarcoma cells (Hofbauer *et al*, 1999b) and immortalized human osteoblastic cells (Hofbauer *et al*, 1998). Initial studies using other interleukins show that they may be also involved in the regulation of OPG, RANKL and RANK expression. IL-6 in combination with its soluble receptor stimulated OPG mRNA in human osteosarcoma cells (Hofbauer *et al*, 1999b). IL-11 treatment of primary murine osteoblasts produced increases in both RANKL and OPG mRNA expression (Horwood *et al*, 1998). IL-18 stimulated the expression of OPG mRNA in murine osteoblastic cells, but had little effect on RANKL (Makiishi-Shimobayashi *et al*, 2001).

Tumor necrosis factor (TNF) α and β have also been tested for their ability to modulate expression of OPG, RANKL and RANK. Both factors stimulated the mRNA levels of OPG (Ljunghall *et al*, 1998; Hofbauer *et al*, 1999b;) and RANKL (Hofbauer *et al*, 1999b) in human osteosarcoma cells and of OPG protein in immortalized human osteoblasts (Hofbauer *et al*, 1998).

Some studies have been performed to examine the effects of combined treatments. In murine osteoblast-like cells, combination treatments of IL-17, IL-11, IL-6 and its soluble receptor, IL-1β or TNFα with calcitriol and prostaglandin E_2 resulted in increased membrane-bound and soluble RANKL expression and decreased OPG mRNA levels. In contrast, co-treatment with IL-4, IL-13, IL-18, interferon-γ or TGFβ_1 inhibited RANKL expression and either had no effect on OPG or produced an increase in its mRNA levels (Nakashima *et al*, 2000).

Other factors

Bisphosphonates are known to inhibit bone resorption. Amongst their other mechanisms, it was recently shown that pamidronate and zoledronic acid stimulate OPG mRNA and protein expression in a dose-dependent manner that can be sustained for up to 3 days (Viereck *et al*, 2002). *Indian hedgehog (Ihh)*, encoding a member of the hedgehog family of signaling factors and expresses in chondrocytes, is documented to enhance RANKL gene expression. This action may be mediated in part through Core-binding factor a1 (Cbfa1), which is a key transcriptional factor for the development of bone as well as cartilage (Takamoto *et al*, 2003).

The regulation of OPG, RANKL and RANK expression in cancer

The regulation of basal OPG expression in osteosarcoma cells involves the protein kinase C and cAMP pathways (Halladay *et al*, 2002; Yang *et al*, 2002). Studies in murine and human osteoblast-like cells show that Cbfa1 is involved in the regulation of OPG transcription, mainly by acting through the proximal Cbfa1 binding site (OSE2 site) (Thirunavukkarasu *et al*, 2000).

Interactions between cancer cells and cells or factors in the bone microenvironment may facilitate tumor cell establishment in the bone. Prostate cancer cells modulate osteoblastogenesis (Yang *et al*, 2001) and in a reciprocal manner, osteoblastic cells influence the metastatic behavior of prostate cancer cells directly or indirectly by production of soluble factors (Festuccia *et al*, 1999; Fu *et al*, 2002), including a soluble form of RANKL (Zhang *et al*, 2001). Co-culture studies have shown that cell-cell contact between melanoma or breast cancer cells and bone marrow cells can induce osteoclasts (Chikatsu *et al*, 2000). In a nude mouse calvarial model, breast cancer cells elicited increased RANKL expression on stromal and osteoblastic cells concomitant with osteoclast induction, implying that the tumor cells had indirectly stimulated bone resorption through transactivation of RANKL (Kitazawa Kitazawa, 2002).

Since the expression of many of these factors is altered in cancer metastasis, preliminary studies have been performed examining the effects of growth factors and hormones on the OPG/RANKL/RANK axis in cancer cells. In one study, treatment with TNFα, TNFβ, dexamethasone or IL-1β dose-dependently increased OPG expression in prostate cancer cells, although this was dependent upon the cell line tested (Penno *et al*, 2002). In our preliminary studies, dihydrotestosterone (DHT) induces OPG mRNA and protein expression in an androgen-responsive prostate cancer cell line LNCaP. This induction is regulated at the transcriptional level (unpublished data).

Taken together, these data suggest that expression of OPG and RANKL may be regulated by these factors in prostate cancer cells in patients, which may influence bone resorption and therefore tumor growth, and may suggest additional targets for therapy.

THERAPEUTIC TARGETING OF THE OPG/ RANKL/ RANK AXIS

It appears that many cancers metastatic to bone express OPG, RANKL and/ or RANK, suggesting that these master regulators of bone resorption provide a checkpoint for metastasis and a therapeutic target that could ameliorate metastasis to bone in a broad range of cancers. Several exciting and provocative studies have examined the therapeutic uses of soluble RANK and OPG in the treatment of hematological and solid tumors in bone.

The development of humoral hypercalcaemia of malignancy (HHM) is a major consequence of bone metastasis. As a fusion protein with human IgG, soluble RANK (sRANK) has proven efficacious in the inhibition of bone resorption in a mouse model of HHM, as induced by PTHrP administration (Oyajobi *et al*, 2001), and in a xenograft cancer model, where SCID mice bearing marrow xenografts from patients with multiple myeloma were treated with 200 μg soluble RANK three times weekly. This regimen effectively prevented myeloma-induced osteoclastic bone destruction (Pearse *et al*, 2001).

In similar rodent HHM models, OPG effectively blocked the actions of the pro-resorptive cytokines and hormones IL-1, PTH, TNFα and PTHrP (Morony *et al*, 1999). Treatment with recombinant human OPG rescued the serum ionized calcium levels of rats that had been thyroparathyroidectomized and treated with exogenous parathyroid hormone and vitamin D_3 (Yamamoto *et al*, 1998). Adenoviral delivery of OPG rescued ovariectomized mice from the decreases in bone volume in the axial and appendicular skeleton normally associated with increased osteoclastic activity as a result of estrogen loss (Bolon *et al*, 2001): a single treatment persisted in abrogating osteoclastic activity for 18 months, although there were side-effects of splenomegaly and hepatomegaly.

Prophylactic treatment of 0.5-2.5 mg/kg OPG injected daily for 7 days and interventional treatment with 2.5 mg/kg OPG administered daily for 4 days reduced serum calcium and phosphate levels in mice bearing syngeneic colon adenocarcinomas (Capparelli *et al*, 2000). Large doses (20 mg/kg) OPG produced hypocalcaemia in normal mice as well as in those carrying FA-6 tumors (Akatsu *et al*, 1998). Treatment of mice bearing syngeneic multiple myeloma cells with recombinant OPG prevented osteolysis and blocked the formation of osteolytic tumors in bone via inhibition of osteoclastogenesis (Croucher *et al*, 2001).

Studies treating immuno-compromised mice bearing human cancer xenografts with OPG resulted in dramatic decreases in the numbers of mature osteoclasts and in the size and/ or number of lesions in bone. OPG prevented the development of osteolytic lesions following treatment of nude mice carrying human MDA-MB-231 breast cancer cells (Morony *et al*, 2001), and inhibited the establishment and progression of human prostate cancer tumors in bone when cancer cells were directly injected into the tibia (Zhang *et al*, 2001) or into human adult bone implanted into severe combined immunodeficient mice (Yonou *et al*, 2003), respectively.

These studies suggest that, even in metastatic tumors that vary in osteolytic/ osteoblastic phenotype, inhibition of the primary resorptive stage may be sufficient to inhibit tumor establishment and growth in bone, and to halt progression of disease. Importantly, treatment with OPG has also been demonstrated to block pain-related behavior in mice carrying bone cancers (Honore *et al*, 2000; Luger *et al*, 2001). While studies are at an early stage at present, it appears that therapeutic targeting of the OPG/ RANKL/ RANK proteins holds great promise for treatment of bone metastases.

One potential drawback to the use of OPG is its inherent ability to bind to tumor necrosis factor-related apoptosis-inducing ligand (TRAIL), another member of the TNF superfamily. This molecule is naturally produced by most tissues and induces apoptosis upon binding to DR4 or DR5, death receptors that contain transmembrane domains and death domains that transduce the death signal via the caspase pathway. Ligation of OPG and TRAIL inhibits the ability of TRAIL to induce apoptosis in Jurkat cells and the anti-osteoclastogenic activities of OPG *in vitro* (Emery *et al*, 1998). Moreover, a recent study shows that OPG can act as a survival factor for human prostate cancer cells treated with TRAIL, although this protective effect was removed upon co-treatment with a molar excess of RANKL (Holen *et al*, 2002). To our knowledge, there are to date no published studies on the effects of OPG on TRAIL-induced apoptosis of bone-metastatic cancer cells *in vivo*, and the formation and biological function of an OPG-TRAIL complex *in vivo* is unknown. However, it is tempting to speculate that use of TRAIL could kill cancer cells and also sequester any available OPG, resulting in an imbalance in resorption that could facilitate establishment of TRAIL-resistant cells in bone.

CONCLUSIONS

Recent developments in the study of cancer metastasis to bone reveal a commonality in the pathways involved. Regardless of the phenotype of lesion produced or of the origin of the cancer cells, it would appear that the bone resorption regulatory molecules OPG, RANKL and RANK play a central role in the mechanisms involved in cancer metastasis to bone. Further investigation of tumor-bone interactions and the factors and signaling cascades that mediate their intercommunication will clarify the mechanisms involved in and may produce novel therapeutic targets for the skeletal metastasis of cancer.

REFERENCES

Akatsu, T., Murakami, T., Ono, K., Nishikawa, M., Tsuda, E., Mochizuki, K., Fujise, N., Higashio, K., Motoyoshi, K., Yamamoto, M. and Nagata, N. (1998) Osteoclastogenesis inhibitory factor exhibits hypocalcemic effects in normal mice and in hypercalcemic nude mice carrying tumors associated with humoral hypercalcemia of malignancy. *Bone* **23**, 495-498.

Anderson, D.M., Maraskovsky, E., Billingsley, W.L., Dougall, W.C., Tometsko, M.E., Roux, E.R., Teepe, M.C., DuBose, R.F., Cosman, D. and Galibert, L. (1997) A homologue of the TNF receptor and its ligand enhance T-cell growth and dendritic-cell function. *Nature* **390**, 175-179.

Arron, J.R., Vologodskaia, M., Wong, B.R., Naramura, M., Kim, N., Gu, H. and Choi, Y. (2001) A positive regulatory role for Cbl family proteins in tumor necrosis factor-related activation-induced cytokine (TRANCE) and CD40L-mediated Akt activation. *Journal of Biological Chemistry* **276**, 30011-30017.

Atkins, G.J., Haynes, D.R., Graves, S.E., Evdokiou, A., Hay, S., Bouralexis, S. and Findlay, D.M. (2000) Expression of osteoclast differentiation signals by stromal elements of giant cell tumors. *Journal of Bone and Mineral Research* **15**, 640-649.

Atkins, G.J., Bouralexis, S., Graves, S.E., Geary, S.M., Evdokiou, A., Zannettino, A.C., Hay, S. and Findlay, D.M. (2001) Osteoprotegerin inhibits osteoclast formation and bone resorbing activity in giant cell tumors of bone. *Bone* **28**, 370-377.

Bekker, P.J., Holloway, D., Nakanishi, A., Arrighi, M., Leese, P.T. and Dunstan, C.R. (2001) The effect of a single dose of osteoprotegerin in post menopausal women. *Journal of Bone and Mineral Research* **16**, 348-360.

Bhatia, P., Sanders, M. and Hansen, M.F. (2003) Expression of RANK and RANKL is altered in invasive carcinoma and bone metastasis of breast cancer. (Abstract). *Oncology* (supplement) **17**, 18.

Bolon, B., Carter, C., Daris, M., Morony, S., Capparelli, C., Hsieh, A., Mao, M., Kostenuik, P., Dunstan, C.R., Lacey, D.L. and Sheng, J.Z. (2001) Adenoviral delivery of osteoprotegerin ameliorates bone resorption in a mouse ovariectomy model of osteoporosis. *Molecular Therapy* **3**, 197-205.

Brändström, H., Jonsson, K.B., Ohlsson, C., Vidal, O., Ljunghall, S. and Ljunggren, Ö. (1998) Regulation of osteoprotegerin mRNA levels by prostaglandin E$_2$ in human bone marrow stroma cells. *Biochemical and Biophysical Research Communications* **247**, 338-341.

Brändström, H., Björkman, T. and Ljunggren, Ö. (2001) Regulation of osteoprotegerin secretion from primary cultures of human bone marrow stromal cells. *Biochemical and Biophysical Research Communications* **280**, 831-835.

Brown, J.M., Vessella, R.L., Kostenuik, P.J., Dunstan, C.R., Lange, P.H. and Corey, E. (2001a) Serum osteoprotegerin levels are increased in patients with advanced prostate cancer. *Clinical Cancer Research* **7**, 2977-2983.

Brown, J.M., Corey, E., Lee, Z.D., True, L.D., Yun, T.J., Tondravi, M. and Vessella, R.L. (2001b) Osteoprotegerin and RANK ligand expression in prostate cancer. *Urology* **57**, 611-616.

Burgess, T.L., Qian, Y., Kaufman, S., Ring, B.D., Van, G., Capparelli, C., Kelley, M., Hsu, H., Boyle, W.J., Dunstan, C.R., Hu, S. and Lacey, D.L. (1999) The ligand for osteoprotegerin (OPGL) directly activates mature osteoclasts. *Journal of Cell Biology* **145**, 527-538.

Capparelli, C., Kostenuik, P.J., Morony, S., Starnes, C., Weimann, B., Van, G., Scully, S., Qi, M., Lacey, D.L. and Dunstan, C.R. (2000) Osteoprotegerin prevents and reverses hypercalcemia in a murine model of humoral hypercalcemia of malignancy. *Cancer Research* **60**, 783-787.

Chikatsu, N., Takeuchi, Y., Tamura, Y., Fukumoto, S., Yano, K., Tsuda, E., Ogata, E. and Fujita, T. (2000) Interactions between cancer and bone marrow cells induce osteoclast differentiation factor expression and osteoclast-like cell formation in vitro. *Biochemical and Biophysical Research Communications* **267**, 632-637.

Chikazu, D., Katagiri, M., Ogasawara, T., Ogata, N., Shimoaka, T., Takato, T., Nakamura, K. and Kawaguchi, H. (2001) Regulation of osteoclast differentiation by fibroblast growth factor 2: stimulation of receptor activator of nuclear factor κB ligand/osteoclast differentiation factor expression in osteoblasts and inhibition of macrophage colony-stimulating factor function in osteoclast precursors. *Journal of Bone and Mineral Research* **16**, 2074-2081.

Coleman, R.E. (1997) Skeletal complications of malignancy. *Cancer* (Supplement) **80**, 1588-1594.

Croucher, P.I., Shipman, C.M., Lippitt, J., Perry, M., Asosingh, K., Hijzen, A., Brabbs, A.C., van Beek, E.J., Holen, I., Skerry, T.M., Dunstan, C.R., Russell, G.R., Van Camp, B. and Vanderkerken, K. (2001) Osteoprotegerin inhibits the development of osteolytic bone disease in multiple myeloma. *Blood* **98**, 3534-3540.

Dougall, W.C., Glaccum, M., Charrier, K., Rohrbach, K., Brasel, K., De Smedt, T., Daro, E., Smith, J., Tometsko, M.E., Maliszewski, C.R., Armstrong, A., Shen, V., Bain, S., Cosman, D. anderson, D., Morrisey, P.J., Peschon, J.J. and Schuh, J. (1999) RANK is essential for osteoclast and lymph node development. *Genes and Development* **13**, 2412-2424.

Emery, J.G., McDonnell, P., Burke, M.B., Deen, K.C., Lyn, S., Silverman, C., Dul, E., Appelbaum, E.R., Eichman, C., DiPrinzio, R., Dodds, R.A., James, I.E., Rosenberg, M., Lee, J.C. and Young, P.R. (1998) Osteoprotegerin is a receptor for the cytotoxic ligand TRAIL. *Journal of Biological Chemistry* **273**, 14363-14367.

Festuccia, C., Bologna, M., Gravana, G.L., Guerra, F., Angelucci, A., Villanova, I., Millimaggi, D. and Teti, A. (1999) Osteoblast conditioned media contain TGF-β1 and modulate the migration of prostate tumor cells and their interactions with extracellular matrix components. *International Journal of Cancer* **81**, 395-403.

Fiumara, P., Snell, V., Li, Y., Mukhopadhyay, A., Younes, M., Gillenwater, A.M., Cabanillas, F., Aggarwal, B.B. and Younes, A. (2001) Functional expression of receptor activator of nuclear factor κB in Hodgkin disease cell lines. *Blood* **98**, 2784-2790.

Fu, Z., Dozmorov, I.M. and Keller, E.T. (2002) Osteoblasts produce soluble factors that induce a gene expression pattern in non-metastatic prostate cancer cells, similar to that found in bone metastatic prostate cancer cells. *The Prostate* **51**, 10-20.

Fuller, K., Wong, B., Fox, S., Choi, Y. and Chambers, T.J. (1998) TRANCE is necessary and sufficient for osteoblast-mediated activation of bone resorption in osteoclasts. *Journal of Experimental Medicine* **188**, 997-1001.

Gao, Y.H., Shinki, T., Yuasa, T., Kataoka-Enomoto, H., Komori, T., Suda, T. and Yamaguchi, A. (1998) Potential role of cbfa1, an essential transcriptional factor for osteoblast differentiation, in osteoclastogenesis: regulation of mRNA expression of osteoclast differentiation factor (ODF). *Biochemical and Biophysical Research Communications* **252**, 697-702.

Giuliani, N., Bataille, R., Mancini, C., Lazzaretti, M. and Barille, S. (2001) Myeloma cells induce imbalance in the osteoprotegerin/osteoprotegerin ligand system in the human bone marrow environment. *Blood* **98**, 3527-3533.

Goltzman, D. (2001) Mechanisms of the development of osteoblastic metastases. *Cancer* **80**, 1581-1587.

Halladay, D.L., Miles, R.R., Thirunavukkarasu, K., Chandrasekhar, S., Martin, T.J. and Onyia, J.E. (2002) Identification of signal transducing pathways and promoter sequences that mediate parathyroid hormone 1-38 inhibition of osteoprotegerin gene expression. *Journal of Cellular Biochemistry* **84**, 1-11.

Hofbauer, L.C., Dunstan, C.R., Spelsberg, T.C., Riggs, B.L. and Khosla, S. (1998) Osteoprotegerin production by human osteoblast lineage cells is stimulated by vitamin D, bone morphogenetic protein-2, and cytokines. *Biochemical and Biophysical Research Communications* **250**, 776-781.

Hofbauer, L.C., Khosla, S., Dunstan, C.R., Lacey, D.L., Spelsberg, T.C. and Riggs, B.L. (1999a) Estrogen stimulates gene expression and protein production of osteoprotegerin in human osteoblastic cells. *Endocrinology* **140**, 4367-4370.

Hofbauer, L.C., Lacey, D.L., Dunstan, C.R., Spelsberg, T.C., Riggs, B.L. and Khosla, S. (1999b) Interleukin-1β and tumor necrosis factor-α, but not interleukin-6, stimulate osteoprotegerin ligand gene expression in human osteoblastic cells. *Bone* **25**, 255-259.

Hofbauer, L.C. and Heufelder, A.E. (2001) Role of receptor activator of nuclear factor-κB ligand and osteoprotegerin in bone cell biology. *Journal of Molecular Medicine* **79**, 243-253.

Holen, I., Croucher, P.I., Hamdy, F.C. and Eaton, C.L. (2002) Osteoprotegerin (OPG) is a survival factor for human prostate cancer cells. *Cancer Research* **62**, 1619-1623.

Honore, P., Luger, N.M., Sabino, M.A., Schwei, M.J., Rogers, S.D., Mach, D.B., O'Keefe, P.F., Ramnaraine, M.L., Clohisy, D.R. and Mantyh, P.W. (2000) Osteoprotegerin blocks bone cancer-induced skeletal destruction, skeletal pain and pain-related neurochemical reorganization of the spinal cord. *Nature Medicine* **6**, 521-528.

Horowitz, M.C., Xi, Y., Wilson, K. and Kacena, M.A. (2001) Control of osteoclastogenesis and bone resorption by members of the TNF family of receptors and ligands. *Cytokine and Growth Factor Reviews* **12**, 9-18.

Horwood, N.J., Elliott, J., Martin, T.J. and Gillespie, M.T. (1998) Osteotropic agents regulate the expression of osteoclast differentiation factor and osteoprotegerin in osteoblastic stromal cells. *Endocrinology* **139**, 4743-4746.

Hsu, H., Lacey, D.L., Dunstan, C.R., Solovyev, I., Colombero, A., Timms, E., Tan, H.-L., Elliot, G., Kelley, M.J., Sarosi, I., Wang, L., Xia, X.-Z., Elliot, R., Chiu, L., Black, T., Scully, S., Caparelli, C., Morony, S., Shimamoto, G., Bass, M.B. and Boyle, W.J. (1999) Tumor necrosis factor receptor family member RANK mediates osteoclast differentiation and activation induced by osteoprotegerin ligand. *Proceedings of the National Academy of Sciences of the United States of America* **96**, 3540-3545.

Huang, L., Xu, J.K., Wood, D.J. and Zheng, M.H. (2000) Gene expression of osteoprotegerin ligand, osteoprotegerin, and receptor activator of NF-κB in giant cell tumor of bone. Possible involvement in tumor cell-induced osteoclast-like cell formation. *American Journal of Pathology* **156**, 761-767.

Huang, L., Cheng, Y.Y., Chow, L.T.C., Zheng, M.H. and Kumta, S.M. (2002) Tumour cells produce receptor activator of NF-κB ligand (RANKL) in skeletal metastases. *Journal of Clinical Pathology* **55**, 877-878.

Ikeda, T., Kasai, M., Utsuyama, M. and Hirokawa, K. (2001) Determination of three isoforms of the receptor activator of nuclear factor-κB ligand and their differential expression in bone and thymus. *Endocrinology* **142**, 1419-1426.

Jung, K., Lein, M., von Hosslin, K., Brux, B., Schnorr, D., Loening, S.A. and Sinha, P. (2001) Osteoprotegerin in serum as a novel marker of bone metastatic spread in prostate cancer. *Clinical Chemistry* **47**, 2061-2063.

Kaneda, T., Nojima, T., Nakagawa, M., Ogasawara, A., Kaneko, H., Sato, T., Mano, H., Kumegawa, M. and Hakeda, Y. (2000) Endogenous production of TGF-β is essential for osteoclastogenesis induced by a combination of receptor activator of NF-κB ligand and macrophage-colony-stimulating factor. *Journal of Immunology* **165**, 4254-4263.

Kitazawa, S. and Kitazawa, R. (2002) RANK ligand is a prerequisite for cancer-associated osteolytic lesions. *Journal of Pathology* **198**, 228-236.

Komori, T., Yagi, H., Nomura, S., Yamaguchi, A., Sasaki, K., Deguchi, K., Shimizu, Y., Bronson, R.T., Gao, Y.-H., Inada, M., Sato, M., Okamoto, R., Kitamura, Y., Yoshiki, S. and Kishimoto, T. (1997) Targeted disruption of Cbfa1 results in a complete lack of bone formation owing to maturational arrest of osteoblasts. *Cell* **89**, 755-764.

Kong, Y.Y., Yoshida, H., Sarosi, I., Tan, H.L., Timms, E., Capparelli, C., Morony, S., Oliveira-dos-Santos, A.J., Van, G., Itie, A., Khoo, W., Wakeham, A., Dunstan, C.R., Lacey, D.L., Mak, T.W., Boyle, W.J. and Penninger, J.M. (1999) OPGL is a key regulator of osteoclastogenesis, lymphocyte development and lymph-node organogenesis. *Nature* **397**, 315-323.

Lacey, D.L., Timms, E., Tan, H.-L., Kelley, M.J., Dunstan, C.R., Burgess, T., Elliott, R., Colombero, A., Elliott, G., Scully, S., Hsu, H., Sullivan, J., Hawkins, N., Davy, E., Capparelli, C., Eli, A., Qian, Y.X., Kaufman, S., Sarosi, I., Shalhoub, V., Senaldi, G., Guo, J., Delaney, J. and Boyle, W.J. (1998) Osteoprotegerin ligand is a cytokine that regulates osteoclast differentiation and activation. *Cell* **93**, 165-176.

Lacey, D.L., Tan, H.L., Lu, J., Kaufman, S., Van, G., Qiu, W., Rattan, A., Scully, S., Fletcher, F., Juan, T., Kelley, M., Burgess, T.L., Boyle, W.J. and Polverino, A.J. (2000)

Osteoprotegerin ligand modulates murine osteoclast survival in vitro and in vivo. *American Journal of Pathology* **157**, 435-448.

Lee, S.K. and Lorenzo, J.A. (1999) Parathyroid hormone stimulates TRANCE and inhibits osteoprotegerin messenger ribonucleic acid expression in murine bone marrow cultures: correlation with osteoclast-like cell formation. *Endocrinology* **140**, 3552-3561.

Lee, Y., Schwartz, E., Davies, M., Jo, M., Gates, J., Wu, J., Zhang, X. and Lieberman, J.R. (2003) Differences in the cytokine profiles associated with prostate cancer cell induced osteoblastic and osteolytic lesions in bone. *Journal of Orthopaedic Research* **21**, 62-72.

Lee, Z.H., Kwack, K., Kim, K.K., Lee, S.H. and Kim, H.H. (2000) Activation of c-Jun N-terminal kinase and activator protein 1 by receptor activator of nuclear factor κB. *Molecular Pharmacology* **58**, 1536-1545.

Lee, Z.H. and Kim, H.-H. (2003) Signal transduction by receptor activator of nuclear factor kappa B in osteoclasts. *Biochemical and Biophysical Research Communications* **305**, 211-214.

Li, J., Sarosi, I., Yan, X.Q., Morony, S., Capparelli, C., Tan, H.L., McCabe, S., Elliott, R., Scully, S., Van, G., Kaufman, S., Juan, S.C., Sun, Y., Tarpley, J., Martin, L., Christensen, K., McCabe, J., Kostenuik, P., Hsu, H., Fletcher, F., Dunstan, C.R., Lacey, D.L. and Boyle, W.J. (2000) RANK is the intrinsic hematopoietic cell surface receptor that controls osteoclastogenesis and regulation of bone mass and calcium metabolism. *Proceedings of the National Academy of Sciences of the United States of America* **97**, 1566-1571.

Lin, D.L., Tarnowski, C.P., Zhang, J., Dai, J., Rohn, E., Patel, A.H., Morris, M.D. and Keller, E.T. (2001) Bone metastatic LNCaP-derivative C4-2B prostate cancer cell line mineralizes in vitro. *Prostate* **47**, 212-221.

Lipton, A., Ali, S.M., Leitzel, K., Chinchilli, V., Witters, L., Engle, L., Holloway, D., Bekker, P. and Dunstan, C.R. (2002) Serum osteoprotegerin levels in healthy controls and cancer patients. *Clinical Cancer Research* **8**, 2306-2310.

Ljunghall, S., Jonsson, K.B., Vidal, O., Ljunghall, S., Ohlsson, C. and Ljunggren, Ö. (1998) Tumor necrosis factor-α and -β upregulate the levels of osteoprotegerin mRNA in human osteosarcoma MG-63 cells. *Biochemical and Biophysical Research Communications* **248**, 454-457.

Luger, N.M., Honore, P., Sabino, M.A., Schwei, M.J., Rogers, S.D., Mach, D.B., Clohisy, D.R. and Mantyh, P.W. (2001) Osteoprotegerin diminishes advanced bone cancer pain. *Cancer Research* **61**, 4038-4047.

Lum, L., Wong, B.R., Josien, R., Becherer, J.D., Erdjument-Bromage, H., Schlöndorff, J., Tempst, P., Choi, Y. and Blobel, C.P. (1999) Evidence for a role of a tumor necrosis factor-α (TNF-α)-converting enzyme-like protease in shedding of TRANCE, a TNF family member involved in osteoclastogenesis and dendritic cell survival. *Journal of Biological Chemistry* **274**, 13613-13618.

Makiishi-Shimobayashi, C., Tsujimura, T., Iwasaki, T., Yamada, N., Sugihara, A., Okamura, H., Hayashi, S. and Terada, N. (2001) Interleukin-18 up-regulates osteoprotegerin expression in stromal/osteoblastic cells. *Biochemical and Biophysical Research Communications* **281**, 361-366.

Matsuzaki, K., Udagawa, N., Takahashi, N., Yamaguchi, K., Yasuda, H., Shima, N., Morinaga, T., Toyama, Y., Yabe, Y., Higashio, K. and Suda, T. (1998) Osteoclast differentiation factor (ODF) induces osteoclast-like cell formation in human peripheral blood mononuclear cell cultures. *Biochemical and Biophysical Research Communications* **246**, 199-204.

Michigami, T., Ihara-Watanabe, M. and Ozono, K. (2001) Receptor activator of nuclear factor κB ligand (RANKL) is a key molecule of osteoclast formation for bone metastasis in a newly developed model of human neuroblastoma. *Cancer Research* **61**, 1637-1644.

Mizukami, J., Takaesu, G., Akatsuka, H., Sakurai, H., Ninomiya-Tsuji, J., Matsumoto, K., Sakurai, N. (2002) Receptor activator of NF-κB ligand (RANKL) activates TAK1 mitogen-activated protein kinase kinase kinase through a signaling complex containing RANK, TB2, and TRAF6. *Molecular and Cellular Biology* **22**, 992-1000.

Mizuno, A., Amizuka, N., Irie, K., Murakami, A., Fujise, N., Kanno, T., Sato, Y., Nakagawa, N., Yasuda, H., Mochizuki, S., Gomibuchi, T., Yano, K., Shima, N., Washida, N., Tsuda, E., Morinaga, T., Higashio, K. and Ozawa, H. (1998) Severe osteoporosis in mice lacking osteoclastogenesis inhibitory factor/osteoprotegerin. *Biochemical and Biophysical Research Communications* **247**, 610-615.

Morinaga, T., Nakagawa, N., Yasuda, H., Tsuda, E. and Higashio, K. (1998) Cloning and characterization of the gene encoding human osteoprotegerin/osteoclastogenesis-inhibitory factor. *European Journal of Biochemistry* **254**, 685-691.

Morony, S., Capparelli, C., Lee, R., Shimamoto, G., Boone, T., Lacey, D.L. and Dunstan, C.R. (1999) A chimeric form of osteoprotegerin inhibits hypercalcemia and bone resorption induced by IL-1β, TNF-α, PTH, PTHrP, and $1,25(OH)_2D_3$. *Journal of Bone and Mineral Research* **14**, 1478-1485.

Morony, S., Capparelli, C., Sarosi, I., Lacey, D.L., Dunstan, C.R. and Kostenuik, P.J. (2001) Osteoprotegerin inhibits osteolysis and decreases skeletal tumor burden in syngeneic and nude mouse models of experimental bone metastasis. *Cancer Research* **61**, 4432-4436.

Mundy, G.R. (1999) Bone remodeling. Primer on the metabolic bone diseases and disorders of mineral metabolism. (ed. by M. J. Favus), pp. 30-38. Lippincott Williams and Wilkins, Philadelphia.

Murakami, T., Yamamoto, M., Ono, K., Nishikawa, M., Nagata, N., Motoyoshi, K. and Akatsu, T. (1998) Transforming growth factor-β1 increases mRNA levels of osteoclastogenesis inhibitory factor in osteoblastic/stromal cells and inhibits the survival of murine osteoclast-like cells. *Biochemical and Biophysical Research Communications* **252**, 747-752.

Nagai, M. and Sato, N. (1999) Reciprocal gene expression of osteoclastogenesis inhibitory factor and osteoclast differentiation factor regulates osteoclast formation. *Biochemical and Biophysical Research Communications* **257**, 719-723.

Nakagawa, N., Kinosaki, M., Yamaguchi, K., Shima, N., Yasuda, H., Yano, K., Morinaga, T. and Higashio, K. (1998) RANK is the essential signaling receptor for osteoclast differentiation factor in osteoclastogenesis. *Biochemical and Biophysical Research Communications* **253**, 395-400.

Nakagawa, N., Yasuda, H., Yano, K., Mochizuki, S., Kobayashi, N., Fujimoto, H., Shima, N., Morinaga, T., Chikazu, D., Kawaguchi, H. and Higashio, K. (1999a) Basic fibroblast growth factor induces osteoclast formation by reciprocally regulating the production of osteoclast differentiation factor and osteoclastogenesis inhibitory factor in mouse osteoblastic cells. *Biochemical and Biophysical Research Communications* **265**, 158-163.

Nakagawa, N., Yasuda, H., Yano, K., Mochizuki, S., Kobayashi, N., Fujimoto, H., Yamaguchi, K., Shima, N., Morinaga, T. and Higashio, K. (1999b) Basic fibroblast growth factor inhibits osteoclast formation induced by 1α,25-dihydroxyvitamin D_3 through suppressing the production of osteoclast differentiation factor. *Biochemical and Biophysical Research Communications* **265**, 45-50.

Nakashima, T., Kobayashi, Y., Yamasaki, S., Kawakami, A., Eguchi, K., Sasaki, H. and Sakai, H. (2000) Protein expression and functional difference of membrane-bound and soluble receptor activator of NF-κB ligand: modulation of the expression by osteotropici factors and cytokines. *Biochemical and Biophysical Research Communications* **275**, 768-775.

Nielsen, O.S., Munro, A.J. and Tannock, I.F. (1991) Bone metastases: pathophysiology andl management policy. *Journal of Clinical Oncology* **9**, 509-524.

Nosaka, K., Miyamoto, T., Sakai, T., Mitsuya, H.,Suda, T.and Matsuoka, M.(2002)o Mechanism of hypercalcemia in adult T-cell leukemia: overexpression of receptor activator of nuclear factor κB ligand on adult T-cell leukemia cells. *Blood* **99**, 634-640.

O'Brien, E.A., Williams, J.H.H. and Marshall, M.J. (2000) Osteoprotegerin ligand regulatesv osteoclast adherence to the bone surface in mouse calvaria. *Biochemical and Biophysical Research Communications* **274**, 281-290.

O'Brien, E.A., Williams, J.H. and Marshall, M.J. (2001) Osteoprotegerin is produced whene prostaglandin synthesis is inhibited causing osteoclasts to detach from the surface of mouse parietal bone and attach to the endocranial membrane. *Bone* **28**, 208-214.

Onyia, J.E., Miles, R.R., Yang, X., Halladay, D.L., Hale, J., Glasebrook, A., McClure, D., j Seno, G., Churgay, L., Chandrasekhar, S. and Martin, T.J. (2000) In vivo demonstration that human parathyroid hormone 1-38 inhibits the expression of osteoprotegerin in bone with the kinetics of an immediate early gene. *Journal of Bone and Mineral Research* **15**, 863-871.

Oyajobi, B.O. anderson, D.M., Traianedes, K., Williams, P.J., Yoneda, T. and Mundy, G.R.i (2001) Therapeutic efficacy of a soluble receptor activator of nuclear factor κB-IgG Fc fusion protein in suppressing bone resorption and hypercalcemia in a model of humoral hypercalcemia of malignancy. *Cancer Research* 61, 2572-2578.

Pearse, R.N., Yaccoby, S., Wong, B.R., Liau, D.F., Colman, N., Michaeli, J., Epstein, J. andl Choi, Y. (2001) Multiple myeloma disrupts the TRANCE/ osteoprotegerin cytokine axis to trigger bone destruction and promote tumor progression. *Proceedings of the National Academy of Sciences of the United States of America* **98**, 11581-11586.

Penno, H., Silfverswärd, C.-J., Frost, A., Brändström, H., Nilsson, O. and Ljunggren, Ö.1 (2002) Osteoprotegerin secretion from prostate cancer is stimulated by cytokines, in vitro. *Biochemical and Biophysical Research Communications* **293**, 451-455.

Quinn, J.M.W., Itoh, K., Udagawa, N., Häusler, K., Yasuda, H., Shima, N., Mizuno, A., Higashio, K., Takahashi, N., Suda, T., Martin, T.J. and Gillespie, M.T. (2001) Transforming growth factor β affects osteoclast differentiation via direct and indirect actions. *Journal of Bone and Mineral Research* **16**, 1787-1794.

Revilla, M., Arribas, I., Sanchez-Chapado, M., Villa, L.F., Bethencourt, F. and Rico, H. (1998) Total and regional bone mass and biochemical markers of bone remodeling in metastatic prostate cancer. *The Prostate* **35**, 243-247.

Rodan, G.A. and Martin, T.J. (1981) Role of osteoblast in hormonal control of bone resorption - a hypothesis. *Calcified Tissue International* **33**, 349-351.

Roland, S. (1958) Calcium studies in ten cases of osteoblastic prostatic metastasis. *Journal of Urology* **79**, 339-342.

Roodman, G.D. (1996) Advances in bone biology: the osteoclast. *Endocrine Reviews* **17**, 308-332.

Roodman, G.D. (1999) Cell biology of the osteoclast. *Experimental Hematology* **27**, 1229-1241.

Roux, S., Meignin, V., Quillard, J., Meduri, G., Guiochon-Mantel, A., Fermand, J.-P., Milgrom, E. and Mariette, X. (2002a) RANK (receptor activator of nuclear factor-κB) and RANKL expression in multiple myeloma. *British Journal of Haematology* **117** , 86-92.

Roux, S., Amazit, L., Meduri, G., Guiochon-Mantel, A., Milgrom, E. and Mariette, X. (2002b) RANK (receptor activator of nuclear factor κB) and RANK ligand are expressed in giant cell tumors of bone. *American Journal of Clinical Pathology* 117, 210-216.

Seidel, C., Hjertner, Ø., Abildgaard, N., Heickendorff, L., Hjorth, M., Westin, J., Nielsen, J.L., Hjorth-Hansen, H., Waage, A., Sundan, A. and Børset, M., The Nordic Myeloma Study Group (2001) Serum osteoprotegerin levels are reduced in patients with multiple myeloma with lytic bone disease. *Blood* **98**, 2269-2271.

Sezer, O., Heider, U., Jakob, C., Eucker, J. and Possinger, K. (2002a) Human bone marrow myeloma cells express RANKL. *Journal of Clinical Oncology* **20**, 353-354.

Sezer, O., Heider, U., Jakob, C., Zavrski, I., Eucker, J., Possinger, K., Sers, C. and Krenn, V. (2002b) Immunocytochemistry reveals RANKL expression of myeloma cells. *Blood* **99**, 4646-4647.

Simonet, W.S., Lacey, D.L., Dunstan, C.R., Kelley, M., Chang, M.-S., Lüthy, R., Nguyen, H.Q., Wooden, S., Bennett, L., Boone, T., Shimamoto, G., DeRose, M., Elliott, R., Colombero, A., Tan, H.-L., Trail, G., Sullivan, J., Davy, E., Bucay, N., Renshaw-Gegg, L., Hughes, T.M., Hill, D., Pattison, W., Campbell, P., Sander, S., Van, G., Tarpley, J., Derby, P., Lee, R., Amgen EST Program and Boyle, W.J. (1997) Osteoprotegerin: a novel secreted protein involved in the regulation of bone density. *Cell* **89**, 309-319.

Takahashi, N., Akatsu, T., Udagawa, N., Sasaki, T., Yamaguchi, A., Moseley, J.M., Martin, T.J. and Suda, T. (1988) Osteoblastic cells are involved in osteoclast formation. *Endocrinology* **123**, 2600-2602.

Takamoto, M., Tsuji, K., Yamashita, T., Sasaki, H., Yano, T., Taketani, Y., Komori, T., Nifuji, A. and Noda, M. (2003) Hedgehog signaling enhances core-binding factor a1 and receptor activator of nuclear factor-κB ligand (RANKL) gene expression in chondrocytes. *Journal of Endocrinology* **177**, 413-421.

Thirunavukkarasu, K., Halladay, D.L., Miles, R.R., Yang, X., Galvin, R.J.S., Chandrasekhar, S., Martin, T.J. and Onyia ,J.E. (2000) The osteoblast-specific transcription factor Cbfa1 contributes to the expression of osteoprotegerin, a potent inhibitor of osteoclast differentiation and function. *Journal of Biological Chemistry* **275**, 25163-25172.

Thirunavukkarasu, K., Miles, R.R., Halladay, D.L., Yang, X., Galvin, R.J.S., Chandrasekhar, S., Martin, T.J. and Onyia, J.E. (2001) Stimulation of osteoprotegerin (OPG) gene expression by transforming growth factor-β (TGF-β). Mapping of the OPG promoter region that mediates TGF-β effects. *Journal of Biological Chemistry* **276**, 36241-36250.

Thomas, G.P., Baker, S.U.K., Eisman, J.A. and Gardiner, E.M. (2001) Changing RANKL/OPG mRNA expression in differentiating murine primary osteoblasts. *Journal of Endocrinology*, **170**, 451-460.

Thomas, R.J., Guise, T.A., Yin, J.J., Elliott, J., Horwood, N.J., Martin, T.J. and Gillespie, M.T. (1999) Breast cancer cells interact with osteoblasts to support osteoclast formation. *Endocrinology*, **140**, 4451-4458.

Tricot, G. (2000) New insights into role of microenvironment in multiple myeloma. *Lancet*, **355**, 248-250.

Tsuda, E., Goto, M., Mochizuki, S., Yano, K., Kobayashi, F., Morinaga, T. and Higashio, K. (1997) Isolation of a novel cytokine from human fibroblasts that specifically inhibits osteoclastogenesis. *Biochemical and Biophysical Research Communications* **234**, 137-142.

Udagawa, N., Takahashi, N., Jimi, E., Matsuzaki, K., Tsurukai, T., Itoh, K., Nakagawa, N., Yasuda, H., Goto, M., Tsuda, E., Higashio, K., Gillespie, M.T., Martin, T.J. and Suda, T. (1999) Osteoblasts/stromal cells stimulate osteoclast activation through expression of osteoclast differentiation factor/RANKL but not macrophage colony-stimulating factor. *Bone* **25**, 517-523.

Vidal, N.O.A., Brändström, H., Jonsson, K.B. and Ohlsson, C. (1998a) Osteoprotegerin mRNA is expressed in primary human osteoblast-like cells: down-regulation by glucocorticoids. *Journal of Endocrinology* **159**, 191-195.

Vidal, O.N.A., Sjögren, K., Eriksson, B.I., Ljunggren, Ö. and Ohlsson, C. (1998b) Osteoprotegerin mRNA is increased by interleukin-1α in the human osteosarcoma cell line MG-63 and in human osteoblast-like cells. *Biochemical and Biophysical Research Communications* **248**, 696-700.

Viereck, V., Emons, G., Lauck, V., Frosch, K.-H., Blaschke, S. and Hofbauer, L.C. (2002) Bisphosphonates pamidronate and zoledronic acid stimulate osteoprotegerin production by primary human osteoblasts. *Biochemical and Biophysical Research Communications* **291**, 680-686.

Wan, M., Shi, X., Feng, X. and Cao, X. (2001) Transcriptional mechanisms of bone morphogenetic protein-induced osteoprotegrin gene expression. *Journal of Biological Chemistry* **276**, 10119-10125.

Weitzmann, M.N., Cenci, S., Brown, C. and Pacifici, R. (2000) Interleukin-7 stimulates osteoclast formation by up-regulating the T-cell production of soluble osteoclastogenic cytokines. *Blood* **96**, 1873-1878.

Wong, B.R., Josien, R., Lee, S.Y., Sauter, B., Li, H.L., Steinman, R.M. and Choi, Y. (1997) TRANCE (tumor necrosis factor [TNF]-related activation-induced cytokine), a new TNF family member predominantly expressed in T cells, is a dendritic cell-specific survival factor. *Journal of Experimental Medicine* **186**, 2075-2080.

Wong, B.R., Josien, R., Lee, S.Y., Vologodskaia, M., Steinman, R.M. and Choi, Y. (1998) The TRAF family of signal transducers mediates NF-κB activation by the TRANCE receptor. *Journal of Biological Chemistry* **273**, 28355-28359.

Wong, B.R., Josien, R. and Choi, Y. (1999a) TRANCE is a TNF family member that regulates dendritic cell and osteoclast function. *Journal of Leukocyte Biology* **65**, 715-724.

Wong, B.R., Besser, D., Kim, N., Arron, J.R., Vologodskaia, M., Hanafusa, H. and Choi, Y. (1999b) TRANCE, a TNF family member, activates Akt/PKB through a signaling complex involving TRAF6 and c-Src. *Molecular Cell* **4**, 1041-1049.

Yamamoto, M., Murakami, T., Nishikawa, M., Tsuda, E., Mochizuki, K., Higashio, K., Akatsu, T., Motoyoshi, K. and Nagata, N. (1998) Hypocalcemic effect of osteoclastogenesis inhibitory factor/osteoprotegerin in the thyroparathyroidectomized rat. *Endocrinology* **139**, 4012-4015.

Yan, T., Riggs, B.L., Boyle, W.J. and Khosla, S. (2001) Regulation of osteoclastogenesis and RANK expression by TGF-β1. *Journal of Cellular Biochemistry* **83**, 320-325.

Yang, J., Fizazi, K., Peleg, S., Sikes, C.R., Raymond, A.K. Jamal, N., Hu, M., Olive, M., Martinez, L.A., Wood, C.G., Logothetis, C.J., Karsenty, G. and Navone, N.M. (2001) Prostate cancer cells induce osteoblast differentiation through a Cbfa1-dependent pathway. *Cancer Research* **61**, 5652-5659.

Yang, X., Halladay, D., Onyia, J.E., Martin, T.J. and Chandrasekhar, S. (2002) Protein kinase C is a mediator of the synthesis and secretion of osteoprotegerin in osteoblast-like cells. *Biochemical and Biophysical Research Communications* **290**, 42-46.

Yasuda, H., Shima, N., Nakagawa, N., Mochizuki, S., Yano, K., Fujise, N., Sato, Y., Goto, M., Yamaguchi, K., Kuriyama, M., Kanno, T., Murakami, A., Tsuda, E., Morinaga, T. and Higashio, K. (1998a) Identity of osteoclastogenesis inhibitory factor (OCIF) and osteoprotegerin (OPG): a mechanism by which OCIF/OPG inhibits osteoclastogenesis in vitro. *Endocrinology* **139**, 1329-1337.

Yasuda, H., Shima, N., Nakagawa, N., Yamaguchi, K., Kinosaki, M., Mochizuki, S.-I., Tomoyasu, A., Yano, K., Goto, M., Murakami, A., Tsuda, E., Morinaga, T., Higashio, K., Udagawa, N., Takahashi, H. and Suda, T. (1998b) Osteoclast differentiation factor is a ligand for osteoprotegerin/osteoclastogenesis-inhibitory factor and is identical to TRANCE/RANKL. *Proceedings of the National Academy of Sciences of the United States of America* **95**, 3597-3602.

Yoneda, T. (1998) Cellular and molecular mechanisms of breast and prostate cancer metastasis to bone. *European Journal of Cancer* **34**, 240-245.

Yonou, H., Kanomata, N., Goya, M., Kamijo, T., Yokose, T., Hasebe, T., Nagai, K., Hatano, T., Ogawa, Y. and Ochiai, A. (2003) Osteoprotegerin/osteoclastogenesis inhibitory factor decreases human prostate cancer burden in human adult bone implanted into nonobese diabetic/severe combined immunodeficient mice. *Cancer Research* **63**, 2096-2102.

Zhang, J., Dai, J., Qi, Y., Lin, D.L., Smith, P., Strayhorn, C., Mizokami, A., Fu, Z., Westman, J. and Keller, E.T. (2001) Osteoprotegerin inhibits prostate cancer-induced osteoclastogenesis and prevents prostate tumor growth in the bone. *Journal of Clinical Investigation* **107**, 1235-1244.

Chapter 8

MATRIX METALLOPROTEINAES AND BONE METASTASIS

R. Daniel Bonfil[1,2], Pamela Osenkowski[2], Rafael Fridman[2], Michael L. Cher[1,2]

[1]*Departments of Urology and* [2]*Pathology, Wayne State University School of Medicine and the Barbara Ann Karmanos Cancer Institute, Detroit, MI*

OVERVIEW ON MMP STRUCTURE AND REGULATION

The degradation of stromal and epithelial extracellular matrices (ECM) is partly mediated by a family of zinc-dependent endopeptidases, the matrix metalloproteinases (MMPs), which have the potential to cleave virtually all structural ECM components and thus are major mediators of extracellular proteolysis in normal and pathological conditions. In humans, the MMP family comprises at least 25 closely homologous multidomain enzymes that share common structural and functional features. Overall, the MMP family has evolved to include both secreted and plasma membrane-tethered members, thus conferring the MMPs with the ability to mediate proteolytic events at both the cell surface and in the immediate peri-cellular milieu. With few exceptions, MMPs comprise four basic domains: a signal peptide, a propeptide domain, a catalytic domain and a C-terminal domain known as the hemopexin-like domain. The propeptide domain is a short stretch of residues containing the conserved PRCG(V/N)PD, which maintains the enzyme in its inactive, zymogen state (referred here as pro-MMP) until its proteolytic removal, via the so-called "cysteine switch" (Nagase, 1999). A cysteine residue within the propeptide domain occupies a coordination site of the catalytic zinc to maintain enzyme latency (Becker et al., 1995; Van Wart and Birkedal-Hansen, 1990). The catalytic domain of MMPs contains two zinc ions, which are important for either structural or catalytic competence, and at least one calcium ion. The catalytic zinc ion is coordinated to three histidine residues, and it is necessary for MMP proteolytic activity (Bode et al., 1994; Salowe et al., 1992). All MMPs, except MMP-7 and MMP-26, contain a hemopexin-like domain, which is connected to the catalytic domain via a hinge region. Depending on the type of MMP, the hemopexin-like domain plays a role in substrate binding and interactions with tissue inhibitors of metalloproteinases (TIMPs), which affect MMP substrate recognition, zymogen activation and inhibition of activity. Structurally, the hemopexin-like domain has an ellipsoid shape, composed of a four-bladed β-propeller structure (Gomis-Ruth et al., 1996). In the case of the zymogenic form of the gelatinases, the hemopexin-like domain can bind TIMPs, a family of endogenous MMP inhibitors, with pro-MMP-2 binding TIMP-2, TIMP-3, and TIMP-4 and pro-MMP-9 binding TIMP-1 and TIMP-3 (Baker et al., 2002). For a long time, the significance of the binding of TIMPs to the latent form of the gelatinases was not understood because the zymogens are devoid of enzymatic activity. It turned out that in the case of pro-MMP-2, binding of TIMP-2 plays a role in zymogen activation by MT-MMPs (described below).

Additions and/or deletions of domains/motifs to the basic structural organization of MMPs are reasons for diversity among members of the MMP family. For example, MMP-2 and MMP-9 (also know as gelatinase A and gelatinase B, respectively) incorporated a fibronectin type II-module in the catalytic domain, which serves to bind the enzymes to denatured collagen and thus is known as the gelatin-binding domain (Allan et al., 1995). MMP-7 (matrilysin) lacks the entire hemopexin-like domain and hence represents the smallest member of the MMP family. The membrane-type MMPs (MT-MMPs) incorporate downstream of the hemopexin-like domain, a transmembrane and cytosolic tail domain in the case of MT1-, MT2-, MT3-, and MT5-MMP or a glycophosphatidylinositol (GPI) anchor in the case of MT4- and MT6-MMP (Itoh et al., 1999; Kojima et al., 2000). The transmembrane domain and the GPI anchor help to target the MT-MMPs to the cell surface were they can mediate pericellular proteolysis, a process that is thought to be critical for cell migration and invasion. Indeed, removal of MT1-, MT2-, or MT3-MMP's transmembrane domain had a detrimental effect on *in vitro* cell invasion (Hotary et al., 2000).

MMP activity is regulated at multiple levels ranging from gene expression to enzyme inhibition. In normal tissues, MMP expression is generally low but it increases significantly under conditions that require ECM degradation such as wound healing and cancer. MMPs are synthesized as latent zymogens, which require activation to acquire proteolytic activity.

Thus, zymogen activation represents an important regulatory step. For activation, limited proteolysis removes the pro-peptide domain generating high enzymatic activity. Some pro-MMPs are activated by MMPs while other proteases such as serine proteases activate other MMPs. A furin-recognition motif, located between the propeptide and the catalytic domains in certain MMPs, is a cleavage site for members of the pro-convertase family of serine proteases (Pei and Weiss, 1995). Non-proteolytic means of pro-MMP activation, via oxidative modification of the cysteine side-chain thiol, which would diminish its ability to serve as an effective ligand to the catalytic zinc ion (Gu et al., 2002; Okamoto et al., 2001), or via conformational changes induced by binding to substrate (Bannikov et al., 2002), have also been reported.

The enzymatic activity of MMPs is inhibited by TIMPs, a family of secreted proteins that includes four members: TIMP-1, TIMP-2, TIMP-3, and TIMP-4 (Gomez et al., 1997). Inhibition of MMP activity by TIMPs is of high-affinity and involves binding of the inhibitor to the active site in a reversible 1:1 stoichometric fashion (Edwards, 2001). All TIMPs can inhibit all active MMPs, but with differing binding affinities. For example, TIMP-1 is a weak inhibitor of MT-MMPs (Butler et al., 1997; Llano et al., 1999; Shimada et al., 1999; Will et al., 1996). Structurally, twelve conserved cysteine residues in the TIMP molecule form six disulfide bonds, which comprise a six-loop, two-domain structure. The N-terminal region of TIMPs is responsible for inhibition of MMP activity, though the C-terminal domain can interact with the catalytic domain of some MMPs, and with the hemopexin-like domain of the latent gelatinases (Brew et al., 2000). The binding of TIMP-2 via its C-terminal region to the hemopexin-like domain of pro-MMP-2 plays a role in the activation of pro-MMP-2 by MT1-MMP on the cell surface. In this process, TIMP-2 acts as a molecular link between an active MT1-MMP on the cell surface and pro-MMP-2. The N-terminal region of TIMP-2 binds to the active site of MT1-MMP, whereas the C-terminal region of the inhibitor binds to the hemopexin-like domain of pro-MMP-2 forming a so-called "ternary complex." The propeptide of the bound pro-MMP-2 is then cleaved at the Asn37-Leu38 peptide bond by a neighboring TIMP-2-free active MT1-MMP molecule. This is followed by a second cleavage event in which the intermediate MMP-2 form is cleaved at the Asn80-Tyr81 peptide bond by a fully active MMP-2 in an autocatalytic manner to achieve full activation (Will et al., 1996). TIMP-2-dependent pro-MMP-2 activation would occur only at low TIMP-2 concentrations relative to MT1-MMP (Albertsson et al., 2000). This would permit availability of enough TIMP-2-free MT1-MMP to hydrolyze the prodomain of the pro-MMP-2 bound in the ternary complex. Thus, under limited conditions,

TIMP-2 would promote activation. On the other hand, high levels of TIMP-2 relative to MT1-MMP would inhibit activation by blocking all free MT1-MMP molecules. Thus, TIMP-2 is a key component of a cascade of zymogen activation initiated by MT1-MMP at the cell surface which generates active MMP-2. In turn, MMP-2 can activate pro-MMP-9 (gelatinase B) (Cowell et al., 1998) and both MT1-MMP and MMP-2 are able to activate pro-MMP-13 (collagenase 3) (Knauper et al., 1996). MMP-13 is also an activator of pro-MMP-9 (Knauper et al., 1997). This cascade of pro-MMP activation in which a protease inhibitor plays a positive role in activation has challenged current views on MMP regulation by TIMPs but most importantly reflects the complicated expression of TIMPs in cancer tissues (discussed below).

MMP SUBSTRATES AND CANCER PROGRESSION

MMPs are classical ECM-degrading proteases in charge of accomplishing the degradation of most ECM components. They are the most efficient collagenolytic proteases in nature, cleaving all members of the collagen family, but they also degrade a large list of non-collagenous ECM substrates including proteoglycans, glycoproteins, elastin, fibronectin, osteonectin, laminin, and vitronectin, just to mention a few (for review, see (Sternlicht and Werb, 2001)). The ECM-degrading activity of MMPs, together with their high levels of expression in tumors, has been the main reason for the association of MMPs with cancer progression. Indeed, ECM degradation, in particular degradation of collagen IV of the basement membranes and collagen I in connective tissues, has long been considered an important requirement for tumor cell invasion. It was found that degradation of ECM components not only serves to break up tissue barriers for migrating cells but also generates ECM cleaved fragments with new biological activities. ECM degradation products can influence cell growth, survival, cell-cell interactions, cell migration, and also regulate tumor angiogenesis. MMP-mediated degradation of collagen XVIII generates endostatin, a peptide fragment with potent anti-angiogenic activity (O'Reilly et al., 1997). MMP cleavage of ECM can also release ECM-bound signaling molecules like growth factors and growth factor binding proteins. For instance, transforming growth factor (TGF)-β strongly binds to the ECM and upon MMP cleavage of the ECM, TGF-β is readily available to the cells. Interestingly, TGF-β can inhibit expression of many MMP genes; thus, the release of TGF-β by MMPs could act as a negative feedback loop to reduce MMP expression and additional TGF-β release (Imai et al., 1997). Fibroblast growth factor (FGF) also has a strong affinity for ECM components, and upon cleavage of such components as proteoglycan perlecan by both MMP-1 and MMP-3, FGF can be released from the ECM (Whitelock et al., 1996). The ability of MMPs to release ECM-bound FGF is considered a major mechanism by which MMPs regulate tumor-induced angiogenesis.

The effect of MMPs extends far beyond regulating the structural integrity of the ECM. In recent years, not only have a variety of non-ECM MMP substrates been identified, the functional consequences of ECM cleavage now indicates that MMPs influence multiple cellular functions by their ability to alter many non-ECM proteins. The list of MMP substrates now includes other proteases, protease inhibitors, cytokines, latent growth factors, growth factor binding proteins, cell-cell and cell-matrix adhesion molecules, and apoptotic ligands (McCawley and Matrisian, 2001). It has been established that the gelatinases, MMP-2 and MMP-9 can cleave and activate growth factor TGF-β (Yu and Stamenkovic, 2000) and the chemokine interleukin 1-β (IL1-β) (Schonbeck et al., 1998). MT4-MMP has also been found to cleave membrane-bound pro-tumor necrosis factor (TNF)-α, generating active TNF-α, (English et al., 2000). Additionally, MMP activity was shown to be responsible for cleavage of the cytokine monocyte chemoattractant protein (MCP)-3 *in vivo*, which resulted in its inactivation (McQuibban et al., 2000). Cell adhesion molecules, like CD44, are also cleaved by MMPs, and this leads to a more invasive phenotype (Kajita et al., 2001). MMPs mediate cleavage of cell surface molecules, like the adherens junction protein E-cadherin. MMP-mediated shedding of E-cadherin has been found to enhance cell invasion by the soluble fragment (Lochter et al., 1997). Integrins are also substrates of MMPs, and MT1-MMP is even considered to be an integrin convertase for the integrin subunit pro-alpha(v) (Ratnikov et al., 2002). Apoptosis can be regulated by MMPs via cleavage of FAS ligand, which binds to the FAS death receptor, or by indirectly cleaving ECM molecules and releasing signals which can stimulate cell survival or death (Powell et al., 1999). Taken together, the broad-spectrum of proteins that can be modified by MMP action demonstrates the complex roles that MMPs may play in tumor progression. Depending on the function of the substrate and/or the cleavage product, MMPs can either elicit positive or negative influences on the tumor cells and their microenvironment.

MMPS IN CANCER: ROLE OF TUMOR-STROMAL INTERACTIONS

Clinical data show that several members of the MMP family are expressed in virtually all types of human cancers. In particular, human malignant tumors contain high levels of expression of gelatinases (MMP-2 and MMP-9) (Forsyth et al., 1999; Kurschat et al., 2002), collagenase-3 (MMP-13) (Etoh et al., 2000), interstitial collagenase (MMP-1) (Yamashita et al., 2001), stromelysin-1 (MMP-3) (P et al., 2001), matrilysin (MMP-7) (Sasaki et al., 2001), stromelysin-3 (MMP-11) (Porte et al., 1995) and MT1-MMP (MMP-14) (Ueno et al., 1997). Overall, the expression and activity of these MMPs have been correlated with increased metastatic potential and poor prognosis in various cancers (for review see (Sternlicht, 2000)), consistent with the roles that MMPs play in degradation of both ECM and non-ECM substrates. Immunohistochemical and in situ hybridization studies have shown that MMP expression in tumor tissues is mostly confined to the malignant areas, particularly at the tumor-stromal interface (Maatta et al., 2000; Yamamura et al., 2002). Interestingly, it was found that MMP production is contributed by both tumor and stromal cells and in some tumors, whereas certain MMPs are produced exclusively by stromal cells. In many carcinomas, tumor-associated fibroblasts produce a desmoplastic response, which is characterized by intense cell proliferation. In addition, the peritumoral fibroblasts express high levels of MMPs, in particular MMP-2, MMP-9, MMP-13, and MT1-MMP (Afzal et al., 1998; Gress et al., 1995). Expression of MMPs in host tissues facilitates tumor cell migration and invasion but may also affect tumor cell survival by promoting angiogenesis. For example, expression of angiogenic factors by tumor cells such as vascular endothelial growth factor (VEGF) induce pro-MMP-2 activation in endothelial cells, which may facilitate endothelial cell migration and degradation of the sub-endothelial basement membrane leading to neovascularization (Zucker et al., 1998). MMP-9 activity has also been associated with tumor angiogenesis (Bergers et al., 2000). Infiltration of macrophages in tumor tissues contributes to the high levels of MMP-9 that is a characteristic of many tumor types.

Expression of MMPs in the tumor stroma appears to be a host response mediated by paracrine signals from the cancer cells (for review, see (Jiang et al., 2002; Sternlicht and Werb, 2001)). The paracrine factors include various cytokines and growth factors. Specific tumor cell-stromal cell interactions are also involved in MMP expression in stromal cells. Among the factors known to upregulate collagen-degrading MMPs in tumor fibroblasts and endothelial cells by cell-cell interactions is the extracellular matrix metalloproteinase inducer (EMMPRIN/CD147) (Guo et al., 1997). EMMPRIN is a membrane-anchored glycoprotein containing two immunoglobulin superfamily domains that is present on the surface of tumor cells and stimulates the production of MMPs by adjacent stromal cells.

In addition to its contribution to MMP synthesis, the tumor stroma is also a major producer of TIMPs, which takes place mostly in fibroblasts. In fact, several studies have shown that certain invasive carcinomas contain high levels of TIMP-1 and TIMP-2 when compared to benign tissues (Jiang et al., 2002). However, studies have also reported a downregulation of TIMP expression in malignant tissues when compared to the levels of MMPs. Thus, the pattern of TIMP expression in cancer is complex and heterogeneous. The high levels of TIMPs found in certain cancers may represent a response of the stroma to high MMP activity. However, TIMPs are multifunctional proteins and thus their role in tumor tissues may not necessarily be limited to MMP inhibition. As discussed above, TIMP-2 can, under certain conditions, stimulate pericellular proteolysis by promoting the MT1-MMP-mediated cascade of pro-MMP activation at the cell surface (Sato et al., 1994; Strongin et al., 1995). Both TIMP-1 and TIMP-2 can inhibit apoptosis of cancer cells, and TIMP-1 can enhance angiogenesis (Egeblad and Werb, 2002). TIMPs also have growth-promoting activity and may also influence cancer cell survival (Bertaux et al., 1991; Hayakawa et al., 1994; Hayakawa et al., 1992). The emerging view of MMPs and TIMPs in cancer is constantly evolving but it is obvious that these proteins play complex roles in cancer progression.

MMPS AND BONE REMODELING

MMP activity is required for normal, physiological bone remodeling. The adult skeletal structure and density are maintained permanently through a highly regulated turnover cycle involving removal (resorption) and replacement (formation) of bone tissue. The bone turnover cycle can be divided into a series of well-described steps (reviewed in (Baron, 1996)). Osteoblasts are normally thought of as bone-forming (matrix-producing) cells. However, according to "Chamber's Hypothesis" (Vaes, 1988), osteoblasts also have a proteolytic function. In the first step of the turnover cycle, osteoblasts or bone lining cells secrete MMPs in order to degrade the thin layer of non-mineralized bone matrix covering all mineralized trabeculae (Chambers et al., 1985). In areas of active bone turnover, this layer is called "osteoid" and is easily seen microscopically. The osteoid layer is composed of type I collagen (the main organic matrix component), glycoproteins, and mucopolysaccharides. The proteolytic generation of collagen fragments induces osteoclast recruitment and activation (Chambers et al., 1985; Holliday et al., 1997). This process involves migration of osteoclast precursors from the hematopoeitic compartment to areas of bone turnover and differentiation and fusion of these cells into functional osteoclasts. In fact, the osteoclast migration process itself also appears to require metalloproteinase secretion (Sato et al., 1998). As a consequence of osteoblast proteolytic activity, the underlying mineralized matrix is exposed, allowing attachment of osteoclasts. Osteoclast remove mineral and organic components (Blair et al., 1986), resulting in depressions known as resorption lacunae or Howship's lacunae. Osteoclasts further degrade bone by secreting acid and proteolytic enzymes into the extracellular resorption lacuna. Initially, cysteine proteases, predominantly cathepsin K, solubilize the inorganic matrix at low pH (Drake et al., 1996), thus making the organic components available for matrix metalloproteinases (MMPs), particularly MMP-9 (Reponen et al., 1994; Tezuka et al., 1994). These MMPs are secreted directly into the lacuna by the osteoclast. Once the resorption process has been completed, osteoblasts re-enter the area to start the bone formation process. They line the resorption lacuna and produce and secrete organic components that fill the bone depression mainly with a network of type I collagen (Kahn and Partridge, 1987; Rodan, 1992). This newly deposited matrix then becomes hardened by mineral deposition, and thus, the destroyed bone mass is recovered. During the completion of bone formation, some of the osteoblasts, which are considered the most mature form of the osteoblastic lineage, become trapped inside the newly formed extracellular matrix, and thus become osteocytes.

Although trabecular (cancellous) bone accounts for only 20 % of the total skeletal mass, it is more metabolically active than cortical bone. It has been estimated that around 25% of the total cancellous bone mass is replaced every year, whereas this happens in only 3% of cortical bone (Dempster and Lindsay, 1993). When there is a pathophysiological impairment of the equilibrium of the bone remodeling process, either more bone resorption or more bone formation takes place, resulting in osteolytic or osteoblastic responses, respectively.

As mentioned above, various matrix proteolytic enzymes, including MMPs, participate in the normal bone remodeling process. Recently, a rare autosomal recessive osteolysis disorder, known as NAO (nodulosis, arthropathy and osteolysis) syndrome, has been linked to inactivating mutations occurring in the MMP-2 gene (Martignetti et al., 2001). The osteolytic response observed in the disease has been suggested to be the result of lack of activation of TGF-β by MMP-2 proteolytic cleavage, which has been described to be necessary to promote osteoblastic activity (Filvaroff et al., 1999).

The phenotype of genetically modified mice allows insight into the role of proteases in the bone remodeling process. Mouse strains deficient in various MMPs, including MMP-2, MMP-3, MMP-7, and MMP-12, have been generated with little or no effect on skeletal development. In contrast, MT1-MMP-deficient mice exhibited severe abnormalities in skeletal development, involving craniofacial, axial, and appendicular bones, growth retardation, and death at very early age (Holmbeck et al., 1999; Zhou et al., 2000). Although some of the MT1-MMP-deficient mice features are similar to those in patients with NAO syndrome, it is unlikely that the anomalies observed in the mice are due to the absence of activation of pro-MMP-2 by MT1-MMP. In fact, MMP-2 knockout mice develop normally and are fertile (Itoh et al., 1997). It is likely that MT1-MMP somehow participates directly in the bone remodeling cycle.

With respect to MMP-9, mice with a null mutation in the MMP-9/gelatinase B gene showed development disorders, including growth and endochondral ossification abnormalities. (Vu et al., 1998). Normally, MMP-9 expression is associated with osteoclasts and mononuclear cells at sites of bone resorption (Bord et al., 1997; Reponen et al., 1994), and has also been localized to osteoclasts during mouse development (Reponen et al., 1994). As described above, it is important to remember that proteases are known to participate in many cellular functions in addition to matrix processing. For example, the angiogenic vascular endothelial growth factor (VEGF) can also contribute to bone development, and MMP-9 has been found to regulate the release of extracellular matrix-bound VEGF in developing bones (Engsig et al., 2000).

Finally, it should be noted that multiple MMPs are involved in the bone turnover process. For example, stromelysins-1 and –2 (MMP-3 and –10, respectively) have been reported to be expressed differentially in human osteophytic and neonatal bones (Bord et al., 1998). While MMP-3 is mostly latent and associated with osteocytes and the matrix surrounding the resorption lacuna, MMP-10 is predominantly produced in its active form and is expressed by osteoblasts, as well as by mononuclear cells and some osteoclasts at resorption sites (Bord et al., 1998).

BONE REMODELING AND BONE METASTASIS

As described elsewhere in this book, bone metastasis is a significant clinical problem associated with tremendous morbidity and mortality. Prostate and breast carcinomas, the most frequent malignant neoplasias in men and women, respectively, are the cancers most commonly associated with bone disease (Rubens, 1991). Although there are no reliable epidemiological data concerning the number of cancer patients that die with bone metastases, it has been estimated to be around 35 % (Mundy, 2002). Multiple myeloma is another cancer associated with intraosseous growth of tumor.

Cancer cells that metastasize to the bone can alter the normal skeletal remodeling process, upsetting the balance between bone formation and bone resorption. Thus, osteolytic or osteoblastic responses can occur in bone as a consequence of skeletal metastasis. It has become clear in recent years that, on a cellular and biochemical level, mixed responses are present even when one response predominates by imaging studies. For example, osteoclast activity is easily demonstrated in prostate cancer patients, even when the x-rays of the pelvic bones and vertebral column show sclerosis (increased density, or "osteoblastic metastasis"). The interaction of cancer cells and elements of the bone microenvironment triggers a "vicious cycle" in which bone cells (osteoblasts, osteoclasts, stromal cells) respond to the presence of tumor cells, and metastatic carcinoma cells react to matrix and stromal cell signals by proliferating and secreting factors that stimulate the bone turnover machinery (Mundy, 1997).

Breast cancer generates predominantly osteolytic bone metastases. Pathways describing this pathophysiologic process have been well described. Bone-resident metastatic tumor cells secrete parathyroid hormone-related peptide (PTHrP) (Powell et al., 1991). PTHrP is one of the main activators of osteoclasts; thus, this pathway thus leads directly to bone destruction. The osteoclastic bone resorption stimulated by PTHrP occurs via osteoblast production of receptor activator of nuclear factor κB ligand (RANKL), also known as osteoclast differentiation factor, osteoprotegerin ligand, and TRANCE (Guise, 2000). Osteolysis can release growth factors stored in the bone matrix, such as TGF-β, that activate autophosphorylation of tumor cell receptors and signaling through pathways that lead to tumor cell proliferation (Mundy, 2002). In this way, a feedback loop is established between breast carcinoma cells and the bone microenvironment that enhances the development and progression of breast carcinoma osteolytic metastases. Other mechanisms, involving proteases, also likely participate in the bone remodeling process in breast cancer (see below).

In the case of multiple myeloma, an osteolytic response is observed in virtually all cases. Although, myeloma grows in bone as a primary tumor, most investigators assume than myeloma behaves similarly to other tumor cells that metastasize to bone from another primary site. The interaction between myeloma cells and bone marrow stromal cells (BMSCs) induces stromal cells to secrete interleukin-6 (IL-6), which stimulates the proliferation of myeloma cells. Conversely, macrophage inflammatory protein-1α (MIP-1α) is an osteoclastogenic factor secreted by myeloma cells that can act in combination with IL-6, PTHrP, and RANKL, causing osteoclast recruitment, activation, and bone destruction (Han et al., 2001).

Although, prostate cancer bone metastases are usually described as "osteoblastic" based on radiographic imaging studies, many investigators have observed that osteolytic and osteoblastic activities coexist in bones colonized by prostate cancer cells. As in breast cancer and multiple myeloma, the establishment of the prostate cancer-bone "vicious cycle" has been partly elucidated. For example, increased bone resorption, associated with the presence prostate cancer cells in bone, can be a consequence of expression of Ca^{2+}-sensing receptor in prostate tumor cells (Sanders et al., 2001). This receptor seems to mediate the secretion of the osteoclast activator PTHrP by prostate cancer cells, facilitating osteolysis. The stimulation of PTHrP production and release by tumor cells can also be caused by TGF-β, which, as mentioned before, activates prostate cancer proliferation, and can be released from bone matrix by osteoclasts.

MMPS AND BONE METASTASIS

A role for MMPs in bone metastasis has long been suspected. Since, as described above, MMPs contribute to the process of normal bone remodeling, and because enhanced turnover of bone matrix occurs when tumor cells metastasize to bone (Cher, 2001), one can predict a role for these enzymes in metastasis-associated bone modification. Several years ago, Stearns and Wang reported that combined administration of a bisphosphonate compound and taxol in SCID mice injected intravenously (iv) with PC-3 ML human prostate cancer cells reduced bone metastases as a consequence of totally blocked production and release of MMPs (Stearns and Wang, 1996). *In vitro* studies carried out with prostate and breast cancer cells later on showed that bisphosphonates, potent inhibitors of bone resorption used for the treatment of osteolytic lesions, can reduce the proteolytic activity of MMPs through chelation of the zinc ion that binds to the active site of those neutral endopeptidases (Boissier et al., 2000).

As might by suspected, MMPs were also found to play a role in breast cancer metastasis. TIMP-2 overexpression in MDA-231 human breast cancer cells, which generate osteolytic lesions when inoculated in the left cardiac ventricle of immunosuppressed mice, reduced bone lytic metastatic burden (Yoneda et al., 1997). The involvement of MMPs in the pathogenesis of osteolytic bone metastases was confirmed by several studies in the same breast cancer model in SCID or nude mice. When broad spectrum MMP inhibitors such as Batimastat (BB-94), GM 6001, or Neovastast (AE-941) were administered, a significant reduction of osteolysis and bone tumor volume was observed (Lee et al., 2001; Weber et al., 2002; Winding et al., 2002).

We demonstrated similar findings in the SCID-human model of prostate cancer bone metastasis. Human prostate cancer cells were injected into human fetal bone fragments previously implanted in SCID mice. Message RNA in situ hybridization and immunohistochemistry revealed prominent signals for MMP-2 and MMP-9 in both cancer cells and neighboring bone stromal cells. Systemic administration of batimastat around the time of intraosseous tumor cell inoculation reduced the degradation of marrow trabeculae within bone implants. This was accompanied by reduced proliferation of prostate tumor cells growing in bone and a decreased number of osteoclasts recruited to the site (Nemeth et al., 2002). Recently, using an ELISA-based assay together with a quenched fluorogenic MMP substrate, we found an upregulation of MMP-9 activity in the experimental bone metastasis tissue, while tissue MMP-2 enzymatic activity was unchanged (unpublished data). In this and other models of bone metastasis, the site(s) of MMP inhibition (ie., cancer cells, bone cells, or both) has not yet been completely described.

Which MMPs are most important in bone metastasis? This is a potentially important clinical question, as targeting the appropriate MMP with a relatively specific inhibitor could improve therapeutic efficacy. Relatively non-specific MMP inhibitors have now been tested in a variety of human clinical trials, and a particularly bothersome side effect of joint pain and stiffness has been found to be a limiting factor. It is thought that the joint-related effects may be associated with agents that inhibit a broad spectrum of MMPs, whereas more selective inhibitors may be less toxic. Although the key proteases associated with bone metastasis have not been conclusively identified, some data are beginning to emerge. As mentioned above, our preliminary data implicate MMP-9 activity in an experimental model of bone metastasis. Others have postulated that MMP-1, produced by osteoblasts, can be induced in response to the presence of breast cancer cells. This, in turn, can facilitate osteoid degradation and homing of breast cancer cells to bone, followed by osteolysis by osteoclasts (Ohishi et al., 1995). Breast cancer cells were also found to stimulate osteoclastic resorptive activity that would be mediated by an enhanced expression of MMP-9 by osteoclasts (Tumber et al., 2001). However, immunohistochemical studies carried out in biopsies from breast cancer patients did not show major differences in MMP/TIMP profiles in osteoclasts and osteoblasts from bone metastases and normal bone. These data suggest that the osteolytic response could result from a dramatic increase in the number and activity of both cell types in regions of tumor cells (Lhotak et al., 2000).

In experimental models, a two-way stimulation of MMPs between the bone microenvironment and cancer cells that preferentially colonize bone was observed. For example, osteoblasts were shown to stimulate MMP-9 secretion by prostate cancer cells (Festuccia et al., 1999), and we demonstrated downregulation of TIMP-1 and –2 expression in bone marrow stromal cells after their co-culture with the tumor cells (Dong et al., 2001). Similarly, myeloma cells induced upregulation of MMP-1 by bone marrow stromal cells (Barille et al., 1997), and matrylisin (MMP-7) secreted by myeloma cells participated in activation of pro-MMP-2 secreted by bone marrow stromal cells (Barille et al., 1999). Conversely, MMP-9 production by myeloma cells has been shown to be upregulated as a consequence of their interaction with bone marrow stromal cells (Van Valckenborgh et al., 2002). Although it is not clear which chemical messengers are involved in this cross-talk, different cytokines and growth factors are presumed to be responsible. For example, in prostate and breast cancer, TGF-β, which in normal cells usually downregulates MMP activity (Orr et al., 2000), induces MMP-9 activity that could contribute to osteoclast-mediated bone resorption (Duivenvoorden et al., 1999).

IN THE FUTURE: MMP ACTIVITY MEASUREMENTS AND PROTEASE ACTIVITY IMAGING

As described above, there is abundant preclinical data suggesting that proteases might be valid therapeutic targets in bone metastasis; surprisingly, however, no protease antagonists have been entered into clinical trials specifically for bone metastasis. In fact, trials in which MMP antagonists have been tested in human cancer have been somewhat disappointing. In retrospect, the MMP inhibitor trials may have been flawed. The protocols used for these trials were similar to those used for traditional cytotoxic agents. Thus, the clinical endpoints were perhaps more appropriate for drugs that kill proliferating cells than for predominantly cytostatic agents like protease inhibitors. Further, the agents were tested in heterogeneous groups of advanced stage cancer patients without regard to bone-related issues; the trials did not examine any biochemical, histologic, or radiographic markers of bone turnover.

New clinical and laboratory approaches are needed to achieve better success in the future. First, it is not clear that the appropriate protease targets have been chosen. Homology searches of the human genome predict that approximately 600 of the approximately 30,000 human genes code for proteases; many of these 600 genes/proteins are still uncharacterized. Moreover, the profile of proteases involved specifically in bone metastasis remains largely undefined. Second, preclinical data predict that the timing of administration of MMP inhibitors must be tailored to the specific disease process. For example, in the RIP1-Tag2 mouse model for pancreatic islet carcinogenesis (Bergers et al., 1999), a broad spectrum MMP inhibitor had little effect on late-stage tumors, while tumor burden was reduced markedly in mice with early-stage tumors. Prevention studies also demonstrated a dramatic reduction in angiogenic islets when the MMP inhibitor was administered prior to the appearance of tumors. Similar data from our laboratory suggest that tissue MMP activity is upregulated early during the colonization of bone by PC cells and downregulated after the bone tumors enlarge suggesting that an MMP inhibitor would work better at lower skeletal tumor burden (unpublished data). Third, it is not clear that drugs with suitable selectivity have been tested in pre-clinical models and clinical trials. Numerous small molecule antagonists of proteases have been produced; however, most are broad-spectrum antagonists that inhibit multiple proteases. As mentioned above, they have side effects that prevent administration of sufficient amounts of drug to drive enzymatic inhibition of the intended target to low, or undetectable, levels. Moreover, the fact that many proteases have only recently been discovered prevents us from knowing the complete inhibition spectrum of the currently available small molecule protease antagonists.

Finally, we must develop systems for monitoring the inhibition of protease activity as a key intermediate endpoint in clinical trials. None of the MMP inhibitor trials have monitored the degree of inhibition of the target proteases *in vivo* as a clinical endpoint. Thus, it is not known if the inhibitor actually reached its target in tumors and reduced protease activity. For clinical trials, the assays must be non-invasive. In other words, there is a need for imaging tools and technologies to non-invasively assess protease activity and its inhibition in cancer patients.

Several laboratories have made progress toward imaging protease activity. One strategy is to use quenched fluorescent protease substrates (Bremer et al., 2001). An *in vivo* protease cleavage event activates the ability of the substrate to emit fluorescence after excitation. While promising, this strategy may be limited by lack of specificity of the substrate for particular enzymes, and the inability to image deep into tissues. Another strategy is to use small molecule activity-based probes as imaging agents. Unlike the substrate-based approaches that require proteolytic activation of the imaging agent by the enzyme, an activity-based probe allows permanent tagging of active enzymes *in vivo* (Bogyo et al., 2000; Greenbaum et al., 2002; Greenbaum et al., 2000). These reagents react only with the active site residues of a catalytically functional enzyme. Currently, these probes are valuable for clinical or experimental work involving tissue sampling, but not for noninvasive imaging. Another approach is to use attenuated luciferase probes. For example, such probes have been developed to image intracellular caspase activity (Laxman et al., 2002). This is done by including protease a cleavage site for caspase-3 within a silenced reporter molecule. Luciferase is activated only after cleavage by caspase-3. The agent was successful in detecting TRAIL-induced apoptosis in a xenograft mouse model. A disadvantage is that luceriferase probes are not appropriate for human use. For human trials, protease-activated magnetic resonance imaging (MRI) contrast agents hold promise. These are modified MRI contrast agents that become activated after a protease enzyme cleavage event. The research that forms the basis for this idea has been described (Louie et al., 2000). Ultimately, these types of non-invasive technologies should result in optimized treatment protocols, tailored to the protease profile of an individual patient's metastasis. Such individualized treatment protocols may improve patient assessment, treatment, and outcome and will be amenable to modification during the course of therapy to match alterations in protease activity.

REFERENCES

Afzal, S., Lalani, E. N., Poulsom, R., Stubbs, A., Rowlinson, G., Sato, H., Seiki, M. and Stamp, G. W. (1998). MT1-MMP and MMP-2 mRNA expression in human ovarian tumors: possible implications for the role of desmoplastic fibroblasts. *Human Pathology* 29, 155-165.

Albertsson, P., Kim, M. H., Jonges, L. E., Kitson, R. P., Kuppen, P. J., Johansson, B. R., Nannmark, U. and Goldfarb, R. H. (2000). Matrix metalloproteinases of human NK cells. *In vivo* 14, 269-276.

Allan, J. A., Docherty, A. J., Barker, P. J., Huskisson, N. S., Reynolds, J. J. and Murphy, G. (1995). Binding of gelatinases A and B to type-I collagen and other matrix components. *Biochemistry Journal* 309 (Pt 1), 299-306.

Baker, A. H., Edwards, D. R. and Murphy, G. (2002). Metalloproteinase inhibitors: biological actions and therapeutic opportunities. *J Cell Sci* 115, 3719-3727.

Bannikov, G. A., Karelina, T. V., Collier, I. E., Marmer, B. L. and Goldberg, G. I. (2002). Substrate binding of gelatinase B induces its enzymatic activity in the presence of intact propeptide. *Journal of Biological Chemistry* 277, 16022-16027.

Barille, S., Akhoundi, C., Collette, M., Mellerin, M. P., Rapp, M. J., Harousseau, J. L., Bataille, R. and Amiot, M. (1997). Metalloproteinases in multiple myeloma: production of matrix metalloproteinase-9 (MMP-9), activation of proMMP-2 and induction of MMP-1 by myeloma cells. *Blood* 90, 1649-1655.

Barille, S., Bataille, R., Rapp, M. J., Harousseau, J. L. and Amiot, M. (1999). Production of metalloproteinase-7 (matrilysin) by human myeloma cells and its potential involvement in metalloproteinase-2 activation. *Journal of Immunology* 163, 5723-5728.

Baron, R. E. (1996). "Anatomy and ultrastructure of bone" In: *Primer on the Metabolic Bone Diseases and Disorders of Mineral Metabolism*, M. J. Favus, ed. (Philadelphia, Lippincott -Raven Publishers), pp. 3-10.

Becker, J. W., Marcy, A. I., Rokosz, L. L., Axel, M. G., Burbaum, J. J., Fitzgerald, P. M., Cameron, P. M., Esser, C. K., Hagmann, W. K., Hermes, J. D. and et al. (1995). Stromelysin-1: three-dimensional structure of the inhibited catalytic domain and of the C-truncated proenzyme. *Protein Science* 4, 1966-1976.

Bergers, G., Brekken, R., McMahon, G., Vu, T. H., Itoh, T., Tamaki, K., Tanzawa, K., Thorpe, P., Itohara, S., Werb, Z. and Hanahan, D. (2000). Matrix metalloproteinase-9 triggers the angiogenic switch during carcinogenesis. *Nat Cell Biol* 2, 737-744.

Bergers, G., Javaherian, K., Lo, K. M., Folkman, J. and Hanahan, D. (1999). Effects of angiogenesis inhibitors on multistage carcinogenesis in mice. *Science* 284, 808-812.

Bertaux, B., Hornebeck, W., Eisen, A. Z. and Dubertret, L. (1991). Growth stimulation of human keratinocytes by tissue inhibitor of metalloproteinases. *Journal of Investigative Dermatolology* 97, 679-685.

Blair, H. C., Kahn, A. J., Crouch, E. C., Jeffrey, J. J. and Teitelbaum, S. L. (1986). Isolated osteoclasts resorb the organic and inorganic components of bone. *Journal Cell Biology* 102, 1164- 1172.

Bode, W., Reinemer, P., Huber, R., Kleine, T., Schnierer, S. and Tschesche, H. (1994). The X-ray crystal structure of the catalytic domain of human neutrophil collagenase inhibited by a substrate analogue reveals the essentials for catalysis and specificity. *Embo J* 13, 1263-1269.

Bogyo, M., Verhelst, S., Bellingard-Dubouchaud, V., Toba, S. and Greenbaum, D. (2000). Selective targeting of lysosomal cysteine proteases with radiolabeled electrophilic substrate analogs. *Chem Biol* 7, 27-38.

Boissier, S., Ferreras, M., Peyruchaud, O., Magnetto, S., Ebetino, F. H., Colombel, M., Delmas, P., Delaisse, J. M. and Clezardin, P. (2000). Bisphosphonates inhibit breast and prostate carcinoma cell invasion, an early event in the formation of bone metastases. *Cancer Research* 60, 2949-2954.

Bord, S., Horner, A., Hembry, R. M. and Compston, J. E. (1998). Stromelysin-1 (MMP-3) and stromelysin-2 (MMP-10) expression in developing human bone: potential roles in skeletal development. *Bone* 23, 7-12.

Bord, S., Horner, A., Hembry, R. M., Reynolds, J. J. and Compston, J. E. (1997). Distribution of matrix metalloproteinases and their inhibitor, TIMP-1, in developing human osteophytic bone. *Journal of Anatomy* 191, 39-48.

Bremer, C., Tung, C. H. and Weissleder, R. (2001). In vivo molecular target assessment of matrix metalloproteinase inhibition. *Nat Med* 7, 743-748.

Brew, K., Dinakarpandian, D. and Nagase, H. (2000). Tissue inhibitors of metalloproteinases: evolution, structure and function. *Biochim Biophys Acta* 1477, 267-283.

Butler, G. S., Will, H., Atkinson, S. J. and Murphy, G. (1997). Membrane-type-2 matrix metalloproteinase can initiate the processing of progelatinase A and is regulated by the tissue inhibitors of metalloproteinases. *European Journal of Biochemistry* 244, 653-657.

Chambers, T. J., Darby, J. A. and Fuller, K. (1985). Mammalian collagenase predisposes bone surfaces to osteoclastic resorption. *Cell Tissue Research* 241, 671-675.

Cher, M. L. (2001). Mechanisms governing bone metastasis in prostate cancer. *Current Opinions in Urology* 11, 483-488.

Cowell, S., Knauper, V., Stewart, M. L., D'Ortho, M. P., Stanton, H., Hembry, R. M., Lopez-Otin, C., Reynolds, J. J. and Murphy, G. (1998). Induction of matrix metalloproteinase activation cascades based on membrane-type 1 matrix metalloproteinase: associated activation of gelatinase A, gelatinase B and collagenase 3. *Biochem J* 331 (Pt 2), 453-458.

Dempster, D. W. and Lindsay, R. (1993). Pathogenesis of osteoporosis. *Lancet* 341, 797-801.

Dong, Z., Nemeth, J. A., Cher, M. L., Palmer, K. C., Bright, R. C. and Fridman, R. (2001). Differential regulation of matrix metalloproteinase-9, tissue inhibitor of metalloproteinase-1 (TIMP-1) and TIMP-2 expression in co-cultures of prostate cancer and stromal cells. *International Journal of Cancer* 93, 507-515.

Drake, F. H., Dodds, R. A., James, I. E., Connor, J. R., Debouck, C., Richardson, S., Lee-Rykaczewski, E., Coleman, L., Rieman, D., Barthlow, R., et al. (1996). Cathepsin K, but not cathepsins B, L, or S, is abundantly expressed in human osteoclasts. *Journal of Biological Chemistry* 271, 12511–12516.

Duivenvoorden, W. C., Hirte, H. W. and Singh, G. (1999). Transforming growth factor beta1 acts as an inducer of matrix metalloproteinase expression and activity in human bone-metastasizing cancer cells. *Clinical Experimental Metastasis* 17, 27-34.

Edwards, D. R. (2001). "The Tissue Inhibitors of Metalloproteinases" In: *Cancer Therapy*, N. J. C. a. K. Appelt, ed. (Totowa, New Jersey, Humana), pp. 67-84.

Egeblad, M. and Werb, Z. (2002). New functions for the matrix metalloproteinases in cancer progression. *Nat Rev Cancer* 2, 161-174.

English, W. R., Puente, X. S., Freije, J. M., Knauper, V., Amour, A., Merryweather, A., Lopez-Otin, C. and Murphy, G. (2000). Membrane type 4 matrix metalloproteinase (MMP17) has tumor necrosis factor-alpha convertase activity but does not activate pro-MMP2. *Journal of Biological Chemistry* 275, 14046-14055.

Engsig, M. T., Chen, Q. J., Vu, T. H., Pedersen, A. C., Therkidsen, B., Lund, L. R., Henriksen, K., Lenhard, T., Foged, N. T., Werb, Z. and Delaisse, J. M. (2000). Matrix metalloproteinase 9 and vascular endothelial growth factor are essential for osteoclast recruitment into developing long bones. *Journal of Cell Biology* 151, 879-889.

Etoh, T., Inoue, H., Yoshikawa, Y., Barnard, G. F., Kitano, S. and Mori, M. (2000). Increased expression of collagenase-3 (MMP-13) and MT1-MMP in oesophageal cancer is related to cancer aggressiveness. *Gut* 47, 50-56.

Festuccia, C., Giunciuglio, D., Guerra, F., Villanova, I., Angelucci, A., Manduca, P., Teti, A., Albini, A. and Bologna, M. (1999). Osteoblasts modulate secretion of urokinase-type plasminogen activator (uPA) and matrix metalloproteinase-9 (MMP-9) in human prostate cancer cells promoting migration and matrigel invasion. *Oncology Research* 11, 17-31.

Filvaroff, E., Erlebacher, A., Ye, J., Gitelman, S. E., Lotz, J., Heillman, M. and Derynck, R. (1999). Inhibition of TGF-beta receptor signaling in osteoblasts leads to decreased bone remodeling and increased trabecular bone mass. *Development* 126, 4267-4279.

Forsyth, P. A., Wong, H., Laing, T. D., Rewcastle, N. B., Morris, D. G., Muzik, H., Leco, K. J., Johnston, R. N., Brasher, P. M., Sutherland, G. and Edwards, D. R. (1999). Gelatinase-A (MMP-2), gelatinase-B (MMP-9) and membrane type matrix metalloproteinase-1 (MT1-MMP) are involved in different aspects of the pathophysiology of malignant gliomas. *British Journal of Cancer* 79, 1828-1835.

Gomez, D. E., Alonso, D. F., Yoshiji, H. and Thorgeirsson, U. P. (1997). Tissue inhibitors of metalloproteinases: structure, regulation and biological functions. *European Journal of Cell Biology* 74, 111-122.

Gomis-Ruth, F. X., Gohlke, U., Betz, M., Knauper, V., Murphy, G., Lopez-Otin, C. and Bode, W. (1996). The helping hand of collagenase-3 (MMP-13): 2.7 A crystal structure of its C-terminal haemopexin-like domain. *Journal of Molecular Biology* 264, 556-566.

Greenbaum, D., Baruch, A., Hayrapetian, L., Darula, Z., Burlingame, A., Medzihradszky, K. F. and Bogyo, M. (2002). Chemical approaches for functionally probing the proteome. *Molecular and Cellular Proteomics* 1, 60-68.

Greenbaum, D., Medzihradszky, K. F., Burlingame, A. and Bogyo, M. (2000). Epoxide electrophiles as activity-dependent cysteine protease profiling and discovery tools. *Chemical Biology* 7, 569-581.

Gress, T. M., Muller-Pillasch, F., Lerch, M. M., Friess, H., Buchler, M. and Adler, G. (1995). Expression and in-situ localization of genes coding for extracellular matrix proteins and extracellular matrix degrading proteases in pancreatic cancer. *International Journal of Cancer* 62, 407-413.

Gu, Z., Kaul, M., Yan, B., Kridel, S. J., Cui, J., Strongin, A., Smith, J. W., Liddington, R. C. and Lipton, S. A. (2002). S-nitrosylation of matrix metalloproteinases: signaling pathway to neuronal cell death. *Science* 297, 1186-1190.

Guise, T. A. (2000). Molecular mechanisms of osteolytic bone metastases. *Cancer* 88, 2892-2898.

Guo, H., Zucker, S., Gordon, M. K., Toole, B. P. and Biswas, C. (1997). Stimulation of matrix metalloproteinase production by recombinant extracellular matrix metalloproteinase inducer from transfected Chinese hamster ovary cells. *Journal of Biological Chemistry* 272, 24-27.

Han, J. H., Choi, S. J., Kurihara, N., Koide, M., Oba, Y. and Roodman, G. (2001). Macrophage inflammatory protein-1alpha is an osteoclastogenic factor in myeloma that is independent of receptor activator of nuclear factor kappaB ligand. *Blood* 97, 3349-3353.

Hayakawa, T., Yamashita, K., Ohuchi, E. and Shinagawa, A. (1994). Cell growth-promoting activity of tissue inhibitor of metalloproteinases-2 (TIMP-2). *J Cell Sci* 107 (Pt 9), 2373-2379.

Hayakawa, T., Yamashita, K., Tanzawa, K., Uchijima, E. and Iwata, K. (1992). Growth-promoting activity of tissue inhibitor of metalloproteinases-1 (TIMP-1) for a wide range of cells. A possible new growth factor in serum. FEBS Lett 298, 29-32.

Holliday, L. S., Welgus, H. G., Fliszar, C. J., Veith, G. M., Jeffrey, J. J. and Gluck, S. L. (1997). Initiation of osteoclast bone resorption by interstitial collagenase. *Journal of Biological Chemistry* 272, 22053-22058.

Holmbeck, K., Bianco, P., Caterina, J., Yamada, S., Kromer, M., Kuznetsov, S. A., Mankani, M., Robey, P. G., Poole, A. R., Pidoux, I., et al. (1999). MT1-MMP-deficient mice develop dwarfism, osteopenia, arthritis and connective tissue disease due to inadequate collagen turnover. *Cell* 99, 81-92.

Hotary, K., Allen, E., Punturieri, A., Yana, I. and Weiss, S. J. (2000). Regulation of cell invasion and morphogenesis in a three-dimensional type I collagen matrix by membrane-type matrix metalloproteinases 1, 2 and 3. *Journal of Cell Biology* 149, 1309-1323.

Imai, K., Hiramatsu, A., Fukushima, D., Pierschbacher, M. D. and Okada, Y. (1997). Degradation of decorin by matrix metalloproteinases: identification of the cleavage sites, kinetic analyses and transforming growth factor-beta1 release. *Biochemistry Journal* 322 (Pt 3), 809-814.

Itoh, T., Ikeda, T., Gomi, H., Nakao, S., Suzuki, T. and Itohara, S. (1997). Unaltered secretion of beta-amyloid precursor protein in gelatinase A (matrix metalloproteinase 2)-deficient mice. *Journal of Biological Chemistry* 272, 22389-22392.

Itoh, Y., Kajita, M., Kinoh, H., Mori, H., Okada, A. and Seiki, M. (1999). Membrane type 4 matrix metalloproteinase (MT4-MMP, MMP-17) is a glycosylphosphatidylinositol-anchored proteinase. *Journal of Biological Chemistry* 274, 34260-34266.

Jiang, Y., Goldberg, I. D. and Shi, Y. E. (2002). Complex roles of tissue inhibitors of metalloproteinases in cancer. *Oncogene* 21, 2245-2252.

Kahn, A. J. and Partridge, N. C. (1987). New concepts in bone remodeling: an expanding role for the osteoblast. *American Journal of Otolaryngology* 8, 258-264.

Kajita, M., Itoh, Y., Chiba, T., Mori, H., Okada, A., Kinoh, H. and Seiki, M. (2001). Membrane-type 1 matrix metalloproteinase cleaves CD44 and promotes cell migration. *Journal of Cell Biology* 153, 893-904.

Knauper, V., Smith, B., Lopez-Otin, C. and Murphy, G. (1997). Activation of progelatinase B (proMMP-9) by active collagenase-3 (MMP-13). *European Journal of Biochemistry* 248, 369-373.

Knauper, V., Will, H., Lopez-Otin, C., Smith, B., Atkinson, S. J., Stanton, H., Hembry, R. M. and Murphy, G. (1996). Cellular mechanisms for human procollagenase-3 (MMP-13) activation. Evidence that MT1-MMP (MMP-14) and gelatinase a (MMP-2) are able to generate active enzyme. *Journal of Biological Chemistry* 271, 17124-17131.

Kojima, S., Itoh, Y., Matsumoto, S., Masuho, Y. and Seiki, M. (2000). Membrane-type 6 matrix metalloproteinase (MT6-MMP, MMP-25) is the second glycosyl-phosphatidyl inositol (GPI)-anchored MMP. FEBS Lett 480, 142-146.

Kurschat, P., Wickenhauser, C., Groth, W., Krieg, T. and Mauch, C. (2002). Identification of activated matrix metalloproteinase-2 (MMP-2) as the main gelatinolytic enzyme in malignant melanoma by in situ zymography. *Journal of Pathology* 197, 179-187.

Laxman, B., Hall, D. E., Bhojani, M. S., Hamstra, D. A., Chenevert, T. L., Ross, B. D. and Rehemtulla, A. (2002). Noninvasive real-time imaging of apoptosis. *Proceedings of the National Academy of Sciences USA* 99, 16551-16555.

Lee, J., Weber, M., Mejia, S., Bone, E., Watson, P. and Orr, W. (2001). A matrix metalloproteinase inhibitor, batimastat, retards the development of osteolytic bone metastases by MDA-MB-231 human breast cancer cells in Balb C nu/nu mice. *European Journal of Cancer* 37, 106-113.

Lhotak, S., Elavathil, L. J., Vukmirovic-Popovic, S., Duivenvoorden, W. C., Tozer, R. G. and Singh, G. (2000). Immunolocalization of matrix metalloproteinases and their inhibitors in clinical specimens of bone metastasis from breast carcinoma. *Clinical Experimental Metastasis* 18, 463-470.

Llano, E., Pendas, A. M., Freije, J. P., Nakano, A., Knauper, V., Murphy, G. and Lopez-Otin, C. (1999). Identification and characterization of human MT5-MMP, a new membrane-bound activator of progelatinase a overexpressed in brain tumors. *Cancer Research* 59, 2570-2576.

Lochter, A., Galosy, S., Muschler, J., Freedman, N., Werb, Z. and Bissell, M. J. (1997). Matrix metalloproteinase stromelysin-1 triggers a cascade of molecular alterations that leads to stable epithelial-to-mesenchymal conversion and a premalignant phenotype in mammary epithelial cells. *Journal of Cell Biology* 139, 1861-1872.

Louie, A. Y., Huber, M. M., Ahrens, E. T., Rothbacher, U., Moats, R., Jacobs, R. E., Fraser, S. E. and Meade, T. J. (2000). In vivo visualization of gene expression using magnetic resonance imaging. *Nat Biotechnol* 18, 321-325.

Maatta, M., Soini, Y., Liakka, A. and Autio-Harmainen, H. (2000). Differential expression of matrix metalloproteinase (MMP)-2, MMP-9, and membrane type 1-MMP in hepatocellular and pancreatic adenocarcinoma: implications for tumor progression and clinical prognosis. *Clinical Cancer Research* 6, 2726-2734.

Martignetti, J. A., Aqeel, A. A., Sewairi, W. A., Boumah, C. E., Kambouris, M., Mayouf, S. A., Sheth, K. V., Eid, W. A., Dowling, O., Harris, J., et al. (2001). Mutation of the matrix metalloproteinase 2 gene (MMP2) causes a multicentric osteolysis and arthritis syndrome. *Nat Genet* 28, 261-265.

McCawley, L. J. and Matrisian, L. M. (2001). Matrix metalloproteinases: they're not just for matrix anymore! *Current Opinions in Cell Biology* 13, 534-540.

McQuibban, G. A., Gong, J. H., Tam, E. M., McCulloch, C. A., Clark-Lewis, I. and Overall, C. M. (2000). Inflammation dampened by gelatinase A cleavage of monocyte chemoattractant protein-3. *Science* 289, 1202-1206.

Mundy, G. R. (1997). Mechanisms of bone metastasis. *Cancer* 80, 1546-1556.

Mundy, G. R. (2002). Metastasis to boen: causes, consequences and therapeutic opportunities. *Nature Rev Cancer* 2, 584-593.

Nagase, H. a. J. F. W., Jr. (1999). Matrix Metalloproteinases. *The Journal of Biological Chemistry* 274, 21491-21494.

Nemeth, J. A., Yousif, R., Herzog, M., Che, M., Upadhyay, J., Shekarriz, B., Bhagat, S., Mullins, C., Fridman, R. and Cher, M. L. (2002). Matrix metalloproteinase activity, bone matrix turnover and tumor cell proliferation in prostate cancer bone metastasis. *Journal of the National Cancer Institute* 94, 17-25.

Ohishi, K., Fujita, N., Morinaga, Y. and Tsuruo, T. (1995). H-31 human breast cancer cells stimulate type I collagenase production in osteoblast-like cells and induce bone resorption. *Clinical Experimental Metastasis* 13, 287-295.

Okamoto, T., Akaike, T., Sawa, T., Miyamoto, Y., van der Vliet, A. and Maeda, H. (2001). Activation of matrix metalloproteinases by peroxynitrite-induced protein S-glutathiolation via disulfide S-oxide formation. *Journal of Biological Chemistry* 276, 29596-29602.

O'Reilly, M. S., Boehm, T., Shing, Y., Fukai, N., Vasios, G., Lane, W. S., Flynn, E., Birkhead, J. R., Olsen, B. R. and Folkman, J. (1997). Endostatin: an endogenous inhibitor of angiogenesis and tumor growth. *Cell* 88, 277-285.

Orr, F. W., Lee, J., Duivenvoorden, W. C. and Singh, G. (2000). Pathophysiologic interactions in skeletal metastasis. *Cancer* 88, 2912-2918.

P, O. C., Rhys-Evans, P. H. and Eccles, S. A. (2001). Expression of matrix metalloproteinases and their inhibitors correlates with invasion and metastasis in squamous cell carcinoma of the head and neck. *Arch Otolaryngol Head Neck Surg* 127, 813-820.

Pei, D. and Weiss, S. J. (1995). Furin-dependent intracellular activation of the human stromelysin-3 zymogen. *Nature* 375, 244-247.

Porte, H., Chastre, E., Prevot, S., Nordlinger, B., Empereur, S., Basset, P., Chambon, P. and Gespach, C. (1995). Neoplastic progression of human colorectal cancer is associated with overexpression of the stromelysin-3 and BM-40/SPARC genes. *International Journal of Cancer* 64, 70-75.

Powell, G. J., Southby, J., Danks, J. A., Stillwell, R. G., Hayman, J. A., Henderson, M. A., Bennett, R. C. and Martin, T. J. (1991). Localization of parathyroid hormone-related protein in breast cancer metastases: increased incidence in bone compared with other sites. *Cancer Research* 51, 3059-3061.

Powell, W. C., Fingleton, B., Wilson, C. L., Boothby, M. and Matrisian, L. M. (1999). The metalloproteinase matrilysin proteolytically generates active soluble Fas ligand and potentiates epithelial cell apoptosis. *Current Biology* 9, 1441-1447.

Ratnikov, B. I., Rozanov, D. V., Postnova, T. I., Baciu, P. G., Zhang, H., DiScipio, R. G., Chestukhina, G. G., Smith, J. W., Deryugina, E. I. and Strongin, A. Y. (2002). An alternative processing of integrin alpha(v) subunit in tumor cells by membrane type-1 matrix metalloproteinase. *Journal of Biological Chemistry* 277, 7377-7385.

Reponen, P., Sahlberg, C., Munaut, C., Thesleff, I. and Tryggvason, K. (1994). High expression of 92-kD type IV collagenase (gelatinase B) in the osteoclast lineage during mouse development. *Journal of Cell Biology* 124, 1091-1102.

Rodan, G. A. (1992). Introduction to bone biology. *Bone* 13, S3-6.

Rubens, R. D. (1991). "The nature of metastatic bone disease" In: *Bone Metastases: diagnosis and treatment*, I. Fogelman, ed. (London, Springer-Verlag), pp. 1-10.

Salowe, S. P., Marcy, A. I., Cuca, G. C., Smith, C. K., Kopka, I. E., Hagmann, W. K. and Hermes, J. D. (1992). Characterization of zinc-binding sites in human stromelysin-1: stoichiometry of the catalytic domain and identification of a cysteine ligand in the proenzyme. *Biochemistry* 31, 4535-4540.

Sanders, J. L., Chattopadhyay, N., Kifor, O., Yamaguchi, T. and Brown, E. M. (2001). Ca^{2+}-sensing receptor expression and PTHrP secretion in PC-3 human prostate cancer cells. *American Journal of Physiol Endocrinol Metab* 281, E1267-E1274.

Sasaki, H., Yukiue, H., Moiriyama, S., Kobayashi, Y., Nakashima, Y., Kaji, M., Kiriyama, M., Fukai, I., Yamakawa, Y. and Fujii, Y. (2001). Clinical significance of matrix metalloproteinase-7 and Ets-1 gene expression in patients with lung cancer. *Journal of Surgical Research* 101, 242-247.

Sato, H., Takino, T., Okada, Y., Cao, J., Shinagawa, A., Yamamoto, E. and Seiki, M. (1994). A matrix metalloproteinase expressed on the surface of invasive tumour cells. *Nature* 370, 61-65.

Sato, T., Foged, N. T. and Delaisse, J. M. (1998). The migration of purified osteoclasts through collagen is inhibited by matrix metalloproteinase inhibitors. *Journal of Bone and Mineral Research* 13, 59-66.

Schonbeck, U., Mach, F. and Libby, P. (1998). Generation of biologically active IL-1 beta by matrix metalloproteinases: a novel caspase-1-independent pathway of IL-1 beta processing. *Journal of Immunology* 161, 3340-3346.

Shimada, T., Nakamura, H., Ohuchi, E., Fujii, Y., Murakami, Y., Sato, H., Seiki, M. and Okada, Y. (1999). Characterization of a truncated recombinant form of human membrane type 3 matrix metalloproteinase. *European Journal of Biochemistry* 262, 907-914.

Stearns, M. E. and Wang, M. (1996). Effects of alendronate and taxol on pc 3 ml cell bone metastases in scid mice. *Invas Metast* 16, 116–131.

Sternlicht, M. D. and Werb, Z. (2001). How matrix metalloproteinases regulate cell behavior. *Annu Rev Cell Dev Biol* 17, 463-516.

Sternlicht, M. D. a. B., G. (2000). Matrix metalloproteinases as emerging targets in anti-cancer therapy: status and prospects. *Emerging Therapeutic Targets* 4, 609-633.

Strongin, A. Y., Collier, I., Bannikov, G., Marmer, B. L., Grant, G. A. and Goldberg, G. I. (1995). Mechanism of cell surface activation of 72-kDa type IV collagenase. Isolation of the activated form of the membrane metalloprotease. *Journal of Biological Chemistry* 270, 5331-5338.

Tezuka, K., Nemoto, K., Tezuka, Y., Sato, T., Ikeda, Y., Kobori, M., Kawashima, H., Eguchi, H., Hakeda, Y. and Kumegawa, M. (1994). Identification of matrix metalloproteinase 9 in rabbit osteoclasts. *Journal of Biological Chemistry* 269, 15006–15009.

Tumber, A., Morgan, H. M., Meikle, M. C. and Hill, P. A. (2001). Human breast-cancer cells stimulate the fusion, migration and resorptive activity of osteoclasts in bone explants. *International Journal of Cancer* 91, 665-672.

Ueno, H., Nakamura, H., Inoue, M., Imai, K., Noguchi, M., Sato, H., Seiki, M. and Okada, Y. (1997). Expression and tissue localization of membrane-types 1, 2 and 3 matrix metalloproteinases in human invasive breast carcinomas. *Cancer Research* 57, 2055-2060.

Vaes, G. (1988). Cellular biology and biochemical mechanism of bone resorption. A review of recent developments on the formation, activation and mode of action of osteoclasts. *Clinical Orthopaedics* 231, 239-271.

Van Valckenborgh, E., Bakkus, M., Munaut, C., Noel, A., St Pierre, Y., Asosingh, K., Van Riet, I., Van Camp, B. and Vanderkerken, K. (2002). Upregulation of matrix metalloproteinase-9 in murine 5T33 multiple myeloma cells by interaction with bone marrow endothelial cells. *International Journal of Cancer* 101, 512-518.

Van Wart, H. E. and Birkedal-Hansen, H. (1990). The cysteine switch: a principle of regulation of metalloproteinase activity with potential applicability to the entire matrix metalloproteinase gene family. *Proceedings of the National Academy of Sciences United States of America* 87, 5578-5582.

Vu, T. H., Shipley, J. M., Bergers, G., Berger, J. E., Helms, J. A., Hanahan, D., Shapiro, S. D., Senior, R. M. and Werb, Z. (1998). MMP-9/gelatinase B is a key regulator of growth plate angiogenesis and apoptosis of hypertrophic chondrocytes. *Cell* 93, 411-422.

Weber, M. H., Lee, J. and Orr, F. W. (2002). The effect of Neovastat (AE-941) on an experimental metastatic bone tumor model. *International Journal of Oncology* 20, 299-303.

Whitelock, J. M., Murdoch, A. D., Iozzo, R. V. and Underwood, P. A. (1996). The degradation of human endothelial cell-derived perlecan and release of bound basic fibroblast growth factor by stromelysin, collagenase, plasmin, and heparanases. *Journal of Biological Chemistry* 271, 10079-10086.

Will, H., Atkinson, S. J., Butler, G. S., Smith, B. and Murphy, G. (1996). The soluble catalytic domain of membrane type 1 matrix metalloproteinase cleaves the propeptide of progelatinase A and initiates autoproteolytic activation. Regulation by TIMP-2 and TIMP-3. *Journal of Biological Chemistry* 271, 17119-17123.

Winding, B., NicAmhlaoibh, R., Misander, H., Hoegh-Andersen, P., Andersen, T. L., Holst-Hansen, C., Heegaard, A. M., Foged, N. T., Brunner, N. and Delaisse, J. M. (2002). Synthetic matrix metalloproteinase inhibitors inhibit growth of established breast cancer osteolytic lesions and prolong survival in mice. *Clinical Cancer Research* 8, 1932-1939.

Yamamura, T., Nakanishi, K., Hiroi, S., Kumaki, F., Sato, H., Aida, S. and Kawai, T. (2002). Expression of membrane-type-1-matrix metalloproteinase and metalloproteinase-2 in nonsmall cell lung carcinomas. *Lung Cancer* 35, 249-255.

Yamashita, K., Mori, M., Kataoka, A., Inoue, H. and Sugimachi, K. (2001). The clinical significance of MMP-1 expression in oesophageal carcinoma. *British Journal of Cancer* 84, 276-282.

Yoneda, T., Sasaki, A., Dunstan, C., Williams, P. J., Bauss, F., De Clerck, Y. A. and Mundy, G. R. (1997). Inhibition of osteolytic bone metastasis of breast cancer by combined treatment with the bisphosphonate ibandronate and tissue inhibitor of the matrix metalloproteinase-2. *Journal of Clinical Investigation* 99, 2509-2517.

Yu, Q. and Stamenkovic, I. (2000). Cell surface-localized matrix metalloproteinase-9 proteolytically activates TGF-beta and promotes tumor invasion and angiogenesis. *Genes Dev* 14, 163-176.

Zhou, Z., Apte, S. S., Soininen, R., Cao, R., Baaklini, G. Y., Rauser, R. W., Wang, J., Cao, Y. and Tryggvason, K. (2000). Impaired endochondral ossification and angiogenesis in mice deficient in membrane-type matrix metalloproteinase I. *Proceedings of the National Academy of Sciences United States of America* 97, 4052-4057.

Zucker, S., Mirza, H., Conner, C. E., Lorenz, A. F., Drews, M. H., Bahou, W. F. and Jesty, J. (1998). Vascular endothelial growth factor induces tissue factor and matrix metalloproteinase production in endothelial cells: conversion of prothrombin to thrombin results in progelatinase A activation and cell proliferation. *International Journal of Cancer* 75, 780-786.

Chapter 9

ENDOTHELINS IN BONE CANCER METASTASES

Theresa A. Guise and Khalid S. Mohammad
Department of Internal Medicine, Division of Endocrinology and Metabolism, University of Virginia, Charlottesville, Virginia

INTRODUCTION

Since their isolation in 1988, endothelins have emerged as modulators of many functions including vasomotor tone, hormone production and cell proliferation. Endothelins and their receptors are expressed by many tissues, thus, it is no surprise that endothelins play an important role in the normal physiological functions and pathological states. Abundant evidence implicates a role for endothelins in cancer. This review will present evidence that endothelins play a major role in the process of cancer metastases to bone.

ENDOTHELIN STRUCTURE AND FUNCTION

Endothelin-1 (ET-1) is a potent vasoconstrictor that belongs to a family of three 21-amino-acid peptides (Yanagisawa et al., 1988, Levin et al., 1995). The endothelins mediate their effects through endothelin A (ET_A) and endothelin B (ET_B) receptors (Levin, 1995; Stern et al., 1995). ET_A receptors bind ET-1 with 10 times greater affinity than ET-3, while the B receptor binds all three endothelins with equal affinity. Most of the activities of ET-1 are mediated via ET_A receptor. The endothelin axis was originally identified in vascular endothelial cells and plays a major role in hypertension, but it is also clearly important in bone and cancer. Each

                                    Endothelins in Bone Cancer Metastases

endothelin is a product of a separate gene that codes for a large precursor-protein mRNA (Lee et al., 1990). All three endothelins bind to two endothelin receptor subtypes, ET_A and ET_B, which have been cloned and isolated and shown to be expressed in a wide variety of tissues (Arai et al., 1990; Cyr et al., 1991; Ogawa et al., 1991). The receptors are members of the superfamily of the seven transmembrane G-protein-coupled receptors linked with guanine-nucleotide-binding G proteins and range from 45,000 to 50,000 daltons in size. ET_A receptors bind ET-1 with 10 times greater affinity than ET-3, while the B receptor binds all three endothelins with equal affinity.

PATHOGENESIS OF OSTEOBLASTIC METASTASES

Osteoblastic metastases occur in most prostate cancer cases and frequently in other common malignancies, such as breast cancer (Guise et al., 1998). Osteoblastic bone lesions are rare in other malignancies, but have been reported in myeloma (Case Records, 1972), colon cancer (Paling et al., 1988), astrocytoma (Kingston et al., 1986), glioblastoma multiforme (Gamis et al., 1990), thymoma (McLennan, 1991), carcinoid (Giordano et al., 1994), nasopharyngeal carcinoma (Liaw et al., 1994), leptomeningial gliomatosis (Pingi et al., 1995), Zollinger-Ellison syndrome (Pederson et al., 1976), and cervical carcinoma (George et al., 1995). Some malignancies that typically cause osteolytic bone destruction rarely cause osteoblastic lesions. For example, patients with multiple myeloma typically develop osteolytic lesions; rarely, they develop osteosclerotic lesions associated with peripheral neuropathy most often in the context of POEMS syndrome (Sternberg et al., 2002). Patients with osteosclerotic myeloma can develop either single or multiple lesions involving the axial skeleton and long bones, but the skull is not usually involved (Lacy et al., 1997). Several factors are shown to be elevated in POEMS syndrome, including IL-1 beta, IL-6 (Gherardi et al., 1996) MMP-1, -2, -3, -9, TIMP-1 (Michizono et al., 2001) and VEGF (Watanabe et al., 1998), which may be responsible for the various manifestations of the disease.

Similar to the pathophysiology of osteolytic metastases, the seed and soil analogy of Paget can be applied to osteoblastic metastases. The tumor cells, as the seeds, secrete factors that stimulate osteoblast activity and bone formation. The bone microenvironment is enriched by osteoblast-derived growth factors, which, in turn, support the local growth of the tumor cells. Consistent with this notion, the histomorphometric studies indicate that prostate cancer osteoblastic metastases are due to tumor-produced factors that stimulate bone formation (Charhon et al., 1983; Koutsilieris, 1995).

Osteoblastic metastases are the result of an overall increase in the bone remodeling process with an imbalance between the osteoclastic bone resorption and the osteoblastic replacement of bone resorption (Boyce et al., 1999, Parfitt, 2000). Prostate cancer metastases to bone are reaction characterized by increased osteoid surface, osteoid volume and mineralization rate (Clarke et al., 1993). The newly formed bone with osteoblastic lesions is a woven bone formed of collagen fibers that are randomly oriented and loosely packed resulting in weak bone that is more susceptible to fracture (Blomme et al., 1999; Rosol, 2000).

Many tumor-associated factors have been proposed as stimulators of the disorganized new bone formation at metastases sites, including insulin-like growth factors (IGF)-1 and -2, transforming growth factor (TGFβ) β, prostate-specific antigen (PSA), urokinase-type plasminogen activator (uPA), fibroblast growth factors (FGF)-1 and -2, bone morphogenetic proteins (BMPs), platelet-derived growth factor (PDGF), and ET-1 (Charhon et al., 1983; Cohen et al., 1992; Koutsilieris et al., 1992; Cohen et al., 1993; Kanety et al., 1993; Koutsilieris et al., 1993; Achbarou et al., 1994; Thalmann et al., 1994; Conover et al., 1995; Nelson et al., 1995; 1996; Gingrich et al., 1996; Tennant et al., 1996; Guise et al., 1998; Nelson et al., 1999; Yi et al., 2002). Some of these factors, such as IGF-1 and -2, TGFβ, BMPs, PDGF, ET-1 and FGFs, directly stimulate osteoblast activity. Others, such as the proteases PSA and UPA, have indirect effects by activating latent TGFβ or by cleaving IGFs from inhibitory binding proteins, such as IGF binding protein 3 (Cohen et al., 1992; Koutsilieris et al., 1992; Cohen et al., 1993; Kanety et al., 1993; Koutsilieris et al., 1993; Conover et al., 1995; Tennant et al., 1996; Yi et al., 2002) (Figure 1). Accumulating evidence suggests a central role for ET-1 in the pathogenesis of osteoblastic metastases.

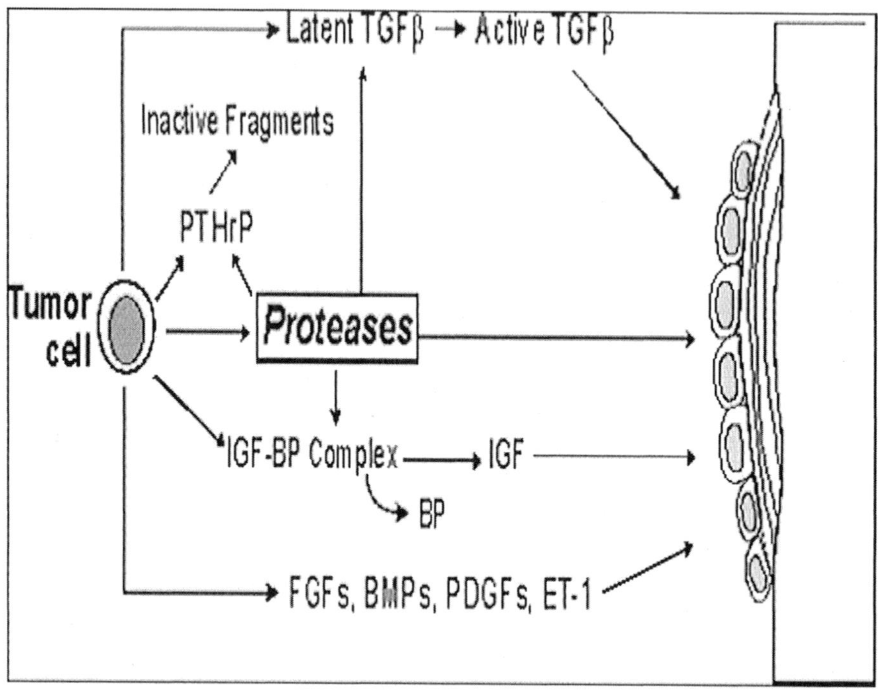

Figure 1. Tumor-produced factors implicated in the pathogenesis of osteoblastic bone metastases. Tumors make growth factors, such as FGFs, BMPs, PDGFs, ET-1 and TGFβ , which stimulate the osteoblast to form new bone. Tumor cells also produce proteases, such as PSA, uPA, prostatin, hepsin, and hK2, which have the capacity to cleave osteolytic factors, such as PTHrP, into inactive fragments or to activate TGFβ or IGFs. Modified from *Guise, T.A. and Mundy, G.R. (1998) Cancer and bone.* Endocrine Review, *19, 18-55.* Reprinted with permission from the Endocrine Society, *Copyright 1998. The Endocrine Society..*

ET-1 and Bone

ET-1 has multiple and diverse effects on bone cells, many of which are not completely understood. ET-1 and ET_A receptor-null mice die shortly after birth from respiratory failure and cardiac abnormalities (Kurihara et al., 1994; Clouthier et al., 2000). The mice also display hypoplasia of the facial bones, but the bone phenotype has not been studied in detail. Nonetheless, other studies demonstrate an active endothelin axis in bone. ET-1 has been detected in osteocytes, osteoblasts, osteoclasts and vascular endothelial cells (Sasaki et al., 1993a; 1993b). It stimulates mitogenesis in osteoblasts, which express both ET_A and ET_B receptors (Takuwa et al., 1990; Stern et al., 1995). ET-1 enhances the effect of other osteoblast-stimulatory factors, such as BMP-7, to induce bone formation (Nelson et al., 1995; Kitten et al., 1997; 2001). ET-1 stimulates phosphate transport, a process important for the initiation of bone matrix calcification, in osteoblast-like MC3T3 cells, by ET_A-mediated activation of PKC (Masukawa et al., 2001). ET-1 enhances expression of osteopontin and osteocalcin in rat osteoblastic osteosarcoma cells (Shioide et al., 1993). Hypoplasia of the facial bones in ET-1 null mice suggests that matrix mineralization of facial bones is disrupted in ET-1 null mice. In situ hybridization studies of ET-1, null mice indicate that ET-1 may regulate proliferation and migration of osteogenic cells in the maxillofacial region, rather than modulate the expression bone matrix proteins (Kitano et al., 1998).

While the stimulatory effects of ET-1 on the osteoblast are clear, its effects on bone resorption are less so. ET-1, in isolated rat osteoclasts, reduced bone resorption and motility (Alam et al., 1992), while in organ cultures it stimulated both bone resorption and bone formation (Tatrai et al., 1992). These differences may be explained by the multiple cell types present in organ cultures compared with purified osteoclast cultures. The endothelin axis may play a role in cartilage development. ET_A receptors are present in chondrocytes, and ET-1 is mitogenic for chondrocytes *in vitro* (Kinoshita et al., 1995; Lodhi et al., 1995; Kimmel et al., 2001).

ET-1 and Cancer

The endothelin axis is also active in cancer (Nelson et al., 2003a), but its role is unclear. The cancers which commonly cause osteoblastic metastases, breast and prostate, express ET-1 and receptors, suggesting that tumor-produced ET-1 may have paracrine (on bone cells) and/or autocrine (on tumor growth and apoptosis) effects. Ovarian (Rosano et al., 2001; Del Bufalo et al., 2002) and colon cancers (Asham et al., 2001) express ET-1; and ET_A receptor blockade decreased tumor growth in an animal model (Asham et al., 2001). The peptide also causes resistance of ovarian carcinoma to paclitaxel-induced apoptosis (Del Bufalo et al., 2002) and induces invasiveness through up-regulation of matrix metalloproteinases (Rosano et al., 2001). Both effects were blocked by ET_A receptor antagonists. Atrasentan (ABT-627) and ET_A receptor antagonist can inhibit both the growth and neoangiogenesis of cervical carcinoma cells allografts in nu^+/nu^+ mice (Bagnato et al., 2002). Another link was made earlier between ET-1 and the progression of neoplastic growth of HPV-associated cervical carcinoma an effect that was inhibited by ET_A receptor antagonist ABT-627 (Venuti et al., 2000; 2002). It was recently suggested that ET_B receptors have a mitogenic or anti-apoptotic effect in melanoma cells (Demunter et al., 2001). When tested in culture, ET_B receptor antagonist (BQ-788) was found to inhibit growth of human melanoma cell lines and slows the growth of human melanoma tumors in nude mice (Lahav et al., 1999).

The role of ET-1 may be different in those tumor types that cause osteoblastic metastases: prostate and breast cancer. In addition to the effects of ET-1 on growth and invasiveness, the paracrine effects of tumor-produced ET-1 on bone cells may predominate, providing a favored growth environment for tumor cells in bone. Prostate epithelium produces ET-1, and both receptors are present throughout the gland (Nelson et al., 1995; 1996; 1999). Prostate cancers express ET-1 and ET_A receptors, but express less ET_B receptors than normal prostate (Nelson et al., 1996). Exogenous ET-1 increases the proliferation of prostate cancer and enhances the mitogenic effects of IGF-1, -2, PDGF, epidermal growth factor (EGF) and FGF-2 on prostate cancer cells. These effects are mediated via ET_A receptors (Nelson et al., 1996). An association between osteoblastic metastases, prostate cancer and ET-1 was first demonstrated by Nelson et al. (Nelson et al., 1995), who showed that plasma ET-1 concentrations were significantly higher in men with advanced, hormone-refractory prostate cancer with bone metastases compared to men with organ-confined prostate cancer or normal controls (Nelson et al., 1995). However, there was no correlation between ET-1 concentrations and tumor burden, or to serum PSA concentrations. In support of this, others have shown that ET-1 production is down-regulated by androgens and up-regulated by the bone-associated factors TGFβ, EGF, IL-1-β, IL-1-α and TNF-α (Nelson et al., 1999; Le Brun et al., 1999). Co-cultures of prostate cancer and bone demonstrate that ET-1 production is increased by prostate cancer cells in contact with bone (Chiao et al., 2000). Recent data from human clinical trials demonstrated that, ET_A receptor antagonist (Atrasentan) suppressed both biochemical and clinical prostate cancer progression markers in bone (Nelson et al., 2003b).

Breast cancers also express ET-1 and are the next most common tumors to cause osteoblastic metastases. Human breast cancer cells MCF-7, T47-D and MDA-MB-231 have been shown to express the endothelin-processing enzyme necessary to convert preproET-1 to ET-1 (Patel et al., 1995; Yorimitsu et al., 1995). Another tumor model, albeit not one of metastases per se, provides evidence that tumor-produced ET-1 induces new bone formation. The WISH human tumor cell line derived from amnion, produces ET-1 and induces abundant local new bone formation when inoculated into the mouse tibia. Stable transfection of WISH with an ET-1 overexpression cDNA construct produced clones that secreted 18-fold more bioactive ET-1 than vector-only controls. After 14 days of growth in the lower leg of nu/nu mice, ET-1 overexpressing tumors produced significantly more new bone than vector-only controls. Conversely, areas of new bone formation were significantly less in animals treated with a selective ET_A receptor antagonist (Nelson et al., 1999).

Thus, substantial data associate ET-1 with osteoblastic metastases due to prostate and breast cancers. However, a direct demonstration of a causal role for ET-1 in bone metastasis has not previously been reported.

EXPERIMENTAL EVIDENCE FOR ET-1 IN THE PATHOGENESIS OF OSTEOBLASTIC METASTASES

Breast Cancer Cell Lines Cause Osteoblastic Bone Metastases in a Mouse Model

Our previous studies utilized a mouse model in which a human breast cancer line, MDA-MB-231, caused osteolytic bone lesions following inoculation into the left cardiac ventricle of nude mice (Guise et al., 1996; Yin et al., 1999). When we assessed the capacity of other cancer lines to cause bone metastases, mice inoculated into the left cardiac ventricle with ZR-75-1 cells developed radiographic-evident osteoblastic lesions over six months. Bone histology demonstrated abundant new bone formation adjacent to metastatic tumor cells. Histomorphometry performed on sections from mice bearing osteoblastic ZR-75-1 tumors and osteolytic MDA-MB-231 tumors, as well as normal control mice indicated that the increased bone matrix associated with the ZR-75-1 tumor was due to increased bone formation rather than decreased bone resorption. Conditioned media from ZR-75-1 and MDA-MB-231 were tested for their capacity to stimulate new bone formation in mouse calvarial organ cultures (Mundy et al., 1999). ZR-75-1 conditioned medium stimulated new bone formation and osteoblast proliferation, while MDA-MB-231 conditioned medium had no effect. Thus, ZR-75-1 tumor cells were secreting a factor (or factors) that stimulated osteoblast proliferation and new bone formation.

Production of Osteoblastic Factors by Breast Cancer Cells

We assayed conditioned medium or RNA from ZR-75-1 cells for: $TGF\beta$-1, -2; BMP-2, -3, -4, -6; IGF-1, -2; PSA; UPA; FGF-2; PTHrP (parathyroid hormone-related protein) and ET-1 and compared them with the osteolytic breast cancer line, MDA-MB-231. Of these factors, only ET-1 was produced in excess by ZR-75-1, compared to MDA-MB-231 cells.

ZR-75-1 Conditioned Medium and ET-1 both Stimulate New Bone formation

To determine if ET-1 was the factor responsible for the new bone formation caused by ZR-75-1, we tested the effect of ET-1 in the neonatal mouse calvarial bone formation assay. ET-1 stimulated new bone formation and osteoblast proliferation in a dose-dependent manner. An ET_A receptor antagonist, BQ-123, blocked this effect. BQ-123 also blocked new bone formation and osteoblast proliferation stimulated by ZR-75-1 conditioned media.

Correlation of Osteoblastic Bone Metastases and ET-1 Secretion by Human Cancer Cell Lines

ET-1 production was measured from other human breast and prostate cancer cell lines *in vitro*. Of the breast cancer lines, T47D, MCF-7 and BT483, both produced ET-1. Furthermore, T47D and MCF-7 caused osteoblastic metastases in the mouse model, while BT483 caused rare mixed osteolytic and osteoblastic lesions detectable only by histology. Conditioned media from MCF-7 and T47D stimulated new bone formation and osteoblast proliferation, which were blocked by ET_A antagonist BQ-123. Of the prostate cancer lines, only DU145 produced significant amounts of ET-1 *in vitro*. However, this cell line failed to cause bone metastases *in vivo*. None of the lines causing osteoblastic metastases produced the osteoclast-stimulatory factor, PTHrP. Consistent with the role of PTHrP as a mediator of osteolytic bone metastases, all cell lines that caused osteolytic bone metastases (MDA-MB-231, BT549, MDA-MB-435, PC-3 and TSU-Pr1) secreted PTHrP *in vitro*.

ET-1-Stimulates New Bone Formation via the A Receptor

To determine the relative contributions of endothelin receptor signaling to new bone formation, we tested three ET receptor antagonists: ET_A antagonist ABT-627 (Opgenorth et al., 1996), ET_B antagonist A-192621 (Von Geldern et al., 1999), and $ET_{A/B}$ antagonist A-182086 (Jae et al., 1997). ET_A selective and $ET_{A/B}$ non-selective antagonists blocked new bone formation and osteoblast proliferation, in a dose-dependent manner, in response to conditioned media from ZR-75-1 cells and ET-1. The ET_B-selective antagonist A-192621 did not do either. ET-1 plus ET_B-selective antagonist A-192621stimulated osteoblast proliferation to a greater level than ET-1 alone. The effect of the ET_A receptor-selective antagonist ABT-

627 to block ET-1-stimulated osteoblast proliferation and new bone formation was specific, since it did not block FGF-2-stimulated new bone formation.

Effects of ET$_A$ Antagonist ABT-627 on Osteoblastic Metastases

These experiments provided evidence *in vitro* that tumor-produced ET-1 caused osteoblastic metastases via the ET$_A$ receptor on osteoblasts. To test the role of ET-1 *in vivo* in the development and progression of osteoblastic metastases, female nude mice were inoculated with ZR-75-1 cells and treated with ET$_A$ antagonist ABT-627 (2 mg/kg/d and 20 mg/kg/d added to drinking water) or vehicle control. MDA-MB-231-inoculated mice were used as negative controls. By 26 weeks post inoculation, all mice in the control group had radiographic evidence of osteoblastic metastases, while no such lesions were detected in mice receiving ABT-627. Histomorphometric analysis of long bones, spine and scapula revealed that both total bone and new bone area were significantly less in the two treatment groups compared to control. ABT-627 had no effect on the development and progression of osteolytic metastases due to MDA-MB-231 cells.

These results indicated that ET$_A$ receptor blockade reduced osteoblastic bone metastases, but did not distinguish whether this was due to direct effects of the compound on tumor cells or an indirect effect to block the effects of ET-1 on the osteoblast. Consistent with the latter notion, there was no effect of ABT-627 on growth of mammary fat pad tumors due to either ZR-75-1 or MDA-MB-231.

SUMMARY AND CONCLUSIONS

Most evidence indicates that osteoblastic bone metastases are due to tumor- produced factors that stimulate the osteoblast. This review supports a causal role for ET-1. Based on our results, we propose a model to explain the tumor cell and bone interactions that are responsible for the osteoblastic response (Figure 2). Tumor cells housed in bone produce factors, such as ET-1, stimulate osteoblast activity. This results in the abundant and disorganized new bone formation that is characteristic of osteoblastic metastases. The effects of ET-1 to stimulate bone formation are mediated by ET$_A$ receptors on the osteoblast. ET$_A$ receptor inhibition successfully blocked osteoblastic bone metastases in a mouse model. These receptor antagonists are currently in clinical trials for advanced prostate cancer and bone metastases (Stephenson, 2001; Carducci et al., 2002; 2003).

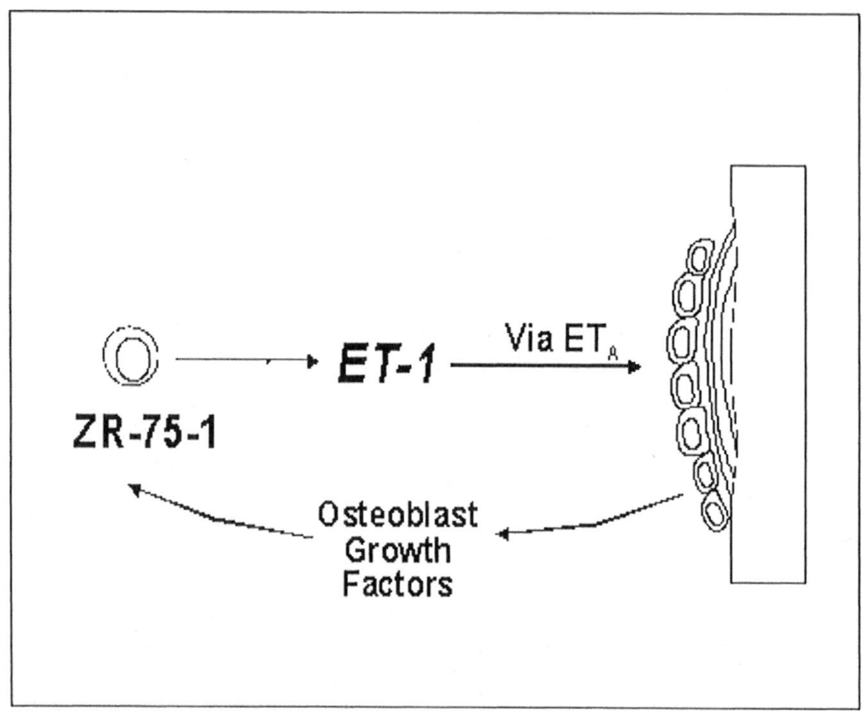

Figure 2. Proposed model for tumor cell-bone interactions that result in osteoblastic metastases. Tumor-produced ET-1 stimulates new bone formation via ET$_A$ receptor on osteoblasts. Growth factors produced by the osteoblast are incorporated into this new bone matrix as well as enrich the local microenvironment. These factors have the potential to stimulate tumor growth as well as further increase tumor production of ET-1.

Therefore, the molecular mechanisms responsible for osteoblastic metastases are complex and involve bi-directional interactions between tumor cells and bone. Elucidation of the interactions at a molecular level can identify therapeutic targets for osteoblastic metastases. Although ET-1 and ET$_A$ receptors are potential targets for this devastating complication of cancer (Remuzzi et al., 2003), they are certainly not the only ones. The rapid pace of metastasis research, will not only expand our therapeutic armamentarium against bone metastases, but will also provide insight into achieving the ultimate goal: the prevention of cancer metastases to bone.

ACKNOWLEDGMENTS

The authors thank Dr. John Chirgwin for critical review of the manuscript.
This work was supported by grants from the National Institutes of Health (CA69158 and CA40035) and the Department of Defense, U.S. Army (DAMD17-99-1-9401).

REFERENCES

Achbarou, A., Kaiser, S., Tremblay, G., Ste-Marie, L-G., Brodt, P., Goltzman, D. and Rabbani, S.A. (1994) Urokinase overproduction results in increased skeletal metastasis by prostate cancel cells in vivo. *Cancer Research*, **54**, 2372-2377.

Alam, A.S., Gallagher, A., Shankar, V., Ghatei, M.A., Datta, H.K., Huang, C.L., Moonga, B.S., Chambers, T.J., Bloom, S.R. and Zaidi, M. (1992) Endothelin inhibits osteoclastic bone resorption by a direct effect on cell motility: implications for the vascular control of bone resorption. *Endocrinology*, **130**, 3617-3624.

Asham, E., Shankar, A., Loizidou, M., Fredericks, S., Miller, K., Boulos, P.B., Burnstock, G. and Taylor, I. (2001) Increased endothelin-1 in colorectal cancer and reduction of tumour growth by ET(A) receptor antagonism. *The British Journal of Cancer*, **85**(11), 1759-1763.

Arai, H., Hori, S., Aramori, I., Ohkubo, H. and Nakanishi, S. (1990) Cloning and expression of a cDNA encoding an endothelin receptor. *Nature*, **348**(6303), 730-732.

Bagnato, A., Cirilli, A., Salani, D., Simeone, P., Muller, A., Nicotra, M.R., Natali, P.G. and Venuti A. (2002) Growth inhibition of cervix carcinoma cells in vivo by endothelin A receptor blockade. *Cancer Research*, **62**(22), 6381-6384.

Blomme, E.A., Dougherty, K.M., Pienta, K.J., Capen, C.C., Rosol, T.J. and McCauley, L.K. (1999) Skeletal metastases of prostate adenocarcinoma in rats: Morphometric analysis and role of parathyroid hormone-related protein. *Prostate*, **39**, 187-197.

Boyce, B.F., Hughes, D.E., Wirght, K.R., Xing, L. and Dai, A. (1999). Recent advances in bone biology provide insight into the pathogenesis of bone diseases. *Laboratory Investigation* **79**, 83-94.

Carducci, M.A., Nelson, J.B., Bowling, M.K., Rogers, T., Eisenberger, M.A., Sinibaldi, V., Donehower, R., Leahy, T.L., Carr, R.A., Isaacson, J.D., Janus, T.J. andre, A., Hosmane, B.S. and Padley, R.J. (2002) Atrasentan, an endothelin-receptor antagonist for refractory adenocarcinomas: safety and pharmacokinetics. *Journal of Clinical Oncology*, **20**(8), 2171-2180.

Carducci, M.A., Padley, R.J., Breul, J., Vogelzang, N.J., Zonnenberg, B.A., Daliani, D.D., Schulman, C.C., Nabulsi, A.A., Humerickhouse, R.A., Weinberg, M.A., Schmitt, J.L. and Nelson, J.B. (2003) Effect of Endothelin-A Receptor Blockade With Atrasentan on Tumor Progression in Men With Hormone-Refractory Prostate Cancer: A Randomized, Phase II, Placebo-Controlled Trial. *Journal of Clinical Oncology*, **15**;21(4), 679-689.

Case Records of the Massachusetts General Hospital (case 29-1972). (1972) *New England Journal of Medicine*, **287**, 138-143.

Charhon, S.A., Chapuy, M.C., Delvin, E.E., Valentin-Opran, A., Edouard ,C.M. and Meunier, P.J. (1983) Histomorphometric analysis of sclerotic bone metastases from prostatic carcinoma special reference to osteomalacia. *Cancer*, **51**, 918-924.

Chiao, J.W., Moonga, B.S., Yang, Y.M., Kancherla, R., Mittelman, A., Wu-Wong, J.R. and Ahmed, T. (2000) Endothelin-1 from prostate cancer cells is enhanced by bone contact which blocks osteoclastic bone resorption. *The British Journal of Cancer*, **83**(3), 360-365.

Clarke, N.W., McClure, J. and George, N.J. (1993) Osteoblast function and osteomalacia in metastatic prostate cancer. *European Urology*, **24**, 286-290.

Clouthier, D.E., Williams, S.C., Yanagisawa, H., Wieduwilt, M., Richardson, J.A. and Yanagisawa, M. (2000) Signaling pathways crucial for craniofacial development revealed by endothelin-A receptor-deficient mice. *Developmental Biology*, **217**(1), 10-24.

Cohen, P., Graves, H.C., Peehl, D.M., Kamarei, M., Giudice, L.C. and Rosenfeld, R.G. (1992) Prostate specific antigen (PSA) is an insulin-like growth factor binding protein-3 (IGFBP-3) protease found in seminal plasma. *The Journal of Clinical Endocrinology and Metabolism*, **75**, 1046-1053.

Cohen, P., Peehl, D.M., Stamey, T.A., Wilson, K.F., Clemmons, D.R. and Rosenfeld, R.G. (1993) Elevated levels of insulin-like growth factor-binding protein-2 in the serum of prostate cancer patients. *The Journal of Clinical Endocrinology and Metabolism*, **76**, 1031-1035.

Conover, C.A., Perry, J.E. and Tindall, D.J. (1995) Endogenous cathepsin D-mediated hydrolysis of insulin-like growth factor-binding proteins in cultured human prostatic carcinoma cells. *The Journal of Clinical Endocrinology and Metabolism*, **80**, 987-993.

Cyr, C., Huebner, K., Druck, T. and Kris, R. (1991) Cloning and chromosomal localization of a human endothelin ETA receptor. *Biochemical and Biophysical Research Communications*, **181**(1), 184-190.

Del Bufalo, D., Di Castro, V., Biroccio, A., Varmi, M., Salani, D., Rosano, L., Trisciuoglio, D., Spinella, F. and Bagnato, A. (2002) Endothelin-1 protects ovarian carcinoma cells against paclitaxel-induced apoptosis: requirement for Akt activation. *Molecular Pharmacology*, **61**(3), 524-532.

Demunter, A., De Wolf-Peeters, C., Degreef, H., Stas, M. and van den Oord, J.J. (2001) Expression of the endothelin-B receptor in pigment cell lesions of the skin. Evidence for its role as tumor progression marker in malignant melanoma. *Virchows Archiv* **438**(5), 485-491.

Gamis, A.S., Egelhoff, J., Roloson, G., Young, J., Woods, G.M., Newman, R. and Freeman, A.I. (1990) Diffuse bony metastases at presentation in a child with glioblastoma multiforme. A case report. *Cancer*, **66**, 180-184.

George, J. and Lai, FM. (1995) Metastatic cervical carcinoma presenting as psoas abscess and osteoblastic and lytic bony metastases. *Singapore Medical Journal*, **36**, 224-227.

Gherardi, R.K., Belec, L., Soubrier, M., Malapert, D., Zuber, M., Viard, J.P., Intrator, L., Degos, J.D. and Authier, F.J. (1996) Overproduction of proinflammatory cytokines imbalanced by their antagonists in POEMS syndrome. *Blood*, 15;87(4), 1458-65.

Gingrich, J.R., Barrios, R.J., Morton, R.A., Boyce, B.F., DeMayo, F.J., Finegold, J.J., Angelopoulou, R. and Rosen, J.M. (1996) Metastatic prostate cancer in a transgenic mouse. *Cancer Research*, **56**, 4096-4102.

Giordano, N., Nardi, P., Vigni, P., Palumbo, F., Battisti, E. and Gennari, C. (1994) Osteoblastic metastases from carcinoid tumor [letter]. *Clinical and Experimental Rheumatology*, **12**, 228-229.

Guise, T.A., Yin, J.J., Taylor, S.D., Dallas, M., Boyce, B.F., Yoneda, T., Kumaga, Y. and Mundy, G.R. (1996) Evidence for a causal role of parathyroid hormone-related protein in breast cancer mediated-osteolysis. *The Journal of Clinical Investigation*, **98**, 1544-1549.

Guise, T.A. and Mundy, G.R. (1998) Cancer and bone. *Endocrine Review*, **19**,18-55.

Jae, H-S., Winn, M., Dixon, D.B., Marsh, K.C., Nguyen, B., Opgenorth, T.J. and von Geldern, T.W. (1997) Pyrrolidine-3-carboxylic acids as endothelin antagonists. 2. Sulfonamide-based ETA/ETB mixed antagonists. *Journal of Medical Chemistry*, **40**, 3217-3227.

Kanety, H., Madjar, Y., Dagan, Y., Levi, J., Papa, M.Z., Pariente, C., Goldwasser, B. and Karasik, A. (1993) Serum insulin-like growth factor-binding protein-2 (IGFBP-2) is increased and IGFBP-3 is decreased in patients with prostate cancer: correlation with serum prostate-specific antigen. *The Journal of Clinical Endocrinology and Metabolism*, **77**, 229-233.

Kimmel, C.B., Miller, C.T. and Moens, C.B. (2001) Specification and morphogenesis of the zebrafish larval head skeleton. *Developmental Biology*, **233**(2), 239-57.

Kinoshita, A., Tamura, T., Aoki. C., Nakanishi, T., Sobue, S., Suzuki, F., Takahashi, K. and Takigawa, M. (1995) Demonstration of endothelin (ET) receptors on cultured rabbit chondrocytes and stimulation of DNA synthesis and calcium influx by ET-1 via its receptors. *Cell Biology International*, **19**(8), 647-54.

Kingston, J.E., Plowman, P.N., Smith, B.F. and Garvan, N.J. (1986) Differentiated astrocytoma with osteoblastic skeletal metastases in a child. *Child's Nervous System*, **2**, 219-221.

Kitano, Y., Kurihara, H., Kurihara, Y., Maemura, K., Ryo, Y., Yazaki, Y. and Harii, K. (1998) Gene expression of bone matrix proteins and endothelin receptors in endothelin-1-deficient mice revealed by in situ hybridization. *Journal of Bone and Mineral Research*, **13**(2), 237-44.

Kitten, A.M, Harvey, S.A., Criscimagna, N., Asher, M., Lee, J.C. and Olson, M.S. (1997) Osteogenic protein-1 downregulates endothelin A receptors in primary rat osteoblasts. *American Journal of Physiology*, **272**(6 Pt 1), E967-975.

Kitten, A.M. and Andrews, C.J. (2001) Endothelin-1 Expression in Long-Term Culture of Fetal Rat Calvarial Osteoblasts: Regulation by BMP-7. *Journal of Cellular Physiology*, 187,218-225.

Koutsilieris, M. and Polychronakos, C. (1992) Proteinolytic activity against IGF-binding proteins involved in the paracrine interactions between prostate adenocarcinoma cells and osteoblasts. *Anticancer Research*, **12**, 905-10.

Koutsilieris, M., Frenette, G., Lazure, C., Lehoux, J.G., Govindan, M.V. and Polychronakos, C. (1993) Urokinase-type plasminogen activator: a paracrine factor regulating the bioavailability of IGFs in PA-III cell-induced osteoblastic metastases. *Anticancer Reseasrch*, **13**, 481-486.

Koutsilieris, M. (1995) Skeletal metastases in advanced prostate cancer: cell biology and therapy. *Critical Reviews in Oncology / Hematology*, **18**, 51-64.

Kurihara, Y., Kurihara, H., Suzuki, H., Kodama, T., Maemura, K., Nagai, R., Oda, H., Kuwaki, T., Cao, W.H. and Kamada, N. (1994) Elevated blood pressure and craniofacial abnormalities in mice deficient in endothelin-1. *Nature*, **368**(6473), 703-710.

Lacy, M.Q., Gertz, M.A., Hanson, C.A., Inwards, D.J. and Kyle, R.A. (1997) Multiple myeloma associated with diffuse osteosclerotic bone lesions: a clinical entity distinct from osteosclerotic myeloma (POEMS syndrome). *American Journal of Hematology*, **56**(4), 288-93.

Lahav, R., Heffner, G. and Patterson, P.H. (1999) An endothelin receptor B antagonist inhibits growth and induces cell death in human melanoma cells in vitro and in vivo. *Proceedings of the National Academy of Science U S A*, **96**(20), 11496-11500.

Le Brun, G., Aubin, P., Soliman, H., Ropiquet, F., Villette, J.M., Berthon, P., Creminon, C., Cussenot, O. and Fiet, J. (1999) Upregulation of endothelin 1 and its precursor by IL-1beta, TNF-alpha, and TGF-beta in the PC3 human prostate cancer cell line. *Cytokine*, **11**, 157-162.

Lee, M.E., Bloch, K.D., Clifford, J.A. and Quertermous, T. (1990) Functional analysis of the endothelin-1 gene promoter. Evidence for an endothelial cell-specific cis-acting sequence. *The Journal of Biological Chemistry*, **265**(18), 10446-10450.

Levin, E.R. (1995) Endothelins. *New England Journal of Medicine*, **333**, 356-365.

Liaw, C.C., Ho, Y.S., Koon-Kwan,N.G., Chen, T.L. and Tzann, W.C. (1994) Nasopharyngeal carcinoma with brain metastasis: a case report. *Journal of Neurooncology*, **22**, 227-230.

Lodhi, K.M., Sakaguchi, H., Hirose, S., Shibabe, S. and Hagiwara, H. (1995) Perichondrial localization of ETA receptor in rat tracheal and xiphoid cartilage and in fetal rat epiphysis. *American Journal of Physiology*, **268**(2 Pt 1), C496-502.

Masukawa, H., Miura, Y., Sato, I., Oiso, Y. and Suzuki, A. (2001) Stimulatory effect of endothelin-1 on Na-dependent phosphate transport and its signaling mechanism in osteoblast-like cells. *Journal of Cellular Biochemistry*, **83**(1), 47-55.

McLennan, M.K. (1991) Case report 657: malignant epithelial thymoma with osteoblastic metastases. *Skeletal Radiology*, **20**, 141-144.

Michizono, K., Umehara, F., Hashiguchi, T., Arimura, K., Matsuura, E., Watanabe, O., Fujimoto, N., Okada, Y. and Osame, M. (2001) Circulating levels of MMP-1, -2, -3, -9, and TIMP-1 are increased in POEMS syndrome. *Neurology*, **27**;56(6),807-810.

Mundy, G., Garrett, R., Harris, S., Chan, J., Chen, D., Rossini, G., Boyce, B., Zhao, M. and Gutierrez, G. (1999) Stimulation of bone formation in vitro and in rodents by statins. *Science*, **286**, 1946-1949.

Nelson, J.B., Hedican, S.P., George, D.J., Reddi, A.H., Piantadosi, S., Eisenberger, M.A. and Simons, J.W. (1995) Identification of endothelin-1 in the pathophysiology of metastatic adenocarcinoma of the prostate. *Nature Medicine*, **1**, 944-949.

Nelson, J.B., Lee, W.H., Nguyen, S.H., Jarrard, D.F., Brooks, J.D., Magnuson, S.R., Opgenorth, T.J., Nelson, W.G. and Bova, G.S. (1996) Endothelin-1 production and decreased endothelin B eceptor expression in advanced prostate cancer. *Cancer Research*, **56**, 663-668.

Nelson, J.B., Nguyen, S.H., Wu-Wong, J.R., Opgenorth, T.J., Dixon, D.B., Chung, L.W. and Inoue, N. (1999) New bone formation in an osteoblastic tumor model is increased by ET-1 overexpression and decreased by ET_A receptor blockade. *Urology*, **53**, 2063-2069.

Nelson, J., Bagnato, A., Battistini, B. and Nisen, P. (2003a) The endothelin axis: emerging role in cancer. *Nature Reviews Cancer*, **3**(2),110-6.

Nelson, J.B., Nabulsi, A.A., Vogelzang, N.J., Breul, J., Zonnenberg, B.A., Daliani, D.D., Schulman, C.C. and Carducci, M.A. (2003b) Suppression of prostate cancer induced bone remodeling by the endothelin receptor A antagonist atrasentan. *The Journal of Urology*, **169**(3),1143-1149.

Ogawa, Y., Nakao, K., Arai, H., Nakagawa, O., Hosoda, K., Suga, S., Nakanishi, S. and Imura, H. (1991) Molecular cloning of a non-isopeptide-selective human endothelin receptor. *Biochemical and Biophysical Research Communications*, **178**(1), 248-55.

Opgenorth, T.J., Adler, A.L., Calzadilla, S.V., Chiou, W.J., Dayton, B.D., Dixon, D.B., Gehrke, L.J., Hernandez, L., Magnuson, S.R., Marsh, K.C., Novosad, E.I., von Geldern, T.W., Wessale, J.L., Winn, M. and Wu-Wong, J.R. (1996). Pharmacological characterization of A-127722: An orally active and highly potent ETA-selective receptor antagonist. *The Journal of Pharmacology and Experimental Theraputics*. **276**, 473-481.

Paling, M.R. and Pope, T.L. (1988) Computed tomography of isolated osteoblastic colon metastases in the bony pelvis. *Journal of Computed Tomography*, **12**, 203-207.

Parfitt, A.M. (2000) The Mechanism of coupling: A role for the vasculature. *Bone*, **26**, 319-323.

Patel, K.V. and Schrey, M.P. (1995) Human breast cancer cells contain a phosphoramidon-sensitive metalloproteinase which can process exogenous big endothelin-1 to endothelin-1: a proposed mitogen for human breast fibroblasts. *The British Journal of Cancer*, **71**, 442-447.

Pederson, R.T., Haidak, D.J., Ferris, R.A., Macdonald, J.S. and Schein, P.S. (1976) Osteoblastic bone metastasis in Zollinger-Ellison syndrome. *Radiology*, **118**, 63-64.

Pingi, A., Trasimeni, G., Di Biasi, C., Gualdi, G., Piazza, G., Corsi, F. and Chiappetta, F. (1995) Diffuse leptomeningeal gliomatosis with osteoblastic metastases and no evidence of intraaxial lesions. *American Journal of Neuroradiology*, **16**, 1018-1020.

Remuzzi, G., Perico, N. and Benigni, A. (2002) New therapeutics that antagonize endothelin: promises and frustrations. *Nature Reviews Drug Discovery*, **1**(12), 986-1001.

Rosano, L., Varmi, M., Salani, D., Di Castro, V., Spinella, F., Natali, P.G. and Bagnato, A. (2001) Endothelin-1 induces tumor proteinase activation and invasiveness of ovarian carcinoma cells. *Cancer Research*, **61**(22), 8340-6.

Rosol, T.J. (2000) Pathogenesis of bone metastases: Role of tumor-related proteins. *Journal of Bone and Mineral Research*, **15**, 844-850.

Sasaki, T. and Hong, M.H. (1993a) Endothelin-1 localization in bone cells and vascular endothelial cells in rat bone marrow. *The Anatomical Record*, **237**, 332-337.

Sasaki, T. and Hong, M.H. (1993b) Localization of endothelin-1 in the osteoclast. *Journal of Electron Microscopy*, **42**, 193-196.

Shioide, M. and Noda, M. (1993) Endothelin modulates osteopontin and osteocalcin messenger ribonucleic acid expression in rat osteoblastic osteosarcoma cells. *Journal of Cellular Biochemistry*, **53**(2), 176-80.

Stephenson, J. (2001) Experimental prostate cancer drugs slow disease progression. *The Journal of the American Medical Association*, **4**;286(1), 34.

Stern, P.H., Tatrai, A., Semler, D.E., Lee, S.K., Lakatos, P., Strieleman, P.J., Tarjan, G. and Sanders, J.L. (1995) Endothelin receptors, second messengers, and actions in bone. *The Journal of Nutrition*, **125**,(suppl), 2028S-2032S.

Sternberg, A.J., Davies, P., Macmillan, C., Abdul-Cader, A. and Swart, S. (2002) Strontium-89: a novel treatment for a case of osteosclerotic myeloma associated with life-threatening neuropathy. *The British Journal of Haematology*, **118**(3), 821-824.

Takuwa, Y., Masaki, T. and Yamashita, K. (1990) The effects of the endothelin family peptides on cultured osteoblastic cells from rat calvariae. *Biochemical and Biophysical Research Communcations*, **170**, 998-1005.

Tatrai, A., Foster, S., Lakatos, P., Shankar, G. and Stern, P.H. (1992) Endothelin-1 actions on resorption, collagen and noncollagen protein synthesis,and phosphatidylinositol turnover in bone organ cultures. *Endocrinology*, **131**(2), 603-607.

Tennant, M.K., Thrasher, J.B., Twomey, P.A., Birnbaum, R.S. and Plymate, S.R. (1996) Insulin-like growth factor-binding protein-2 and -3 expression in benign human prostate epithelium, prostate intraepithelial neoplasia, and adenocarcinoma of the prostate. *The Journal of Clinical Endocrinology and Metabolism*, **81**, 411-420.

Thalmann, G.N., Anezinis, P.E., Chang, S., Zhau, H., Kim, E.E., Hopwood, V.L., Pathak, S., von Eschenbach, A.C. and Chung, L.W.K. (1994) Androgen-independent cancer progression and bone metastasis in the LNCaP model of human prostate cancer. *Cancer Research*, **54**, 577-2581.

Venuti, A., Salani, D., Manni, V., Poggiali, F. and Bagnato, A. (2000) Expression of endothelin 1 and endothelin A receptor in HPV-associated cervical carcinoma: new potential targets for anticancer therapy. *FASEB Journal*, **14**, 2277-2283.

Venuti, A., Salani, D., Cirilli, A., Simeone, P., Muller, A., Flamini, S., Padley, R. and Bagnato, A. (2002) Endothelin receptor blockade inhibits the growth of human papillomavirus-associated cervical carcinoma. *Clinical Science* (Lond), 103 Suppl **48**,3 10S-313S.

Von Geldern, T.W., Tasker, A.S., Sorensen, B.K., Winn, M., Szczepankiewicz, B.G., Dixon, D.B., Chiou, W.J., Wang, L.,. Wessale, J.L., Adler, A., Marsh, K.C., Nguyen, B. and Opgenorth, T.J. (1999) Pyrrolidine-3-carboxylic acids as endothelin antagonists. 4. Side chain conformational restriction leads to ETB selectivity. *Journal of Medical Chemistry*, **42**, 3668-3678.

Watanabe, O., Maruyama, I., Arimura, K., Kitajima, I., Arimura, H., Hanatani, M., Matsuo, K., Arisato, T. and Osame, M. (1998) Overproduction of vascular endothelial growth factor/vascular permeability factor is causative in Crow-Fukase (POEMS) syndrome. *Muscle and Nerve*, **21**(11), 1390-7.

Yanagisawa, M., Kurihara, H., Kimura, S., Tomobe, Y., Kobayashi, M., Mitsui, Y., Yazaki, Y., Goto, K. and Masaki, T. (1988) A novel potent vasoconstrictor peptide produced by vascular endothelial cells. *Nature*, **332**, 411-415.

Yi, B., Williams, P.J., Niewolna, M., Wang, Y. and Yoneda, T. (2002) Tumor-derived platelet-derived growth factor-BB plays a critical role in osteosclerotic bone metastasis in an animal model of human breast cancer. *Cancer Research*, **62**, 917-23.

Yin, J.J., Selander, K.S., Chirgwin, J.M., Dallas, M., Grubbs, B.G., Wieser, R., Massagué, J., Mundy, G.R. and Guise, T.A. (1999) TGFβ signaling blockade inhibits parathyroid hormone-related protein secretion by breast cancer cells and bone metastases development. *The Journal of Clinical Investigation*, **103**, 197-206.

Yorimitsu, K., Moroi, K., Inagaki, N., Saito, T., Masuda, Y., Masaki, T., Seino, S. and Kimura, S. (1995) Cloning and sequencing of a human endothelin converting enzyme in renal adenocarcinoma (ACHN) cells producing endothelin-2. *Biochemical and Biophysical Research Communications*, **208**, 721-727.

Chapter 10

BISPHOSPHONATE ACTIONS ON BONE AND VISCERAL METASTASES

Toshiyuki Yoneda[1], Nobuyuki Hashimoto[1], and Toru Hiraga[2]
[1]*Endocrine Research, Department of Medicine, The University of Texas Health Science Center at San Antonio, TX;* [2]*Department of Biochemistry, Osaka University Graduate School of Dentistry, Osaka, Japan*

INTRODUCTION

Bone abundantly stores a variety of growth factors and thus provides migrating cancer cells with fertile soil. Osteoclastic bone resorption releases these growth factors providing fertile environment, which allows colonizing cancer cells to proliferate and survive. Consequently, cancer cells produce a variety of factors that in turn influence bone metabolism. This intimate partnership between cancer cells and bone will be a driving force to develop and progress bone metastases. Accordingly, suppression of osteoclastic bone resorption should be a logic approach to inhibit bone metastases. Bisphosphonates (BPs), specific inhibitors of osteoclasts, have been widely used for the treatment of bone metastases in cancer patients. In addition, recent studies suggest the possibility that BPs can reduce visceral metastases by inhibiting cell growth and inducing apoptosis in cancer cells. In this chapter, the authors will review the recent experimental results regarding the effects of BPs on bone and visceral metastases and also show their own data obtained using animal models of breast cancer metastasis. Accumulating data suggest that there is no doubt that BPs are beneficial for the treatment of existing bone metastases, while the beneficial effects of BPs on visceral metastases are not warranted yet.

CURRENT UNDERSTANDINGS OF THE MECHANISM OF OSTEOLYTIC AND OSTEOSCLEROTIC BONE METASTASES

Bone is a preferential secondary site of breast, prostate and lung cancers (Coleman, 1997). Although the precise mechanism of bone metastases is to be elucidated, it has been recognized that interactions between metastatic cancer cells and bone microenvironment are critical to the development and progression of bone metastases based on the "Seed and Soil" theory proposed by Paget (1887) (Figure 1). Bone is a storehouse of a variety of growth factors including insulin-like growth factors (IGFs), transforming growth factor β (TGFβ), fibroblast growth factors (FGFs), platelet-derived growth factors (PDGFs) and bone morphogenetic proteins (BMPs) (Hauschka et al., 1986). In physiological conditions, bone continually remodels through osteoclastic bone resorption, followed by osteoblastic bone formation to maintain its mass constant. Upon osteoclastic bone resorption, the bone-stored growth factors are released into bone marrow cavity and facilitate the subsequent osteoblastic bone formation. In bone metastases, cancer cells colonizing the marrow cavity utilize these growth factors to promote their growth and metabolic activity. Consequently, osteoblasts are supplied with limited amounts of growth factors, resulting in reduced bone formation. Under these circumstances, osteolysis progresses when cancer cells are stimulated to produce osteoclast-activating factors whereas osteosclerosis progresses when cancer cells are stimulated to produce osteoblast-activating factors. In a representative case of the osteolytic bone metastases in breast cancer, we have reported that bone-derived IGF-1 and TGFβ stimulate the growth and production of parathyroid hormone-related protein (PTH-rP) in metastatic breast cancer cells (Yin et al., 1999), respectively. PTH-rP produced by these cancer cells in turn likely to increase the expression of the receptor-activated NF-κB ligand (RANKL) in osteoblasts. RANKL subsequently binds to its cognitive receptor RANK that is expressed in cells of osteoclast lineage and enhances osteoclast activity (Thomas et al., 1999).

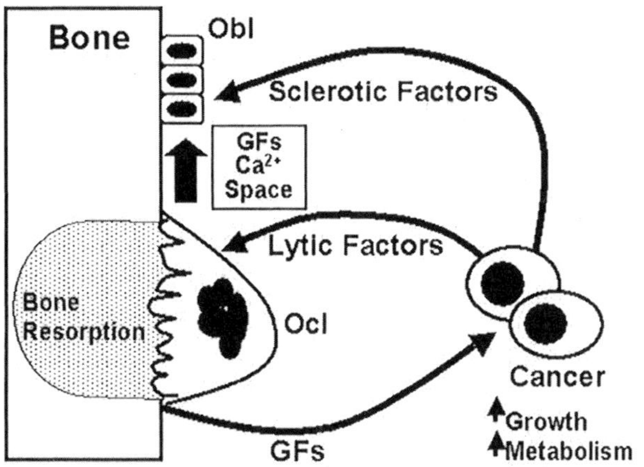

Figure 1. Cross-talk between osteoclasts (Ocl), metastatic cancer cells and osteoblasts (Obl) during the development and progression of osteolytic and osteosclerotic bone metastases. In osteolytic bone metastases, growth factors (GFs) such as IGFs and TGF released as a consequence of osteoclastic bone resorption stimulate metastatic breast cancer cells to proliferate and produce lytic factors that in turn stimulate osteoclast formation and activation. In osteosclerotic bone metastases, GFs, Ca^{2+} and space that become available following osteolysis are utilized by osteoblasts for developing sclerotic lesions. In addition, cancer cells also produce osteosclerotic factors that enhance osteoblast activity.

Most (>80%) of prostate cancers (Milch et al., 1956; Adami, 1997; Carlin and Andriole, 2000) and breast cancers (>20%) occasionally (Kamby et al., 1988) develop osteosclerotic bone metastases. Although much less is known about the mechanisms underlying osteosclerotic bone metastases than osteolytic bone metastases, it has long been recognized that blood or urinary levels of biochemical markers of bone resorption are elevated during the advancement of osteosclerotic bone metastases in prostate cancer patients (Pecherstorfer et al., 1995; Berutti et al, 2000; Garnero et al., 2000). These clinical observations suggest that osteoclastic bone resorption is involved in the pathophysiology of osteosclerotic bone metastases (Milch et al., 1956; Urwin et al., 1985; Clarke et al., 1991). It has been speculated that bone-stored growth factors and calcium that are released as a consequence of bone resorption stored in bone in turn facilitate osteoblasts to proliferate, differentiate and mineralize. In addition, tumor-derived osteosclerotic factors further promote osteosclerosis (Figure 1). We have recently reported that tumor-derived PDGF-BB is critical to the osteosclerotic bone metastases caused by the MCF-7 human breast cancer cells overexpressing the proto-oncogene *Neu* (Yi et al., 2002). Time-dependent histological examinations of this model revealed that osteoclastic bone resorption preceded osteosclerosis. Collectively, it is likely that osteoclasts play a key role in the pathophysiology of both osteolytic and osteosclerotic bone metastases. Accordingly, suppression of osteoclasts would be a logic and primary approach to inhibit bone metastases.

BISPHOSPHONATES (BPS) AND CANCER

BPs have characteristic chemical properties that confer strong affinity to bone and selective accumulation of BP in bone (Fleisch et al., 2001). BPs deposited in bone are then preferentially incorporated by osteoclasts by yet-unknown mechanisms and inhibit bone resorption through suppression of osteoclastogenesis and promotion of apoptosis in existing osteoclasts (Fleisch et al., 2001). Because of these unique properties, BPs have been widely used for cancer-related bone diseases and complications in which osteoclasts play primary roles such as bone metastases, bone pain and hypercalcemia. BPs are thus beneficial for patients with breast cancer (Hortbagyi et al., 1996; Lipton, 1997; Rosen et al., 2001a), prostate cancer (Adami, 1997; Saad et al., 2002), lung cancer (Rosen et al., 2001b) and multiple myeloma (Bataille, 1996 Berenson et al., 1996, 2002, Bloomfield, 1998 Rosen et al., 2001a, Croucher et al., 2003) who are frequently associated with these bone diseases. These accumulating results have induced the proposal that BPs are given in preventative manners to those patients who are most likely to eventually develop bone metastases. Considering preferential deposition of BPs in bone and selective inhibitory effects of BPs on osteoclasts (Fleisch et al., 2001), this proposal is tempting. There is, however, no clinical evidence that indicates that the preventative administration of BPs causes little unwanted adverse effects.

Recent in vitro studies show that BPs have direct actions on cancer cells (van der Pluijm et al., 1996; Boisser et al., 1997, 2000, Shipman et al., 1997, 1999 Fromigue et al., 2000; Lee et al., 2001). These results raise the possibility that BPs can inhibit cancer cell colonization not only in bone but also visceral organs. This is an important issue to be clarified, because most cancer patients with bone metastases usually have also developed metastases in visceral organs (Coleman and Ruben 1987, Koenders et al., 1991; Diel et al., 1998) that are the major direct cause of death. Clinical studies showed that BPs did not affect survival despite that BPs markedly reduce bone metastases (Hortobagyi et al., 1996a; Body et al., 1998; Theriault et al., 1998). These results suggest that bone metastases are not directly associated with survival and that BPs have little effects on visceral organ metastases. In contrast, a recent study described by Diel et al. (1998) suggests that the BP clodronate possesses direct anti-cancer effects on metastases in non-bone organs, thereby affecting survival. However, subsequent analogous clinical studies failed to show the beneficial effects of clodronate on visceral metastases and survival (Saart et al., 2001; Powles et al., 2002). Thus, whether BPs possess anti-cancer effects and inhibit visceral organ metastases are still controversial. Because cancer patients with bone and non-bone metastases usually receive varieties of anti-cancer treatments together with BPs, the effects of BPs alone on visceral metastases and survival are difficult to evaluate in systematic well-controlled manners in clinical studies. These studies are readily done using animal models.

In this chapter, the results of the studies in which we addressed these two important but yet-unclear issues using animal models of breast cancer metastasis will be described.

EFFECTS OF BPS ON CANCER CELLS IN BONE METASTASES

It is established that BPs inhibit the colonization of metastatic tumor cells in bone. BPs significantly decreased bone metastases and delayed the onset of skeletal events such as bone pain and hypercalcemia in patients with breast, prostate, lung cancer and multiple myeloma (Bataille, 1996; Hortobagyi et al., 1996a; Berenson et al., 1996, 2002; Lipton, 1997; Adami, 1997; Bloomfield, 1998; Body et al., 1998; Theriault et al., 1998; Mundy and Yoneda, 1998; Rosen et al., 2001a, 2001b; Croucher et al., 2001; Saad et al., 2002). There is, therefore, little doubt that BPs are beneficial agents for the treatment of patients with these bone-seeking tumors. The primary underlying mechanism of suppression of bone metastases by BPs is an inhibition of osteoclastic bone resorption. Using an animal model of the MDA-MB-231 human breast cancer, we have shown that the BP risedronate (Sasaki et al., 1995; Hughes et al., 1995) and ibandronate (Hiraga et al., 2001) suppresses bone metastases with increased apoptosis in osteoclasts. Moreover, apoptosis in MDA-MB-231 breast cancer cells in bone metastases was also promoted in BP-treated animals (Figure 2). The promotion of apoptosis in MDA-MB-231 cells could be due to either restriction of the supply of bone-stored growth factors due to an inhibition of osteoclastic bone resorption by BPs or direct effects of BPs (Figure 3). We observed that high concentrations of BPs (10^{-5} to 10^{-4}M) increased apoptosis in MDA-MB-231 cells (Hiraga et al., 2001) and the 4T1 mouse breast cancer cells in culture (Hiraga et al., in press). However, these concentrations of BPs also induced apoptosis in bone marrow cells in culture (Hiraga et al., in press).

Since apoptosis in bone marrow cells is not increased despite that cancer cells showed enhanced apoptosis in bone metastases in BP-treated animals, it seems that apoptosis-inducing effects of BPs on cancer cells in bone metastases are indirect rather than direct.

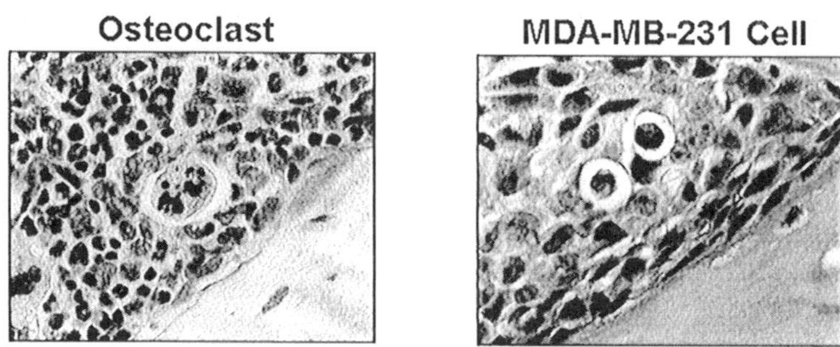

Figure 2. Apoptosis of osteoclasts (left) and the MDA-MB-231 human breast cancer cells (right) in bone metastases in BP-treated animals. A multinucleated osteoclast detaches from the endosteal bone surface and shows apoptosis with nuclear condensation (left) (HE, x100). Two MDA-MB-231 cells in the vicinity of the endosteal bone surface show apoptosis (right) (HE, x200). Because of rapid shrinkage of cell body, apoptotic MDA-MB-231 cells are usually surrounded by characteristic amorphous space.

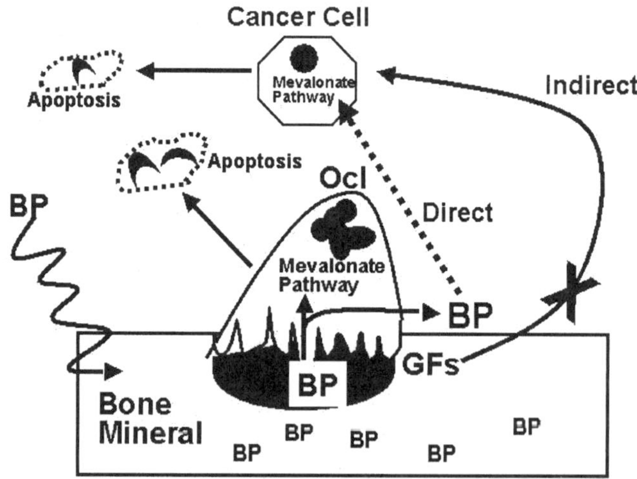

Figure 3. BP actions in bone metastasis. BPs preferentially deposit in bone due to strong affinity to bone minerals. BPs are then selectively incorporated by osteoclasts (Ocl) through yet-unknown mechanism and induce apoptosis partly through inhibiting mevalonate pathway. Extra BPs are moved to the basolateral side of osteoclasts presumably by transcytosis and released into the marrow cavity. (Continued on next page)

(Fig. 3 legend continued)
The released BPs may directly induce apoptosis in metastatic cancer cells through an inhibition of mevalonate pathway. Alternatively, inhibition of osteoclastic bone resorption by BPs restricts the supply of bone-stored growth factors (GFs) to metastatic cancer cells, thereby inducing apoptosis.

EFFECTS OF PREVENTATIVE ADMINISTRATION OF BPS ON BONE METASTASES

Preventative administration of BPs for breast cancer patients who have predisposition to bone metastases later in their clinical course has been suggested. Considering preferential accumulation of BPs in bone (Fleisch et al., 2001), BPs likely cause little adverse effects in non-bone organs. However, several experimental in vivo studies have reported increased visceral metastases following BP administration (Kostenuik et al., 1993; Sasaki et al., 1995; Stearns et al., 1996). We studied the effects of preventative administration of the BP ibandronate using two different animal models of bone metastases (Michigami et al., 2002). In the orthotopic model of the 4T1 mouse breast cancer that spontaneously develops metastases to bone, lung and liver following intramammary inoculation of cells (Yoneda et al., 2000), the preventative administration of ibandronate markedly inhibited the development of new bone metastases with reduced osteoclastic bone resorption (Michigami et al., 2002). On the other hand, lung and liver metastases were not reduced by ibandronate, demonstrating that ibandronate had no effects on visceral metastases of 4T1 tumors. ON the other hand, in the heart inoculation model of the MDA-MB-231 human breast cancer that develops bone and adrenal metastases, the preventative administration of ibandronate increased adrenal metastases with a profound reduction in bone metastases. In contrast, the therapeutic administration in which ibandronate was given for established bone metastases showed no effects on the adrenal metastases. Although the mechanism underlying increased adrenal metastases by the preventative administration is unknown, these results suggest that the preventative administration of BPs may promote visceral metastases of breast cancer in certain situations. In these particular experiments, mice received ibandronate alone (no anti-cancer treatments) by daily sc injections for longer than 4 weeks. In the clinical settings, breast cancer patients receive BPs at much less frequency and always have been treated with anti-cancer agents while BPs are given. In fact, we observed no increases in the adrenal metastases when a potent anti-cancer agent doxorubicin was co-administered with ibandronate (Michigami et al., 2002). These results suggest that BPs definitely inhibit bone metastases of breast cancer regardless of the administration protocols. However, it still remains possible that the preventative administration of BPs causes adverse effects on visceral metastases. The American Society for Clinical Oncology (ASCO) guideline proposes that BP administration is not recommended for the treatment of breast cancer patients without clinical evidence of bone metastases (Hillner et al., 2000). Collectively, the current situation suggests that the preventative administration of BPs may not be feasible for cancer patients with visceral metastases and no clinically-detectable bone metastases. Since our experimental data suggest that co-administration of anti-cancer agents blocks an increase in visceral metastases, the usefulness of preventative administration of BPs can be evaluated in clinical studies.

EFFECTS OF COMBINATION OF BPS AND ANTI-CANCER AGENTS ON BONE METASTASES

In the most experiments described above, tumor-bearing mice were treated with only BPs and no anti-cancer therapies were given. This therapeutic regimen is far different from that in breast cancer patients with bone metastases who are primarily treated with anti-cancer agents and given BP as an adjuvant agent only when necessary. In fact, most clinical studies have been performed using BP in combination with conventional anti-cancer therapies (Hortobagyi et al., 1996a; Diel et al., 1998 Body et al., 1998; Theriault et al., 1998). We examined the effects of one of the most potent BPs zoledronic acid (ZOL) combined with an oral anti-cancer agent UFT on bone metastases using an orthotopic bone metastasis model of the 4T1 mouse breast cancer (Yoneda et al., 2000). The fluoropyrimidine 5-fluorouracil (5-FU) is one of the most widely-used chemotherapeutic agents for the treatment of breast cancer (Hortobagyi et al., 1996b). Recently, several oral fluoropyrimidines with improved safety profile and equivalent/superior efficacy compared with intravenous 5-FU have been developed (Ho et al., 1998). UFT is one of the oral anticancer agents consisting of tegafur, a prodrug of fluorouracil, and uracil that inhibits the degradation of fluorouracil at a molar ration of 1:4 (Takiuchi et al., 1998). Although UFT is shown to have therapeutic effects in breast cancer patients (Tashiro et al., 1994), the effects on bone metastasis are unknown. ZOL is one of the newest generation BPs with the most potent inhibitory effects on osteoclastic bone resorption among currently-existing BPs (Green et al., 1994; Fleisch et al., 2001). Phase III clinical trials in cancer patients have recently been completed and the compound is now registered in the U.S. and Europe for the treatment of bone metastases associated with a wide variety of tumors (Rosen et al., 2001a). However, the effects of ZOL combined with anti-cancer agents on bone metastases in breast cancer are unknown.

In these experiments, ZOL was administered by single bolus iv injection and UFT was given orally once a day from 7 days after 4T1 tumor inoculation to the end of the experiments (Hiraga et al., in press). UFT alone significantly suppressed tumor formation at the orthotopic inoculation site. UFT also inhibited bone metastases probably through inhibiting primary tumor development. As expected, ZOL alone markedly reduced bone metastases and, to our surprise, it decreased lung and liver metastases as well. Moreover, combination of ZOL and UFT decreased not only bone metastases but also lung and liver metastases in an additive fashion (Hiraga et al., in press, manuscript in preparation). It is speculated that ZOL has direct effects on 4T1 cells and thus is different from other BPs.

EFFECTS OF BPS ON OSTEOSCLEROTIC BONE METASTASES

Prostate cancer has a predilection for spreading to bone and almost all of bone metastases of prostate cancer are osteosclerotic (Milch et al., 1956; Adami, 1997; Carlin and Andriole, 2000). The well-recognized clinical observations that biochemical and histomorphometrical indicators of bone resorption are increased during the advancement of osteosclerosis (Pecherstorfer et al., 1995; Berruti et al., 2000; Garnero et al., 2000) suggest that osteoclasts contribute to the pathophysiology of osteosclerotic bone metastases in prostate cancer. In support of this notion, a recent clinical study has reported that ZOL significantly reduces skeletal-related events in prostate cancers (Saad et al., 2002). To study the mechanism of action of BPs on osteosclerotic bone metastases in prostate cancer, animal models are useful. Unfortunately, however, there are currently few animal models of prostate cancer that reproducibly develop osteosclerotic bone metastases. Lack of consistent animal models is one of the major reasons for our limited understandings of the mechanism of osteosclerosis in bone metastasis in prostate cancers. We have recently found that the MCF-7 human estrogen-dependent breast cancer cells form osteosclerotic bone metastases following heart inoculation into female nude mice (Yi et al., 2002). Of note, histological examinations revealed that osteoclastic bone resorption was predominant at the early stages and that these osteolytic lesions are progressively replaced by osteosclerotic lesions as a function of time. Thus, although MCF-7 cancer is not a prostate cancer, this model appears to be suitable to test the effects of BP on the development of osteosclerotic bone metastases and to examine the longstanding notion that precedence of osteolysis is necessary for the development of osteosclerotic bone metastases (Milch et al., 1956). Using this newly-established model of osteosclerotic bone metastasis of breast cancer, we examined the effects of the BP ibandronate. One group of mice received daily subcutaneous ibandronate injections from 7 days before cell inoculation to 4 weeks after the inoculation to inhibit the osteolysis at the early stage, left untreated thereafter and sacrificed 10 weeks after inoculation (early treatment). Another group of mice received ibandronate from 6 to 10 weeks after cell inoculation during which period osteosclerosis predominantly takes place and sacrificed at week 10 (late treatment). Both group of mice received the same total amount of ibandronate. Our data showed that early treatment inhibited the development of the osteosclerotic bone metastases, whereas late treatment failed to inhibit them. These results demonstrate that inhibition of early osteoclastic bone resorption by ibandronate inhibits the following development of osteosclerotic bone metastases and thus suggest that bone resorption is necessary for the subsequent development of osteosclerotic bone metastases in this model. They also suggest that BPs may have therapeutic effects on osteosclerotic bone metastases in prostate cancer when administered at the stage of predominant osteolysis. These results need to be verified using prostate cancer models that consistently develop osteosclerotic bone metastases.

EFFECTS OF BPS ON CANCER CELLS IN NON-BONE SITES

Recent studies have reported that BPs reduce cell growth, induce apoptosis and inhibit invasion and attachment to bone matrix in various types of tumor cells in culture (van der Pluijm et al., 1996; Boisser et al., 1997, 2000; Fromigue et al., 2000; Lee et al., 2001), demonstrating direct effects of BPs on tumor cells. BPs are found to inhibit the mevalonate pathway, leading to a suppression of prenylation of small G proteins (Shipman et al., 1997, 1999; Luckman et al., 1998; Fisher et al., 1999). However, it should be pointed that the effective concentrations in these studies are relatively high. Consistent with these reports, our data showed that ibandronate increased apoptosis in MDA-MB-231 cells in culture only at concentrations as high as 10^{-4}M (Hiraga et al., 2001). Although the concentration of BPs could reach this level in bone (Sato et al., 1991), it is unlikely that BPs deposit at such high levels in visceral organs in vivo given their chemical properties (Fleisch et al., 2001). Furthermore, the effect is unlikely specific for MDA-MB-231 cells, since 10^{-4}M ibandronate also increased apoptosis in bone marrow cells (Hiraga et al., in press) and inhibited cell growth in osteoblasts, stromal cells and fibroblasts in culture (unpublished observations). Thus, the in vitro results should be cautiously interpreted and are not conclusive enough to propose direct anti-cancer effects of BPs.

As a piece of clinical evidence for anti-cancer action of BPs, Diel et al. (1998) have reported that breast cancer patients treated with the BP clodronate together with the conventional anti-cancer therapies show not only decreased bone metastases but also reduced visceral metastases and improved survival compared with the patients treated with the conventional anti-cancer therapies alone. This report caused a sensation in the field, because BPs will be then further beneficial for breast cancer patients who, in most cases, have developed visceral metastases when bone metastases are detected. Three years later, however, Saarto et al. (2001) published a contrasting report describing that clodronate increased visceral metastases and decreased survival in breast cancer patients. As an unexpected result in this study is that clodronate showed little effects on bone metastases. Subsequently, Powles et al. (2002) have reported that clodronate significantly inhibits bone metastases, whereas visceral metastases are not decreased but survival is prolonged. To make story more complicated, Diel et al. (2000) later found no significant effects of clodronate on the visceral metastases in the same populations of patients in their extended follow-up study. These apparently conflicting results suggest that anti-cancer effects of clodronate are marginal, if any. Prolonged survival in clodronate-treated breast cancer patients in the studies of Diel et al. (1998) and Powles et al. (2002) could be due to improved performance status and quality of life resulting from an inhibition of bone metastases. In support of this notion, we observed that a suppression of bone metastases by the BP risedronate significantly extended survival of MDA-MB-231 tumor-bearing animals (Sasaki et al., 1995). In summary, the results to date does not show compelling evidence that BPs possess direct anti-cancer actions. Moreover, from oncological points of view, even if BPs are proved to directly inhibit cell growth and promote apoptosis in cancer cells, these effects of BPs are probably much less potent than conventional anti-cancer agents. Accordingly, it is most reasonable to use BPs as an ajuvant in the treatments of cancer patients with bone and visceral metastases.

CONCLUSION

Inhibitory effects of BPs on bone metastases are established. The effects are in most of the part due to an inhibition of osteoclast activity, which secondarily suppresses cell growth and promotes apoptosis in cancer cells in bone metastases. In contrast, direct effects of BPs on cancer cells are still unclear. Although in vitro data that BPs have direct effects on various types of tumor cells are accumulating, requirement of relatively high concentrations and BP inhibition of cell growth and promotion of apoptosis in bone marrow cells, osteoblasts and stromal cells at these concentrations suggest that these effects are non-specific. In addition, BP potency of inhibition of cell growth and promotion of apoptosis is marginal, if any, compared with conventional chemotherapeutic agents. Thus, it is unlikely that BPs significantly suppress cancer cells in non-bone sites where BPs do not deposit as high levels as in bone and osteoclasts are absent. Meanwhile, our in vivo results using ZOL raise the possibility that modification of the chemical structure endows BPs with yet-unknown additional actions. To search for such actions, new assay systems based on the concepts apart from what we know about bone biology may need to be developed. In this context, it should be noted that recent studies have reported previously-unknown effects of BPs using unique assay systems (Sawada et al., 2002; Fournier et al., 2002). Development of new study models should also be useful to differentiate the action of individual BP. It is anticipated that such approaches will allow us to identify novel beneficial effects of BPs and expand the use of BPs for not only bone-related diseases non-bone diseases.

ACKNOWLEDGMENTS

The authors thank Roche, Novartis, and Taiho Pharmaceutical Company for providing us with ibandronate, zoledronic acid and UFT, respectively. The authors also thank Miss Hisako Takeuchi for her excellent secretarial assistance.

This work was supported by NIH Grants PO1-CA40035, RO1-AR28149 and RO1-DK45229

REFERENCES

Adami, S. (1997) Bisphosphonates in prostate carcinoma. *Cancer*, **80**, 1674-1679.
Bataille, R. (1996) Management of myeloma with bisphosphonates. *New England Journal of Medicine*, **334**, 529-535.

Berenson, J.R., Lichtehstein, A., Porter, L., Dimopoulos, M.A., Bordoni, R., George, S., Lipton, A., Keller, A., Ballester, O., Kovacs, M.J., Blacklock, H.A., Bell, R., Simeone, J., Reitsman, D.J., Heffernan, M., Seaman, J. and Knight, R.D. (1996) Efficacy of pamidronate in reducing the skeletal events in patients with advanced multiple myeloma. *New England Journal of Medicine*, **334**, 488-493.

Berenson, J.R., Hillner, B.E., Kyle, R.A., Anderson, K., Lipton, A., Yee, G.C. and Biermann, J.S. (2002) American Society of Clinical Oncology Bisphosphonates Expert Panel American Society of Clinical Oncology clinical practice guidelines: the role of bisphosphonates in multiple myeloma. *Journal of Clinical Oncology*, **20**, 3719-3736.

Berruti, A., Dogliotti, L., Bitossi, R., Fasolis, G., Gorzegno, G., Bellina, M., Torta, M., Porpiglia, F., Fontana, D. and Angeli, A.l. (2000) Incidence of skeletal complications in patients with bone metastatic prostate cancer and hormone refractory disease: predictive role of bone resorption and formation markers evaluated at baseline. *Journal of Urology*, **164**, 1248-1253.

Bloomfield, D.J. (1998) Should bisphosphonates be part of the standard therapy of patients with multiple myeloma or bone metastases from other cancers? An evidence-based review. *Journal of Clinical Oncology*, **16**, 1218-1225.

Body, J.J., Bartl, R., Burckhardt, P., Delmas, P.D., Diel, I.J., Fleish, H., Kanis, J.A., Kyle, R.A., Mundy, G.R. and Paterson, A. H. G. Rubens, R. D. (1998) Current use of bisphosphonates in oncology. *Journal of Clinical Oncology*, **16**, 3890-3899.

Boisser, S., Magnetto, S., Frappart, L., Cuzin, B., Ebetino, F.H., Delmas, P.D. and Clezardin, P. (1997) Bisphosphonates inhibit prostate and breast carcinoma cell adhesion to unmineralized and mineralized bone extracellular matrices. *Cancer Research*, **57**, 3890-3894.

Boissier, S., Ferreras, M., Peyruchaud, O., Magnetto, S., Ebetino, F.H., Colombel, M., Delmas, P., Delaisse, J.M. and Clezardin, P. (2000) Bisphosphonates inhibit breast and prostate carcinoma cell invasion, an early event in the formation of bone metastases. *Cancer Research*, **60**, 2949-2954.

Carlin, BI. and Andriole, GL. (2000) The natural history, skeletal complications, and management of bone metastases in patients with prostate carcinoma. *Cancer*, **88**, (12 Suppl), 2989-2994.

Clarke, N.W., McClure, J. and George, N.J.R. (1991) Morphometric evidence for bone resorption and replacement in prostate cancer. *British Journal of Urology*, **68**, 74-80.

Coleman, R.E. and Rubens, R.D. (1987) The clinical course of bone metastases from breast cancer. *British Journal of Cancer*, **55**, 61-66.

Coleman, R.E. (1997) Skeletal Complications of malignancy. *Cancer*, **80**, 1588-1594.

Croucher, P.I., De, Hendrik. R., Perry, MJ., Hijzen, A., Shipman, C.M., Lippitt, J., Green, J., Van, Marck. E., Van, Camp. B. and Vanderkerken, K. (2003) Zoledronic acid treatment of 5T2MM-bearing mice inhibits the development of myeloma bone disease: evidence for decreased osteolysis, tumor burden and angiogenesis, and increased survival. *Journal of Bone and Mineral Research*, **18**, 482-492.

Diel, I.J., Solomayer, E-F., Costa, S.D., Gollan, C., Goerner, R., Wallwiener, D., Kaufmann, M. and Bastert, G.. (1998) Reduction in new metastases in breast cancer with adjuvant clodronate treatment. *New England Journal of Medicine*, **339**, 357-363.

Diel, I.J., Solomayer, E-F., Gollan, C., Shutz, F. and Bastert, G. (2000) Bisphosphonates in the reduction of metastases in breast cancer-Results of the extended follow-up of the first study population. *Proceedings of the American Society for Clinical Oncology (ASCO)* Abst # 314

Fisher, J.E., Rogers, M.J., Halasy, J.M., Luckman, S.P., Hughes, D.E., Masarachia, P.J., Wesolowski, G., Russel, R.G.G., Rodan, G.A. and Reszka, A.A. (1999) Alendronate mechanism of action: geranylgeraniol, an intermediate in the mevalonate pathway, prevents inhibition of osteoclast formation, bone resorption, and kinase activation in vitro. *Proceedings of the National Academy of Sciences of the United States of America*, **96**, 133-138.

Fleisch, H., Reszka, A., Rodan, G., Rogers, M. (2001) Bisphosphonates: Mechanism of action. In Principles of Bone Biology (Eds. Bilezikian JP, Raisz LG, Rodan GA), Academic Press, San Diego, pp.1361-1385.

Fournier, P., Boissier, S., Filleur, S., Guglielmi, J., Cabon, F., Colombel, M. and Clezardin, P. (2002) Bisphosphonates inhibit angiogenesis in vitro and testosterone-stimulated vascular regrowth in the ventral prostate in castrated rats. *Cancer Research*, **62**, 6538-6544.

Fromigue, O., Lagneaux, L. and Body, J.J. (2000) Bisphosphonates induce breast cancer cell death in vitro. *Journal of Bone and Mineral Research*, **45**, 2211-2221.

Garnero, P., Buchs, N., Zekri, J., Rizzoli, R., Coleman, RE. and Delmas, P.D. (2000) Markers of bone turnover for the management of patients with bone metastases from prostate cancer. *British Journal of Cancer*, **82**, 858-864.

Green, J.R., Muller, K. and Jaeggi, K.A. (1994) Preclinical pharmacology of CGP 42'446, a new, potent, heterocyclic bisphosphonate compound. *Journal of Bone and Mineral Research*, **9**, 745-751.

Hauschka, PV., Manrakos, A.E., Iafrati, M.D., Doleman, S.E. and Klagsbrun, M. (1986) Growth factors in bone matrix. Isolation of multiple types of affinity chromatography on heparin sepharose. *Journal of Biological Chemistry*, **261**, 12665-12674.

Hillner, B.E., Ingle, J.N., Berenson, J.R., Janjan, N.A., Albain, K.S., Lipton, A., Yee, G., Biermann, J.S., Chlebowski, RT. and Pfister, D.G. (2000) American society of clinical oncology guideline on the role of bisphosphonates in breast cancer. *Journal of Clinical Oncology*, **18**, 1378-1391.

Hiraga, T., Williams, P.J., Mundy, G..R. and Yoneda, T. (2001) The bisphosphonate ibandronate promotes apoptosis in MDA-231 human breast cancer cells in bone metastases. *Cancer Research*, **61**, 4418-4424.

Hiraga, T., Ueda, A., Tamura, D., Hata, K., Williams, P.J., Ikeda, F., Yoneda, T. Effects of oral UFT combined with or without zoledronic acid on distant metastasis in the 4T1/luc mouse breast cancer. *Cancer* (in press).

Ho, DH., Pazdur, R., Covington, W., Brown, N., Huo, Y.Y., Lassere, Y. and Kuritani, J. (1998) Comparison of 5-fluorouracil pharmacokinetics in patients receiving continuous 5-fluorouracil infusion and oral uracil plus N1-(2'-tetrahydrofuryl)-5-fluorouracil. *Clinical Cancer Research*, **4**, 2085-2088.

Hortobagyi, G.N., Theriault, R.L., Porter, L., Blayney, D., Lipton, A., Sinoff, C., Wheeler, H., Simeone, J.F., Seaman, J., Knight, R.D., Heffernan, M. and Reitsman, D.J. (1996a) Efficacy of pamidronate in reducing skeletal complications in patients with breast cancer and lytic bone metastases. *New England Journal of Medicine*, **335**, 1785-1791.

Hortobagyi, GN. and Piccart-Gebhart, MJ. (1996b) Current management of advanced breast cancer. *Seminars in Oncology*, **23** (Suppl. 11), 1-5.

Hughes, D.E., Wright, K.R., Uy, H.L., Sasaki, A., Yoneda, T., Roodman, G.D., Mundy, G.R. and Boyce, B.F.(1995) Bisphosphonates promote apoptosis in murine osteoclasts in vitro and in vivo. *Journal of Bone and Mineral Research*, **10**, 1478-1487.

Kamby, C., Andersen, J., Ejlertsen, B., Birkler, N.E., Rytter, L., Zedeler, K., Thorpe, S.M., Norgaard, T., Rose, C. (1988) Histological grade and steroid receptor content of primary breast cancer – impact on prognosis and possible modes of action. *British Journal of Cancer*, **58**, 480-486.

Koenders, P.G., Beex, L.V.A.M., Langens, R., Kloppenborg, P.W.C., Smals, A.G.H. and Benraad, T.H.J. (1991) Breast cancer study group. *Breast Cancer Research and Treatment*, **18**, 27-32.

Kostenuik, P.J., Orr, F.W., Suyama, K. and Singh, G. (1993) Increased growth rate and tumor burden of spontaneously metastatic Walker 256 cancer cells in the skeleton of bisphosphonates-treated rats. *Cancer Research*, **53**, 5452-5457.

Lee, M.V., Fong, E.M., Singer, F.R. and Guenette, R.S. (2001) Bisphosphonate treatment inhibits the growth of prostate cancer cells. *Cancer Research*, **61**, 2602-260.

Lipton, A. (1997) Bisphosphonates and breast cancer. *Cancer*, **80**, 1668-1673.

Luckman, S.P., Hughes, D.E., Coxon, F. P., Russell, R.G.G. and Rogers, M.J. (1998) Nitrogen-containing bisphosphonates inhibit the mevalonate pathway and prevent post-transitional prenylation of GTP-binding proteins, including Ras. *Journal of Bone and Mineral Research,* **13**, 581-589.

Michigami, T., Hiraga, T., Williams, P.J., Nishimura, R., Mundy, G.R. and Yoneda, T. (2002) The effect of the bisphosphonate ibandronate on breast cancer metastasis to visceral organs. *Breast Cancer Research and Treatment*, **75**, 249-258.

Milch, R.A. and Changus, G.W. (1956) Response of bone to tumor invasion. *Cancer*, **9**, 340-351.

Mundy, G.R. and Yoneda, T. (1998) Bisphosphonates as anticancer drug. *New England Journal of Medicine*, **339**, 357-363.

Paget, S. (1889) The distribution of secondary growths in cancer of the breast. *Lancet*, **1**, 571-573.

Pecherstorfer, M., Ludwig, H., Zimmer-Roth, H., Schiling, T., Woitge, H.W., Schmidt, H., Baumgartner, G., Thiebaud, D., Ludwig, H. and Seibel, M.J. (1995) The diagnostic value of urinary pyridinium cross-links of collagen, alkaline phosphatase and urinary calcium excretion in neoplastic bone disease. *The Journal of Clinical Endocrinology and Metabolism*, **121**, 542-548.

Powles, T., Paterson, S., Kanis, J.A., McCloskey, E., Ashley, S., Tidy, A., Rosenqvist, K., Smith, I., Ottestad, L., Legault, S., Pajunen, M., Nevantaus, A., Männistö, E., Suovuori, A., Atula, S., Nevalainen, J. and Pylkkänen, L. (2002) Randomized, placebo-controlled trial of clodronate in patients with primary operable breast cancer. *Journal of Clinical Oncology*, **20**, 3219-3224.

Rosen, L.S., Gordon, D., Kaminski, M., Howell, A., Belch, A., Mackey, J.A., Apffelstaedt, J., Hussein, M., Coleman, RE., Reitsma, D.J., Seaman, J.J., Chen, B.L., Ambros, Y. (2001a) Zoledronic acid versus pamidronate in the treatment of skeletal metastases in patients with breas cancer or osteolytic lesions of multiple myeloma: a phase III, double-blind, comparative trial. *Cancer*, **7**, 377-387.

Rosen, L., Gordon, D. and Tchekmedyian, S. (2001b) Zometa significantly increased the median time to first skeletal related event (SRE) in patients with osteolytic bone metastases from non-small cell lung cancer (NSCLC) and other solid tumors (OST). *Lung Cancer*, **34**, Suppl 1.

Saad, F., Gleason, DM., Murray, R., Tchekmedyian, S., Venner, P., Lacombe, L., Chin, J.L., Vinholes, J.J., Goas, J.A. and Chen, B. (2002) Zoledronic Acid Prostate Cancer Study Group. A randomized, placebo-controlled trial of zoledronic acid in patients with hormone-refractory metastatic prostate carcinoma. *Journal of the National Cancer Institute*, **94**, 1458-1468.

Saarto, T., Blomqvist, C., Virkkunen, P. and Elomaa, I.I. (2001) Adjuvant clodronate treatment does not reduce the frequency of skeletal metastases in node-positive breast cancer patients: 5-year results of a randomized controlled trial. *Journal of Clinical Oncology,* **19**, 10-17.

Sasaki, A., Boyce, B.F., Story, B., Wright, K.R., Chapman, M., Boyce, R., Mundy, G.R. and Yoneda, T. (1995) Bisphosphonate risedronate reduces metastatic human breast cancer burden in bone in nude mice. *Cancer Research,* **55**, 3551-3557.

Sato, M., Grasser, W., Endo, N., Akins, R., Simmons, H., Thompson, D.D., Golub, E. and Rodan, G.A. (1991) Bisphosphonate action. Alendronate localization in rat bone and effects on osteoclast ultrastructure. *Journal of Clinical Investigation,* **88**, 2095-2105.

Sawada, K., Morishige, K., Tahara, M., Kawagishi, R., Ikebuchi, Y., Tasaka, K. and Murata, Y. (2002) Alendronate inhibits lysophosphatidic acid-induced migration of human ovarian cancer cells by attenuating the activation of Rho. *Cancer Research,* **62**, 6015-6020.

Shipman, C.M., Rogers, M.J., Apperley, J.F., Russell, R.G.G. and Croucher, P.I. (1997) Bisphosphonate induces apoptosis in human myeloma cell lines: a novel anti-tumour activity. *British Journal of Haematology,* **98**, 665-672.

Shipman, C.M., Croucher, P.I., Russell, R.G.G., Helfrich, M.H. and Rogers, M.J. (1999) The bisphosphonate incadronate (YM175) causes apoptosis of human myeloma cells in vitro by inhibiting the mevalonate pathway. *Cancer Research,* **58**, 5294-5297.

Stearns, M.E. and Wang, M. (1996) Effects of alendronate and taxol on PC-3ML cell bone metastases in SCID mice. *Invasion and Metastasis,* **16**, 116-131.

Takiuchi, H. and Ajani, JA. (1998) Uracil-tegafur in gastric carcinoma: A comprehensive review. *Journal of Clinical Oncology,* **16**, 2877-2885.

Tashiro, H., Nomura, Y. and Ohsaki, A. (1994) A double blind comparative study of tegafur (FT) and UFT (a comibantion of tegafur and uracil) in advanced breast cancer. *Japanese Journal of Clinical Oncology,* **24**, 212-217.

Theriault, R.L., Hortobagyi, G.N., Leff, R., Gluck, S., Stewart, J.F., Costello, S., Kennedy, I., Simeone, J., Seaman, J.J., Knight, R.D., Mellars, K., Heffernan, M. and Reitsman, D.J. (1999) Pamidronate reduces skeletal morbidity in women with advanced breast cancer and lytic bone lesions: A randomized, placebo-controlled trial. *Journal of Clinical Oncology,* **17**, 846-854.

Thomas, R.J., Guise, T.A., Yin, J.J., Elliott, J., Horwood, N.J., Martin, T.J. and Gillespie, M.T. (1999) Breast cancer cells interact with osteoblasts to support osteoclasts formation. *Endocrinology,* **140**, 4451-4458.

Urwin, G.H., Percival, R.C., Harris, S., Beneton, M.N.C., Williams, J.L. and Kanis, S.A. (1985) Generalized increase in bone resorption in carcinoma of the prostate. *European Journal of Urology,* **57**, 721-723.

Van der Pluijm, G., Vloedgraven, H., van Beek, E., van der Wee-Pals, L., Lowik, C. and Papapoulos, S. (1996) Bisphosphonates inhibit the adhesion of breast cancer cells to bone matrices in vitro. *Journal of Clinical Investigation,* **98**, 698-705.

Yi, B., Williams, P.J., Niewolna, M., Wang, Y. and Yoneda, T. (2002) Tumor-derived PDGF-BB plays a critical role in osteosclerotic bone metastasis in an animal model of human breast cancer. *Cancer Research,* **62**, 917-923.

Yin, J.J., Selander, K., Chirgwin, J.M., Dallas, M., Grubbs, B.G., Wieser, R., Massague, J., Mundy, G.R. and Guise, T.A. (1999) TGFβ signaling blockade inhibits PTH-rP secretion by breast cancer cells and bone metastasis development. *Journal of Clinical Investigation,* **103**, 197-206.

Yoneda, T., Michigami, T., Yi, B., Williams, P.J., Niewolna, M. and Hiraga, T. (2000) Actions of bisphosphonate on bone metastasis in animal models of breast cancer. *Cancer*, **88**, 2979-2988.

Chapter 11

GENE THERAPY FOR PROSTATE CANCER BONE METASTASIS
Gene Therapy Targeting Bone Metastasis

Chia-Ling Hsieh, Hiroyuki Kubo and Leland W.K. Chung
Molecular Urology and Therapeutics Program, Department of Urology, Winship Cancer Institute, Emory University School of Medicine, Atlanta, GA

INTRODUCTION

Cancer is not a single cell disease but involves complex interaction between cancer cells and their microenvironment (Ingber, 2002; Liotta and Kohn, 2001; Quaranta, 2002; Shekhar et al., 2003; Sung and Chung, 2002). It has been widely recognized that the growth, survival and invasion of cancer cells require the participation of vascular endothelial component of the host (Folkman, 2001; Monsky et al., 2002), the inflammatory and neuroendocrine cells and their cytokine repertoire (Aprikian et al., 1994; Coussens and Werb, 2002; Murakami et al., 2002), and the inductive fibromuscular stromal cells (Aumuller, 1989; Franks et al., 1970; Tuxhorn et al., 2002). Experimental model systems to determine the molecular and cellular basis of prostate cancer progression to androgen independence and metastasis to bone revealed that intimate interaction between cancer cells and prostate or bone stromal cells is required (Chung et al., 1989; Gleave et al., 1991; Gleave et al., 1992; Olumi et al., 1998; Olumi et al., 1999). Under the inductive influence of prostate or bone stromal cells, the human LNCaP prostate cancer cell line can be driven to express both androgen-independent (AI) and bone metastatic potential when co-cultured in vitro as 3-dimensional (3-D) prostate organoids or allowed to form chimeric tumors when co-inoculated in vivo in castrated hosts (Rhee et al., 2001; Thalmann et al., 1994; Wu et al., 1994). These experiments demonstrated a fundamental principle that governs prostate cancer progression, the reciprocal interaction between genetically modified prostate cancer cells and the relevant fibromuscular stromal environment under androgen-deprived and 3-dimensional (3-D) growth conditions. Only in the presence of such interactions can the AI and bone metastatic progression of human prostate cancer cells be achieved. Apparently, permanent phenotypic and genotypic changes are induced in both prostate cancer and interactive stromal compartments (Hyytinen et al., 1997; Pathak et al., 1997). The consequences of cellular interaction include changes observed in the stroma, which becomes "reactive" and drives further progression of human prostate cancer cells to the AI and metastatic state (Sung and Chung, 2002). To tackle the molecular mechanisms underlying the progression of prostate cancer cells to androgen independence and bone metastasis under the influence of fibromuscular stromal cells, we and others have proposed that both soluble factors and insoluble extracellular matrices (ECMs) are likely to be involved through cellular communication or "cross-talk" between these mosaic factors, their receptors and downstream signaling pathways (Sung and Chung, 2002; Tuxhorn et al., 2001; Varani et al., 1999; Wong and Wang, 2000). In this review, we will focus our discussion on three areas: first, the development of the gene therapy concept and strategies to co-target prostate cancer growth in bone; second, the application of local-regional and systemic gene therapy in human clinical trials; and third, a discussion of the future development of effective gene therapy approaches for the treatment of prostate cancer bone metastasis.

STROMAL-EPITHELIAL INTERACTIONS

Cellular interaction between prostate luminal epithelial cells and their underlying fibromuscular stroma has been recognized as a crucial determinant supporting fetal prostate development, growth maintenance and the differentiation status of the adult prostate gland (Chung et al., 1984; Hayashi et al., 1993; McNeal, 1990). Aberrant interaction between stroma and epithelium through the acquisition of inductive influence from "reawakening" embryonic mesenchymes has been proposed to contribute to the development of benign enlargement of the prostate gland {BPH, (Chung et al., 1984; McNeal, 1990; Miller et al., 1985)). By introducing fetal urogenital sinus mesenchyme directly to adult prostate gland, we have shown a marked enlargement of the mouse prostate gland with histomorphologic and androgen-dependency profiles mimicking human BPH (Chung and Auble, 1988; Miller et al., 1985). Isoenzymatic profiles of mouse strain-specific glucose dehydrogenase activity in the enlarged mouse prostate gland reveal not only the growth of inductive fetal urogenital sinus tissues but also the growth of the responding adult prostate epithelial cells. These results suggest that adult prostate epithelial cells are not quiescent and are competent to respond to growth inductive signals from fetal tissues (Chung and Auble, 1988; Chung et al., 1984; Miller et al., 1985). An understanding of the molecular regulatory mechanisms of such interactions could result in the development of reagents to treat of human BPH by interrupting cellular interactions. The fundamental biology of tissue and cell interactions apparently is highly conserved and operative also in such conditions as the loss of growth control in neoplastic tissues. For example, organ-specific and tumor-associated (Camps et al., 1990; Gleave et al., 1992) stromal cells were demonstrated to promote human prostate tumor growth and/or support progression to the AI state and exhibit bone metatastic potential (Thalmann et al., 1994; Wu et al., 1994; Wu et al., 1998). Using a human prostate cancer cell line, LNCaP, as a model, we have shown that both the genotype and phenotype of this cell line can be altered permanently in a non-random manner by cellular interaction with prostate and bone stroma (Thalmann et al., 1994; Thalmann et al., 2000; Wu et al., 1994; Wu et al., 1998). The resultant LNCaP sublines acquired AI growth potential and the propensity to metastasize to bone. Clearly cellular interaction is reciprocal; not only are tumor cells responsive to the "inductive cue" emanating from the stroma, but the phenotype and genotype of the stromal cells surrounding tumor epithelium also underwent permanent alterations when co-cultured or in close contact with tumor epithelium (Elenbaas and Weinberg, 2001; Rhee et al., 2001; Ronnov-Jessen et al., 1995; Tuxhorn et al., 2001; Tuxhorn et al., 2002) or when harvested directly from tumor xenografts in vivo (Pathak et al., 1997). These observations are consistent with the proposal that a "vicious cycle" between tumor and stroma ultimately cascades into the malignant progression of prostate tumors {(Sung and Chung, 2002), see Figure 1}. Intimate and dynamic interactions between tumor cells and their local and systemic microenvironment are requisite molecular steps for cancer growth, progression and metastasis. Understanding the molecular mechanisms of this interaction could help in designing novel diagnostic and therapeutic strategies.

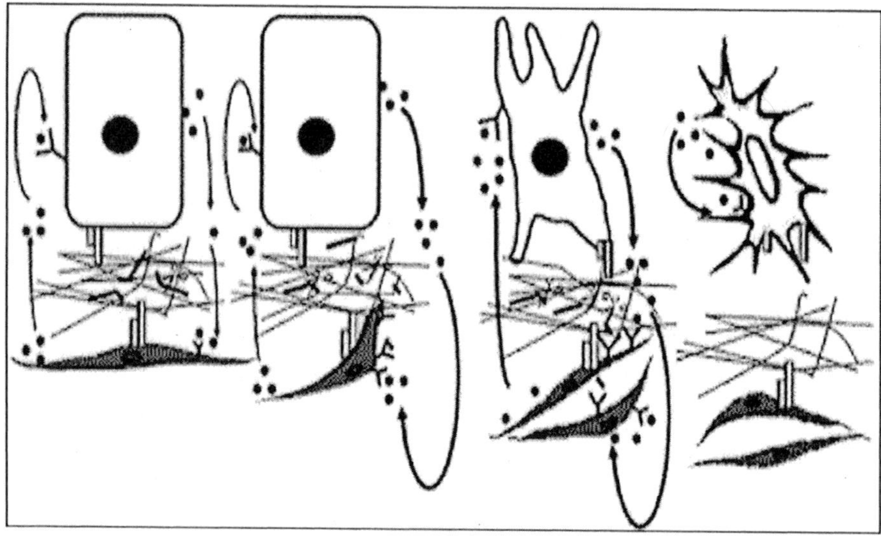

Figure 1. A "vicious cycle" is proposed as the underlying molecular basis of local prostate cancer growth and its distant bone and visceral metastases. Normal prostate gland loses its homeostatic control through aberrant growth factor and extracellular matrix-mediated signaling. Tissue interaction and cellular response to microenvironment changes results in altered gene expression profiling and behavioral changes by the cancer cells and their associated stromal component, characterized as "reactive" stroma and "reactive" epithelium. This is likely due to altered growth factor or ECM mediated signaling as the consequence of transcription factor activation of "switching" (Yeung and Chung, 2002). The "vicious cycle" may be initiated by the aberrant growth factor/ECM milieu in prostate cancer which up-regulates key transcription factors that modulate further growth factor, ECM and metalloproteinase expression in stromal cells. Increased expression of these soluble, insoluble matrix-associated factors and metalloproteinases can cause additional abnormalities characterized by the loss of growth control and enhanced cancer cell migration, invasion and metastasis (Sung and Chung, 2002). Because of the phenotypic and genotypic changes detected in cancer cells and their microenvironment, analysis of the molecular signatures of tumor cells and the stromal compartment could yield new diagnostic and treatment strategies.

RATIONALES OF SYSTEMIC GENE THERAPY FOR THE TREATMENT OF PROSTATE CANCER BONE METASTASIS

Innovative therapeutic strategies need to be developed for the treatment of advanced forms of prostate cancer, such as bone metastasis, for which there is no effective therapy. While it is well accepted that small-sized pharmaceuticals can penetrate tissue and cells efficiently and are effective against the growth of solid tumors, unfortunately the toxicity to normal cells and tissues from most of the pharmacologic agents are significant and drug resistance often develops. Delivery of therapeutic genes to tissues and cells using viral or non-viral vectors is an attractive alternative that has been in rapid development in recent years. Gene-based therapeutics are generally non-toxic and can induce tumor cell death through cytotoxic mechanisms, induction of host immune response, or oncolytic and anti-angiogenic mechanisms. This area of therapeutic development is particularly relevant given the fact that increasing numbers of genes have been cloned in recent years and their actions have been characterized as controlling cell growth and differentiation. Moreover, once a prototype gene is shown to be effective, rapid molecular engineering can alter the sequence of such genes and improve their relative therapeutic efficacy. Among existing gene therapy protocols, the adenovirus (Ad)-based vector system appears to be most popular and extensively tested. One important consideration to achieve successful delivery of therapeutic gene(s) to relevant cancer tissues or cells is the degree of infectivity by the Ad vector system upon cell contact. The entry of Ad vector into tumor cells has been shown to depend on the expression of coxsackie and adenovirus receptor (CAR) and the RGD sequences within viral penton protein (Bergelson et al., 1997; Tomko et al., 1997; Wickham et al., 1993). In practice, it is not possible to infect all cancer cells with Ad vector. As tumor cells become progressively more invasive in some of tumor types (such as human bladder cancer), their level of CAR decreases, which hinders viral entry and transgene expression (Li et al., 1999; Okegawa et al., 2000). Strategies have been developed to re-target Ad vectors by the use of bi-functional antibody conjugates (Wickham et al., 1996) genetically modifying viral fiber protein to alter its tropism toward the designed epitope (Krasnykh et al., 1996), or the use of different Ad vector subtypes to bypass the CAR requirement (Schoggins et al., 2003). Alternatively, increased specificity and amplification of cytotoxicity by Ad vector can be achieved by the use of an appropriately engineered Ad vector with transgene expression under the control of tissue-specific promoters {reviewed in Kanai,(Kanai, 2001)}, further amplified by powerful enhancing agents (Hsieh et al., 2002; Rodriguez et al., 1997) or modified by the use of alternative DNA elements (Lee et al., 2002; Wu et al., 2001). Finally, it is recognized that the lethal phenotype of cancer is distinguished by its ability to metastasize; thus, to have an impact on survival, cancer gene therapy most likely needs to be delivered by a systemic route.

ADENOVIRUS-MEDIATED GENE DELIVERY AND CO-TARGETING STRATEGY

Recombinant adenovirus is a potential candidate vector for clinical gene therapy based on several key attributes, including ease of production to high titer, infection of both dividing and nondividing cells of different lineage relationships, and systemic stability, which together allow efficient *in vivo* gene expression. However, virus has several important limitations including its widespread tropism to normal and tumor cells, dependence of viral infection on the availability of viral surface receptors on target cells, and the stimulation of host inflammatory and immune responses thus result in short-term transgene expression. Despite these limitations, the basic advantages of adenoviral vector and its demonstrated *in vivo* efficacy have made it particularly attractive as a starting point for future development of this vector system (Figure 2). In this section, we emphasize current improvement in the efficiency and specificity of adenoviral vectors and restricted transgene expression in target cells. This strategy may be also useful to achieve selective and persistent co-targeting effects for the treatment of prostate cancer bone metastasis, wherein both prostate cancer and bone stromal cells are co-targeted with minimized host organ toxicity. This strategy could also be further developed to co-target prostate cancer cells and their associated fibromuscular stromal cells for enhanced efficiency of transgene expression to treat localized prostate cancers.

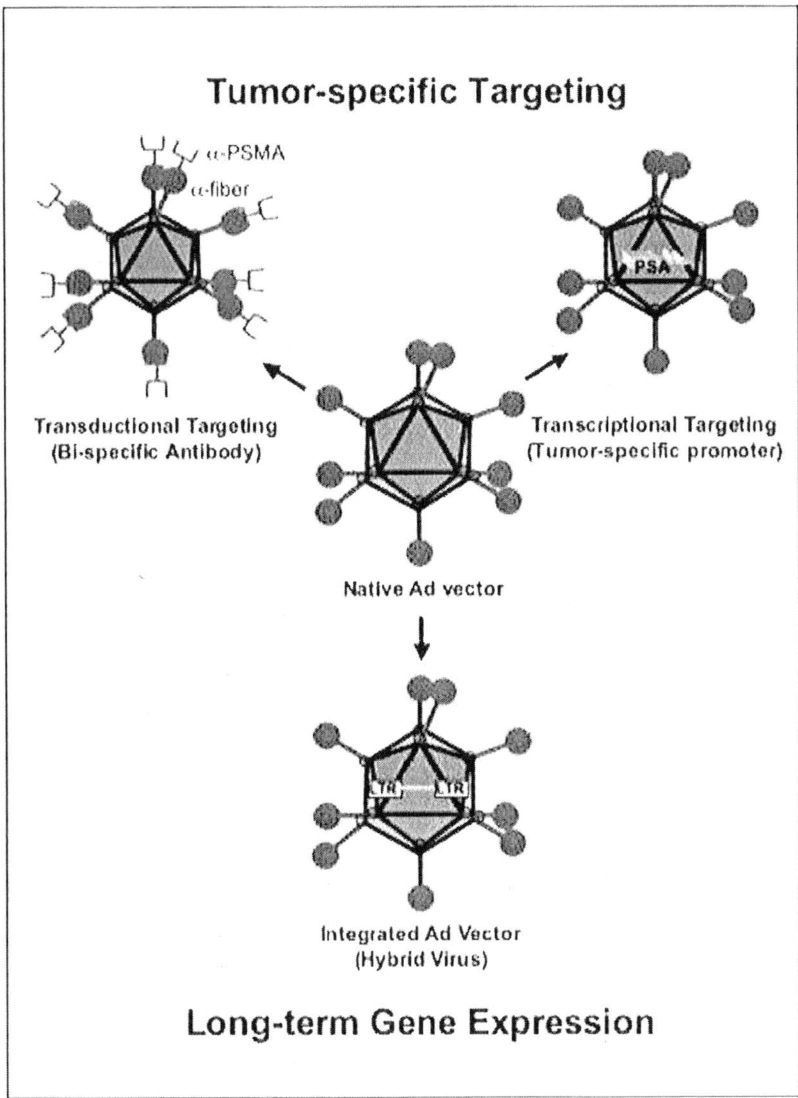

Figure 2. Strategies for developing tumor-specific and long-term transgene expressing adenoviral vector for cancer therapy. Native Ad vectors preferentially bind to the native receptor, CAR, and use a universal promoter to direct nonspecific expression of the transgene. Transcriptional targeting Ad vectors by using a tumor-specific promoter (E.g. PSA promoter) can selectively express transgene only in cells that express PSA. Transductional targeting Ad vectors by using a bispecific antibody can redirect Ad vectors binding to a cell surface receptor (e.g. PSMA) expressed more abundantly on the cell surface of androgen-independent prostate tumors. Long-term transgene expression in cancer cells by Ad vectors can be improved using hybrid vectors combining the highly efficient DNA delivery of adenovirus with the integrating machinery of retroviruses or AAV.

TRANSCRIPTIONAL TARGETING

The ultimate success of cancer gene therapy will depend on the ability to deliver transgene to target cells efficiently, whilst minimizing expression in other tissues. A variety of techniques exist to achieve this goal, including loco-regional administration, manipulation of tumor blood supply and transcriptional targeting useing of cell-specific promoters to drive gene expression limited to cells that express a certain specific transcription factor repertoire (Nettelbeck et al., 2000). Although some promoters placed in the Ad genome have been found to lose specificity, promoters that do retain specificity in this setting are emerging (Adachi et al., 2000; Yamamoto et al., 2001). These strategies have allowed cell-specific gene delivery via adenoviral vectors and have the potential to enhance the utility of this vector for targeting tumor but without damaging the normal cells.

Based on observations that noncollagenous bone matrix proteins such as osteopontin (OPN), osteocalcin (OC), bone sialoprotein (BSP) and osteonectin (ON) are expressed at high levels in primary and metastatic prostate cancer specimens (Curatolo et al., 1992; Jacob et al., 1999; Matsubara et al., 2001; Thalmann et al., 1999; Waltregny et al., 1998), Koeneman *et al.* hypothesized that in order to thrive and grow in the bone environment, prostate cancer cells must acquire "bone-like" or osteomimetic properties (Koeneman et al., 1999). A recent study using the osteotropic prostate cancer cells (C4-2B) demonstrated that in addition to having an osteoblastic phenotype, C4-2B cells could produce hydroxyapatite mineral *in vitro*; and stimulate osteoblasts to initiate mineralization in the bone (Lin et al., 2001). The increased expression of bone matrix proteins by prostate cancer cells in skeletal metastatic sites may underlie the predilection of prostate cancer for bone and explain the osteotrophic characteristics of prostate cancer bone metastasis. Because of the osteomimetic properties of prostate tumor epithelial cells in bone, we proposed a novel co-targeting strategy incorporating an adenoviral gene therapy approach to the treatment metastatic prostate cancers. Several previous publications demonstrated that an Ad vector-mediated toxic gene, hsv-TK, expression driven by osteoblasts-specific mouse OC promoter, inhibited the growth of osteosarcoma and its metastasis (Ko et al., 1996; Shirakawa et al., 1998) and blocked the growth of localized prostate tumors and their skeletal xenografts (Chung et al., 1997). A phase I OC dose-escalation trial has demonstrated the safety of an intratumoral delivery of the tumor-restricted gene therapy (Ad-OC-TK) followed by an oral acyclovir or valacyclovir administration (Koeneman et al., 2000; Kubo et al., 2003). In addition, our laboratory also demonstrated substantial efficacy of systemic Ad-OC-E1a, a replication competent Ad vector carrying mouse OC promoter driven the viral early *E1a* gene for the treatment of androgen-independent prostate cancer skeletal xenografts (Matsubara et al., 2001). In this study, forty percent of the mice were "cured" by systemic Ad-OC-E1a without subsequent PSA rebound or tumor cells found in the skeleton. These results imply that a gene therapy approach using bone matrix protein promoters such as OC to drive the expression of therapeutic genes co-targeting tumor epithelium and its supporting stroma may be an effective strategy for destroying human prostate tumor skeletal metastasis.

Because protein-DNA and protein-protein interactions control the extent to which the gene is activated or suppressed, knowledge of the promoter properties and specific domains required for maximal levels of expression and cell type-restricted transcriptional activity would allow for modifications of the promoter size to accommodate current options for selective gene transfer into target cells. Unlike mouse OC gene, human OC expression is transcriptionally regulated by vitamin D and was thought to be limited to cells of the osteoblast lineage. We recently constructed an 800-bp human OC (hOC) promoter, which contains a vitamin D responsive element and its activity can be induced by vitamin D_3. Concomitant Ad-hOC-E1 (a novel replication-competent Ad vector) and vitamin D_3 treatment markedly reduced the growth of DU145 tumor xenografts by a single systemic administration of Ad-hOC-E1 (Hsieh et al., 2002). Furthermore, three groups of transcription factors, Runx2, JunD/Fra-2, and Sp-1 has been demonstrated to be responsible for the high hOC promoter activity in PC3 cells, a cell line derived from skeletal metastatic prostate tumors, by binding to the OSE2, AP-1/VDRE, and OSE1 elements, respectively (Yeung et al., 2002). These upregulated transcriptional factors in prostate cancer cells may be potential therapeutic targets. To enhance hOC promoter activity without losing its specificity, we generated an artificial hOC promoter consisting of dimers of the three elements designed as supra-hOC promoter with significantly higher activity than the wild type promoter. Supra-hOC provides an additional level of molecularly-engineered promoter to target prostate tumor and prostate or bone stromal cells, in which they express significant OC activity. Ad-hOC promoter driven therapeutic approaches may be used for the management of both localized and metastatic prostate cancers to bone.

TRANSDUCTIONAL TARGETING

The promiscuous tropism of Ad is due to the widespread distribution of a native primary cellular receptor, CAR, on the cell surface. Normal tissues such as airway epithelia (Zabner et al., 1997) and bone marrow mesenchymal stem cells (Conget and Minguell, 2000) lack accessible CAR and are therefore poorly transduced. Down-regulation of the CAR gene in several malignant cancer cell lines including melanoma, glioma, bladder and prostate cancer cells has also been documented (Li et al., 1999; Okegawa et al., 2000). This variability may have a significant impact on the outcome of adenovirus-based gene therapy. Recent advances in the biological understanding of adenovirus structure and adenovirus receptor interactions have fueled the rapid development of targeted adenovirus vectors. In one approach to the development of cancer cell-specific vectors, Ad has been targeted at the level of transduction to achieve selective delivery of the therapeutic gene. Transductional targeting of Ad is accomplished by retargeting binding of the knob domain of the fiber capsid protein away from CAR to an alternative, cell-selective receptor, with subsequent internalization mediated by the interaction of the capsid penton base protein with the cellular integrin $\alpha v\beta 3$ and $\alpha v\beta 5$. In this regard, both immunologic and genetic methods to alter viral tropism have been developed (Curiel, 1999; Wickham, 2000). Immunologic retargeting has been achieved via conjugates a bispecific molecule comprised of an antifiber knob Fab and a targeting moiety consisting of a ligand or antireceptor antibody. The bispecific component simultaneously blocks native receptor binding and redirects virus binding to a tissue-specific receptor. Restrictive gene delivery into tumors by this approach has been accomplished via a variety of cellular pathways including receptors for FGF and EGF (Kleeff et al., 2002; van der Poel et al., 2002). Genetic strategies to alter adenoviral tropism have included both fiber modification and fiber replacement. In the former, Curiel and his colleagues identified the HI loop of fiber as a propitious locale for introduction of heterologous peptides. Incorporation of a cyclic RGD peptide which has affinity for tumor vasculature at this locale allowed gene delivery via cellular integrins with dramatic efficiency in pancreatic carcinoma (Wesseling et al., 2001). This immunologic approach offers great flexibility for rapidly validating the feasibility of targeting via a particular receptor, whereas the genetic system offers the best advantages in producing a manufacturable therapeutic and more completely ablating all native adenovirus receptor interactions. To date, 51 human adenovirus serotypes belonging to six species, A–F, have been recognized. They show a wide range of tissue tropism and are associated with several clinical syndromes, such as respiratory, cardiac, gastrointestinal, ocular and urinary tract diseases. Their tropism can be modified by genetically replacing the knob domain. This initial "proof of principle" study was conducted by Krasnykh and colleagues (Krasnykh et al., 1996) using a chimeric Ad vector containing the serotype 3 knob on the Ad5 fiber shaft and capsid to access a viral tropism switch from Ad5 to Ad3. Recently, Zhang et al. screened the binding affinity of representatives from every species of human adenovirus for established cell lines from different origin. They found that Ad11 from species B2 showed an impressively high binding efficiency for several types of cells including human endothelial cell line and hepatoma, breast cancer, prostatic cancer and laryngeal human cancer cell lines (Zhang et al., 2003) that are less permissive for commonly-used adenovirus vector Ad5. It would be useful to modify adenovirus vector with high affinity for both prostate cancer epithelial and bone stroma cells based on this same principle to develop bone-targeting Ad vectors for the treatment of prostate cancer bone metastasis. Ultimately, a higher degree of specificity for cancer cells could be achieved by combining the complementary approaches of transcriptional and transductional targeting, each of which might be imperfect by itself. Barnett *et al.* have recently reported that the use of OC promoter, which has specificity for osteoblasts and osteoblastic metastatic lesion, combined with a bispecific antibody conjugate with specificity for both the fiber knob domain and EGFR, resulted in a markedly improvement in the selectivity of transgene expression in cancer cells compared to transductionally or transcriptionally targeted Ad vector alone (Barnett et al., 2002). This dual-targeting Ad vector approach has the potential to enhance the utility of this vector agent for a co-target gene therapy strategy to treat prostate cancer bone metastasis.

TARGETING THROUGH "BYSTANDER" EFFECTS BY EMPLOYING SPECIFIC ENZYME/PRO-DRUG SYSTEM

Another effective way to circumvent the low transduction efficiency of the currently available vectors is the delivery of therapeutic genes encoding intracellular enzymes for the conversion of a pro-drug to a cytotoxic drug, which can then spread to neighboring non-transduced cells ("bystander" effect) via prior established intercellular communication network. The local production of the biologically active cytotoxic drugs from their pro-drugs within the tumor should result in greater therapeutic effects and wider therapeutic indices than systemic delivery of drugs in the absence of gene therapy. Importantly, the local spread of active drugs following pro-drug activation by cells which express the pro-drug activation enzymes can kill adjacent non-transduced cells, obviating requirement to achieve gene transfer to *all* tumor cells, which appears unrealistic with current technology. Many different potential enzyme/pro-drug combinations have been described (Table 1) and the most frequently used systems are HSV thymidine kinase with ganciclovir (tk/GCV), and *E. coli* cytosine deaminase with 5-fluorocytosine (CD/5-FC). All of these enzyme/pro-drug gene therapy strategies have demonstrated an ability to affect tumor regression through both direct and bystander mechanisms in murine models (Chen et al., 1994; Eastham et al., 1996; Ko et al., 1996; Topf et al., 1998). The bystander effect has been proposed to results from transfer of the activated drugs from pro-drugs between cells via either gap junctions or as apoptotic vesicles engrafted by surrounding cells. Although the enzyme/pro-drug system has been shown to be highly active within homospecific tumors, the heterospecific bystander effect between different cell types which lack gap junctional intercellular communication (such as stroma-epithelium) is limited. One possible way to improve the heterospecific bystander effect between stroma and cancer epithelium by enzyme/pro-drug therapy could be the extracellular conversion of a hydrophilic pro-drug to a lipophilic, cell-permeable cytotoxic drug. An extracellular cytotoxic effector system composed of a secreted form of the normally lysosomal human beta-glucuronidase (s-betaGluc) was designed to convert an inactivated glucuronidated derivative of doxorubicin (HMR 1826) to the cytotoxic drug, doxorubicin, which is taken up by both transduced and non-transduced cells in a gap junction-independent manner (Weyel et al., 2000). Instead of secreted form of the enzyme, a more stringent retention of the enzyme at the site of the producer cell, such as its attachment to the cell surface, would be desirable. A hybrid enzyme composed the transmembrane domain of the human PDGF receptor fused with a C-terminally truncated form of s-betaGluc has been made and revealed a high steady-state level of accumulation on cell surface. A doxorubicin pro-drug, doxorubicin beta-glucuronide, is effectively cleaved by the transduced s-betaGluc to release the active drug doxorubicin locally and produce a strong bystander antitumor activity *in vivo* (Heine et al., 2001).

Table 1. Enzymes and pro-drugs for gene therapy.

Enzyme	Pro-drug	Reference
Cytosine deaminase	5-Fluorocytosine	(Huber et al., 1993; Huber et al., 1994)
Thymidine kinase	Ganciclovir/ Acyclovir	(Link et al., 1997; Nishihara et al., 1997; Rosolen et al., 1998)
Nitroreductase	5-(Aziridin-1-yl)-2,4-dinitrobenzamide (CB1954)	(Bailey and Hart, 1997; Bailey et al., 1996)
Carboxypeptidase G2	4-([2-chloroethyl][2-mesyloxyethyl]amino)benzoyl-L-glutamic acid (CMDA)	(Friedlos et al., 2002; Stribbling et al., 2000)
Cytochrome 450	oxazaphosphorine	(Chen et al., 1996; Chen et al., 1997; Waxman et al., 1999)
β-glucuronidase	doxorubicin (DOX-GA3)	(Fonseca et al., 1999; Heine et al., 2001; Weyel et al., 2000)

The effectiveness of these strategies for human prostate cancer therapy may be blunted by of their limited effect on slowly dividing cells that require prolonged expression of the therapeutic genes and long-term administration of the pro-drug to increase the proportion of cells transduced with greater bystander effects. Recent studies have demonstrated that tumor cells transfected with other therapeutic genes such as p53 and Ad5 E1A exhibit bystander effects inhibiting tumor growth by alternative mechanism, such as suppressing angiogenesis and inducting apoptosis (Dong et al., 1999; Nishizaki et al., 1999; Shao et al., 2000; Wei et al., 1995). In addition, the tumor cell-killing efficacy of suicide genes such as TK and CD has been improved using these genes encoded within replication-competent Ad vectors (Lee et al., 2001; Rogulski et al., 2000; Wildner et al., 1999). In these cases the therapeutic suicide genes are amplified through viral replication, accomplished by the availability of E1 gene product for adenoviral replication and supplied by the replicating virus.

HYBRID VIRAL VECTORS

One of the main obstacles to the practical implementation of human gene therapy has been the lack of a single-vector system capable of highly efficient delivery and stable integration of therapeutic genes *in vivo*. Non-viral gene delivery systems exhibit minimal toxicity and little antigenicity, but the *in vivo* transduction efficiency and frequency of genomic integration is extremely low. Viral gene delivery systems exploit the natural mechanisms evolved by different viruses for cellular entry and gene transfer. However, of the virus-based vector systems developed thus far, none are optimal and each system displays advantages and disadvantages characteristic of each virus (Table 2). Thus, retrovirus and adeno-associated virus (AAV) vectors are each capable of stable integration into the host cell genome, but achieving high production titers and adequate levels of *in vivo* transduction with these vectors has proven difficult (Anderson, 1998; Dong et al., 1996). Conversely, adenovirus-based vectors can achieve extremely high titers and efficient transduction of many cell types *in vivo*, but genomic integration is extremely rare (Harui et al., 1999). Additionally, high titers of standard E1/E3-deleted Ad vectors elicit a robust immune response, resulting in transient expression of delivered genes *in vivo* (Kaplan et al., 1997; Yang et al., 1996). In contrast to standard Ad vectors, which retain more than two-thirds of the adenoviral genome, helper dependent adenovirus vectors (HDAd) are deleted of all viral coding sequences and contain only the Ad inverted terminal repeats (ITRs) and packaging signal, φ, required for replication and packaging (Mitani et al., 1995). Transgene expression from HDAd vectors is prolonged *in vivo* compared with standard Ad vectors, presumably because of a reduced cellular immune response against HDAd-infected cells. Nonetheless, as the Ad lacks specific machinery for genomic integration, the HDAd episome is eventually lost from the transduced cells. Thus, one of the fundamental problems associated with the use of Ad based vectors remains: the difficulty of obtaining permanent expression of transferred genes. To improve the integration frequencies of adenoviral vectors, a variety of hybrid vectors combining the highly efficient DNA delivery of adenovirus with the integrating machinery of retroviruses, AAV, have emerged. Permanent target cell transduction by chimeric Ad vectors carrying retroviral structural genes and vector sequences inserted separately into standard E1/E3-deleted or E1/E3/E4-deleted Ad vectors has been reported by several laboratories (Bilbao et al., 1997; Caplen et al., 1999; Feng et al., 1997; Torrent et al., 2000). A high-capacity AAV/Ad hybrid vector system that combines, in a single particle, the large cloning capacity and efficient cell cycle-independent nuclear gene delivery of Ad vectors with the long-term transgene expression and lack of viral genes of AAV vectors has also been recently developed (Goncalves et al., 2002). These hybrid vectors have shown promise *in vitro*. Moreover, the use of the HDAd as an expression platform represents a significant advantage over previous Ad–retrovirus systems, since both retroviral structural genes and transfer vector constructs can be contained in the same Ad carrier {up to 38 kb of total cloning capacity (Morsy and Caskey, 1999)}, dramatically enhancing the efficiency of viral production. These developments should eventually lead to more effective gene therapy vectors while minimizing and improving the previously recognized deficiencies of these vectors for future gene therapy in the clinic.

Table 2. Gene transfer vectors used against cancer.

Delivery System	Non-viral vectors	Retro-virus	Lentivirus	Adenovirus (Ad)	Adeno-associated virus (AAV)	Vaccinia virus
Titer	No	10^7	10^5 pseudo-type:10^9	$>10^{11}$	10^4	$>10^{12}$
Maximum size of transgene	Unlimited	8kb	10kb	7-8 kb HDAd:38 kb	4.8 kb	Almost unlimited
Genomic integration	No	Yes	Yes	No	Yes	No
Duration of gene expression	Transient	Pronged	Pronged	Transient	Pronged	Transient
Cell mitosis required	No	Yes	No	No	No	No
Trans-fection efficiency	Poor	Variable	Variable	High	High	High
Toxicity	Yes	No	Yes	Yes	No	Yest

NOVEL MOLECULAR TARGETS FOR CANCER GENE THERAPY

To develop rational new therapeutic approaches for targeting prostate cancer bone metastasis, we must first understand the multi-step processes that lead to prostate cancer metastasis to bone. The molecular machinery of metastasis formation is a prime target for intervention. As depicted in Figure 3, at the site of primary tumor growth cancer cells interact with stroma and gain the ability to extravasate into the bloodstream. In the blood, prostate cancer cells are expected to survive and move as an embolus prior to adhering to bone marrow-associated endothelial cells. The attachment and interaction of prostate cancer cells to marrow endothelial ECMs could activate the invasive properties of prostate cancer cells by increasing ECM-integrin signaling, production of matrix metalloproteinases (MMPs), and extravasation of prostate cancer cells into the marrow space. At the final step

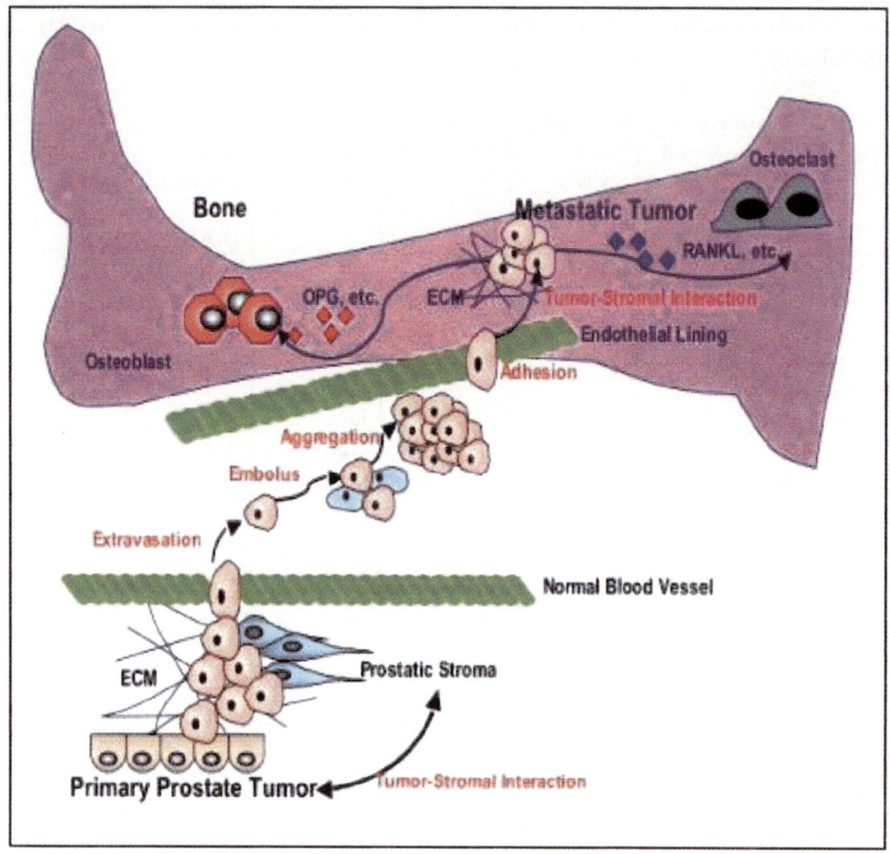

Figure 3. The multi-step processes of prostate cancer metastasis to bone. Once prostate cancer cells gain the ability to extravasate into the bloodstream, prostate cancer cells move as an embolus prior to adhering to bone marrow-associated endothelial cells. Attachment and interaction between prostate cancer cells and marrow endothelial ECMs could activate the invasive properties of prostate cancer cells and allow their extravasation into the marrow space. Prostate cancer cells then interact directly and reciprocally with osteoblasts and osteoclasts through a series of soluble factors via cell surface receptors (e.g., RANK) to gain additional invasive, migratory and adhesive properties, to anchor onto additional bone sites made available by osteoclast-induced bone "pitting", to induce osteoblastic reactions and eventually to replace the bone marrow components.

of this progression, prostate cancer cells interact directly and reciprocally with osteoblasts and osteoclasts through a series of soluble factors (e.g., receptor activator of NF-kB ligand, RANKL, PTHrP, endothelin-1) via cell surface receptor (e.g., RANK, PTHrP and endothelin receptors) to allow prostate cancer cells to survive, proliferate, migrate and invade and eventually replace the entire bone marrow components. The proliferating prostate cancer cells secrete factors that cause osteoblastic reaction which is characterized by accelerated osteoblast proliferation and bone turnover (Brown et al., 2001; Guise et al., 2003; Lee et al., 2003; Lin et al., 2001; Mundy, 1997; Nemeth et al., 2002). At the molecular level, the metastatic phenotype of prostate cancer cells is generated by the expression of homing receptors with associated signaling molecules, their ligands, and extracellular matrix-degrading proteases. In this section, we discuss current understanding of the molecular interactions involved in the dissemination of cancer cells. Leading to the identification of promising molecular targets of cancer gene therapy.

Chemokines/chemokine receptors

Chemokines are a superfamily of small, cytokine-like proteins that induce cytoskeletal rearrangement, firm adhesion to endothelial cells and directional migration through their interaction with G-protein-coupled receptors. These secreted proteins act in a coordinated fashion with cell-surface proteins, including integrins, to direct the specific homing of various subsets of hematopoietic cells to specific anatomical sites. Many patho-physiological conditions require the participation of chemokines, including inflammation, infection, tissue injury, allergy, cardiovascular diseases, and malignant tumors. The role of chemokines in malignant tumors is complex. While some chemokines may enhance innate or specific host immunity against tumor implantation, others may favor tumor growth and metastasis by promoting tumor cell proliferation, migration or neovascularization in tumor tissue (Wang et al., 1998). Understanding the functional role of chemokines and their receptors in tumorigenesis and metastasis, including prostate cancer, could lead to the development of novel therapeutic approaches.

Prostate and breast neoplasms have a striking tendency to metastasize or home to bone. The mechanisms responsible for selecting the bone marrow as a preferential metastatic site have not yet been elucidated but may include a "chemoattraction" pathway that organ-specific attractant molecules enter the circulation, stimulating the migrating tumor cells to invade the walls of blood vessels and enter the organs. The coordinated secretion of chemokines, and their binding to receptors on the cell surface, directs leukocyte cell homing to specific tissue sites. The secretion of stromal-derived factor-1 (SDF-1, as known as CXCL12) by bone marrow stromal cells and its receptor CXCR4 expression by hematopoietic stem cells during maturation and migration into bone marrow provides an elegant example of this homing process, as reviewed by Lapidot and Kollet (Lapidot and Kollet,

2002). Similar processes have been suggested in the homing of transformed cells to specific organ sites. Müller and colleagues (Muller et al., 2001) recently reported the involvement of the CXCR4 in the metastasis of breast cancer to the SDF-1-rich environment of the bone marrow and lymph nodes. The investigators demonstrated that malignant cells express distinct and nonrandom patterns of chemokine receptors that guide their metastatic destination, determined by the expression levels of chemokines by target organs. The metastatic spread of the tumors to the lung and lymph nodes can be successfully blocked by CXCR4 antibody. Taichman *et al.* (Taichman et al., 2002) recently reported similar findings in prostate cancer cells lines. These authors demonstrated that the level of CXCR4 increased (as detected by both RT-PCR and Western blot analysis) with enhanced malignant potential of prostate cancer cell lines which presumable will migrate across bone marrow endothelial cell monolayers in response to SDF-1. These results suggest that metastatic prostate carcinomas may also use the SDF-1/CXCR4 pathway to localize to bone. In this regard, it is conceivable that SDF-1/CXCR4 axis in the metastatic cascades of prostate carcinoma may include novel targets for therapeutic intervention to prevent prostate cancer bone metastasis.

Osteoclastogenesis

Skeletal deposits of metastatic prostate cancer alter the normal physiology of the bone, leading to disruption of normal remodeling cycles. Although often characterized as osteoblastic, histomorphometric studies of prostate cancer bone metastases have shown that some of the sclerotic lesions are actually mixed in nature, with both increased osteoblastic and osteolytic reactions. A number of studies have shown that patients with advanced prostate cancer exhibit elevated levels of osteolytic bone resorption markers in urine and blood (Coleman et al., 1992). The preponderance of evidence indicates that osteolysis is present in prostate cancer bone metastasis even when the overall character appears to be osteoblastic. Roland (Roland, 1958) introduced the hypothesis that every primary or metastatic cancer in bone begins with osteolysis. The release of growth factors from the mineralized matrix during bone resorption may facilitate the initial seeding and growth of tumor cells in the bone. Therefore, modulation of the altered bone remodeling observed with prostate cancer bone metastasis offers an attractive target for therapeutics intervention.

Several factors have been found to be important in tumor-induced enhancement of osteoclast activity. One key factor is the protein receptor activator of nuclear factor-κB ligand (RANKL), which is required to induce osteoclastogenesis in healthy bone. Increased expression of this critical bone resoption regulator was observed in prostate cancer bone metastases compared with nonosseous metastases or primary tumors (Brown et al., 2001). This suggests a mechanism whereby prostate cancer cells may modulate bone turnover through osteoclast activation and increased bone "pitting". This phenomenon could have profound implications for the establishment of additional sites of cancer growth and metastasis in bone in patients with advanced prostate and breast cancer. Zhang *et al.* (Zhang et al., 2001) recently demonstrated that prostate cancer cells directly induce osteoclastogenesis from osteoclast precursors in the absence of underlying stroma *in vitro* by producing a soluble form of RANKL. Their hypothesis is supported by the evidence that human prostate tumor burden in bone, but not subcutaneous, is highly responsive to the administration of a decoy receptor for RANKL, osteoprotegerin (OPG) (Zhang et al., 2001), which is expected to decrease osteoclastogenesis, or by zoledronic acid, a new-generation of bisphosphonates that decrease osteoclast life span by promoting apoptosis (Corey et al., 2003). These results, taken together, support the important role of enhanced osteoclast activity in the establishment of primary and secondary prostate cancer skeletal metastasis. Targeting bone turnover by modulating osteoclastogenesis could lead to the development of rationale therapy for slowing prostate cancer metastatic progression. In addition to RANKL, other potential targets for prostate cancer bone metastasis are parathyroid hormone-related protein (PTHrP), interleukin-6, endothelin-1, and matrix metalloproteinases (MMPs) which are produced by prostate cancer cells, and stimulating bone turnover by enhancing osteolytic reactions in the bone.

Tumor-host adhesive interactions

The process of tumor metastasis is a complex cascade of adhesive interactions between tumor cells and host tissues (Reviewed in Chapter 1). The endothelium of blood vessels constitutes a physical barrier to cells in the circulatory system and metastatic cells must penetrate the interendothelial junctions to invade the underlying tissue. Cell adhesion molecules (CAMs) are important for the preferential metastasis of prostate cancer to bone (Cooper et al., 2000). CAMs mediate the initial adhesion to the human bone marrow endothelium and then to the underlying bone matrix. The adhesion of cancer cells to the vascular endothelium is a critical step in the metastaic cascade and is mediated by integrins (Honn and Tang, 1992). Integrin $\alpha v \beta 3$ is known to be involved in a variety of cell biological activities, including angiogenesis, cell adhesion, and migration on several extracellular matrix components. Angiogenesis facilitates the growth and metastasis of solid tumors by, providing nutrients to the expanding tumor mass and providing a pathway for tumor cell dissemination. The expression of αvβ3 on endothelial cell surface plays an important role in this process (Varner and Cheresh, 1996). Endothelial cells stimulated by tumor-derived angiogenic factors enter the cell cycle and express the integrin αvβ3, which allows endothelial cells to interact with a wide variety of ECM proteins as they invade the tissue surrounding the tumors. In several malignancies, however, the tumor cells express αvβ3, and this expression correlates with tumor progression in melanoma, glioma, and ovarian and breast cancers. In breast cancer, αvβ3 characterizes the metastatic phenotype, as this integrin is up-regulated in invasive tumors and distant metastases (Felding-Habermann et al., 2001; Liapis et al., 1996). Similar to breast cancer cells, prostate cancer cells preferentially metastasize to the bone. The role of integrin αvβ3 in prostate cancer progression is also currently reviewed by Cooper *et al.* (Cooper et al., 2002). Expression or increased utilization of αvβ3 by prostate cancer cells has been linked to the progression of the disease (Edlund et al., 2001). αvβ3, in part, facilitates prostate cancer cell adhesion to and migration on osteopontin and vitronectin, which are common proteins in the bone microenvironment. Interestingly, osteopontin was detected in greater amounts in androgen-independent prostate cancer cell lines, suggesting that it contributes to androgen-independent growth of tumors in the bone (Thalmann et al., 1999). These observations implicate that prostate cancer cells, after entering the bone environment, are surrounded by osteopotin from sources including the bone matrix, osteoblasts, and the cancer cells themselves. Osteopontin can mediated preferential cell adhesion, migration, and growth of prostate cancer cells expressing αvβ3. Thus, it is reasonable to suggest that integrin αvβ3 and osteopontin may be highly attractive targets for treatment of prostate cancer skeletal metastasis. Small molecular drugs such as antibodies, synthetic peptides and soluble receptors are frequently used for therapeutic interference with receptor-ligand interaction and are also available for the inhibition of integrin αvβ3 ligation by osteopontin (Kerr et al., 2000; Weber, 2001). Suppression of integrin αvβ3 and osteopontin gene expression has been also demonstrated by gene therapy strategies such as ribozyme, antisense oligonucleotides (Behrend et al., 1995; Su et al., 1995) and intracellular single chain antibodies (Koistinen et al., 1999). These strategies may provide insight in the future development of gene therapy for the treatment of prostate cancer bone metastasis.

Ets factors: a mediator of ECM remodeling

Tumor invasion and metastasis depend on the ability of tumor cells to break through the surrounding connective tissue barriers. Degradation of

ECM by tissue serine proteases and the large family of MMPs is crucial to this process (Johansson et al., 2000). The human Ets family includes 25 genes that code for positively and negatively acting transcription factors involved in various aspects of cell proliferation and differentiation. A large number of genes, including genes for transcription factors, MMPs, cell cycle regulators, extracellular matrix receptors and growth factors, are known to contain Ets binding sites (Sementchenko and Watson, 2000). There is increasing evidence, currently reviewed by Singh *et al.* (Singh et al., 2002), that Ets factors correlated with invasive phenotype and that the role of Ets factors in tumor invasion is mainly related to transcriptional activation of enzymes involved in ECM degradation, such as serine proteases, MMPs and their inhibitors (TIMPs). Expression of Ets1 was shown to be limited to stromal cells in the vicinity of the tumors, whereas surrounding uninvolved tissue was negative for Ets1 expression (Calmels et al., 1995; Wernert, 1997). Immunohistochemical and *in situ* mRNA analyses of various human tumor tissues have also demonstrated upregulation of Ets1 in invasive tumors whereas Ets1 transcripts are rarely detected in benign and non-invasive tumors (Kitange et al., 1999a; Naito et al., 2000; Nakayama et al., 1996; Nakayama et al., 2001; Ozaki et al., 2000). Recent studies suggest, however, that the function of Ets factors may not be limited to regulating genes involved in the degradative pathways. Ets factors may regulate a wider spectrum of ECM-related target genes including matrix proteins such as tenascin, collagen, and fibronectin as well as other cellular components involved in cell-matrix interactions. Two gene therapy strategies, antisense oligonucleotides (Kitange et al., 1999b) and dominant-interference Ets 1 mutants (Delannoy-Courdent et al., 1998; Kim et al., 2000) have been successfully employed to inhibit the expression of Ets1 in tumor cells and block their migration and invasion. A novel prostate epithelium-specific Ets transcription factor, PDEF (prostate-derived Ets factor), was recently discovered, functioning as an androgen-independent transcriptional activator of the PSA promoter in hormone-refractory prostate cancer cells and possibly involved in prostate cancer development and progression (Oettgen et al., 2000). Therefore, targeting PDEF may be a valid therapeutic strategy for hormone refractory and bone metastatic prostate cancer.

Angiogenesis: VEGF pathway

Tumor growth and metastasis depend on the ability of a tumor to recruit blood vessels for delivery of oxygen and nutrients (Folkman, 1971). This process, angiogenesis, is driven by various growth factors (VEGF, bFGF, insulin-like growth factor-1, angiopoietin-1, and epidermal growth factor), and cytokines (IL-8), facilitated by collagenase activity {reviewed by Kumar and Fidler (Kumar and Fidler, 1998)}. In prostate cancer, microvessel density is correlated with the development of metastases and overall patient survival (Lissbrant et al., 1997). Of these factors, VEGF is one of the most potent facilitators of angiogenesis identified to date, with effects on endothelial cell proliferation, motility, and vascular permeability (Gerber et al., 1998; Keck et al., 1989). The use of antibodies that neutralize VEGF, VEGFR blockers, dominant-negative receptor strategies, and tyrosine kinase inhibitors have helped elucidate the central role of VEGF in tumor angiogenesis (Asano et al., 1995; Goldman et al., 1998; Kim et al., 1993; Millauer et al., 1996). Recent studies have confirmed that constitutive expression of VEGF in human prostate tumor cells whereas VEGFR-1 and VEGFR-2 expression is increased in PIN and prostate cancer compared with normal epithelial cells (Jackson et al., 2002). These data suggest that VEGF may regulate both angiogenesis and tumor cell growth via autocrine and/or paracrine mechanisms in prostate cancer. Sweeney *et al.* demonstrated reduced tumorigenicity and metastasis in prostate cancer orthotropic and tibial xenografts in nude mice treated with DC101, a neutralizing antibody that binds to the murine VEGFR-2/flk-1 receptor (Sweeney et al., 2002). Recombinant adenovirus encoding the ligand-binding ectodomain of the VEGF receptor 2 (Flk1) fused to an Fc domain has been shown to reduce vascular density and prostate tumor growth and prolong survival time in orthotopically implanted tumors as well as in spontaneous prostate tumors in TRAMP transgenic animals (Becker et al., 2002). In addition, the expression of 150-kDa oxygen-regulated protein ORP150, a new member of the heat shock protein family that functions as a molecular chaperone in the endoplasmic reticulum, was found to increase in infiltrating cancer cells and coordinated with the presence of vascular VEGF in human prostate cancer tissues. Secretion of VEGF by prostate cancer cells *in vitro* and tumor formation in the xenograft model were markedly reduced by adenoviral-mediated antisense ORP150 treatment (Miyagi et al., 2002). These proof-of-principle studies have led the way for the evaluation of targeting the VEGF pathway for the treatment of prostate cancer bone metastasis.

GENE THERAPY TARGETING HOST IMMUNE SYSTEM

Patients with malignant diseases often have deficiencies in their cellular immunity independent of the immunosuppressive effects of chemotherapy and radiotherapy. Immunosuppression is expressed during embryonic development (Sotomayor et al., 1996). This phenomenon could be the result of a lack of tumor-associated antigen (TAA) specific T-cells (Sotomayor et al., 1996) or from a lack of costimulatory signals as a consequence of generalized immunodeficiency through a low-efficiency major histocompatibility complex (MHC) presentation to effector cells (Lenschow and Bluestone, 1993), or alternatively through the production of immunosuppressive factors, such as transforming growth factor-β (TGF-β) and IL-10 (Mocellin et al., 2001; Wojtowicz-Praga, 1997) by tumors that leads to the impairment of the host immune response to tumor antigens (Kavanaugh and Carbone, 1996) Immunotherapy mediated through cytotoxic T lymphocytes (CTL) offers a promising treatment avenue, because T cells, in principle, can migrate throughout the body and specifically recognize and destroy metastatic tumor cells in an antigen-specific manner (see Figure 4). CTLs recognize a complex of self-MHC and endogenously synthesized peptide on the surface of cells. Thus, any endogenously synthesized protein, whether cytoplasmic, membrane-bound, or secreted, can serve as the source of antigenic peptide, which is then displayed on the cell surface. Immune-based strategies for treating prostate cancer have recently been facilitated by the identification of a number of prostate tissue/tumor antigens that can be targeted, either by antibody or T cells, to promote prostate tumor cell injury or death. These same prostate antigens can also be used for the construction of vaccines to induce prostate-specific T cell-mediated immunity. As a result of the limited efficacy of conventional radiotherapy and chemotherapy regimens for treating advanced prostate cancer and the significant morbidities associated with surgical treatment of localized disease, immunotherapeutics offer a spectrum of alternative modalities that have proven to be effective in other forms of malignancies such as renal cell carcinoma and malignant melanoma (Glaspy, 2002; Parmiani et al., 2002).

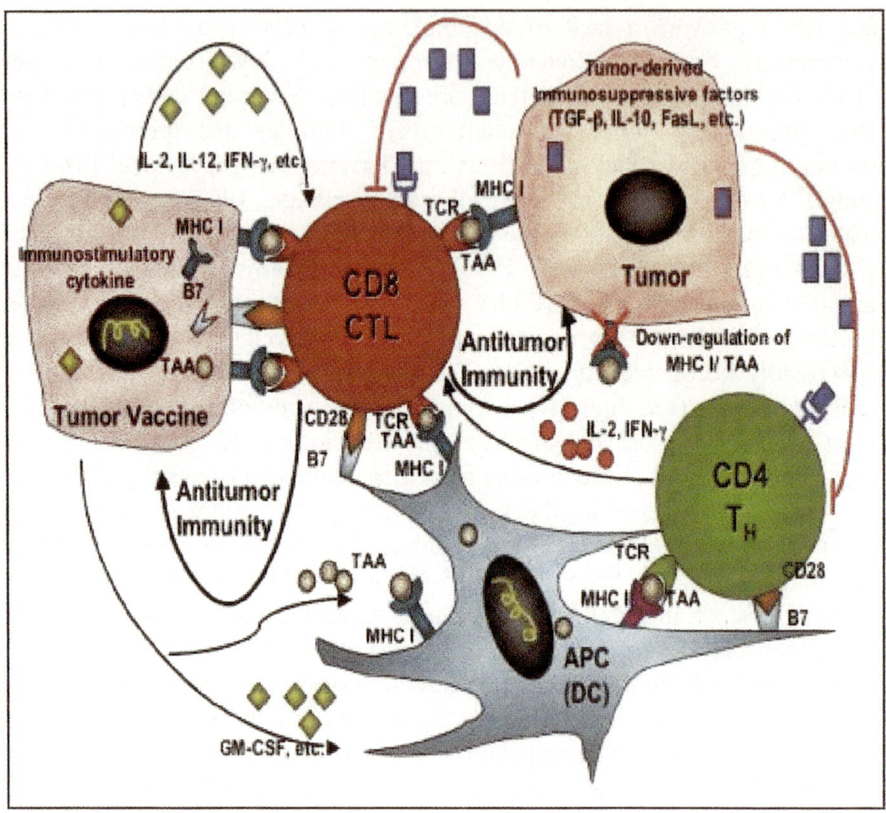

Figure 4. Strategy for immunotherapy to overcome tumor-induced immune tolerance Tumor cells produce immunosuppressive mediators, such as TGF-β, IL-10, and Fas ligand (FasL) or down regulate TAA and MHC molecular expression on their cell surface that leads to the impairment of the CTL immune response to tumors. One strategy to augment the antitumor immune response is to modify tumor cells (tumor vaccine) by transfer of a variety of genes, including target antigen, cytokines such as IL-2, IL-12, IFN-γ, and GM-CSF, costimulatory molecules such as B7, and MHC molecules to facilitate the start of a robust immune response. Alternative approach is using dentritic cells (DCs) pulsed with peptides from TAA or transduced with TAA genes leading to prolonged antigen presentation.

Novel Targets of Prostate Cancer Immunotherapy

Much of the work on tumor immunotherapy has implicitly assumed that it is necessary to identify and characterize antigens specifically and uniquely expressed in tumors but not normal tissues because of nonresponsiveness to self-antigens (Nossal, 1994). However, recent work has revealed that many targets for anti-melanoma CTL, such as tyrosinase, MART-1, gp100, and gp75, are normal self-antigens specific to the melanocyte lineage (Bakker et al., 1994; Brichard et al., 1993; Kawakami et al., 1994; Wang et al., 1995).

Further, the existence of a number of tissue-specific autoimmune diseases supports the concept that self-reactive immune effectors can be activated under appropriate conditions. To date, the most extensively studied antigens enrolled in clinical trials for prostate cancer immunotherapy have been prostate-specific antigen (PSA) (Murphy et al., 1996; Salgaller et al., 1998b; Tjoa et al., 1997), prostate acid phosphatase (PAP) (Burch et al., 2000; Fong et al., 2001), and prostate-specific membrane antigen (PSMA) (Murphy et al., 1996; Salgaller et al., 1998a; Tjoa et al., 1999). Several other genes and protein have been identified with prostate restricted or enhanced expression profiles. While not prostate cancer-specific, the high expression levels of these proteins in normal and neoplastic prostate epithelial cells, relative to all other normal human tissues, has propelled studies designed to exploit this tissue compartmentalization to therapeutic purposes.

Prostate stem cell antigen (PSCA) was identified by PCR-based subtractive hybridization (Reiter et al., 1998). PSCA is predominantly expressed on the surface of prostate cells and overexpressed by both androgen-dependent and androgen-independent prostate tumors. Elevated PSCA expression has been shown to correlate with increased tumor stage, grade, and progression to androgen-independence (Gu et al., 2000). *In situ* hybridization (ISH) and immunohistochemical (IHC) studies demonstrated PSCA expression in more than 80% of the localized prostate cancers and in all prostate cancer bone metastatic lesions examined (Gu et al., 2000; Reiter et al., 1998). Two recent studies demonstrated the suitability of PSCA as an appropriate target for T cell-based immunotherapy. Firstly, anti-PSCA monoclonal antibody therapy inhibited prostate tumor growth and metastasis, and prolonged survival of mice bearing human prostate cancer xenografts (Ross et al., 2002; Saffran et al., 2001). Secondly, *in vitro* stimulation with PSCA-derived peptide induced a tumor-specific CTL response (Dannull et al., 2000). Based upon these preclinical studies, PSCA represents another attractive prostate-specific antigen that may be suitable for immunotherapeutic targeting.

Studies employing combinations of subtractive hybridization and microarray analysis have identified and confirmed the expression of several additional prostate-specific genes including prostase/KLK4 (Nelson et al., 1999b), prostein (Xu et al., 2001), STEAP (Hubert et al., 1999), and p504S/Alpha-Methylacyl-CoA-Racemase (Xu et al., 2000). The enhanced pattern of prostate-specific expression of these genes makes them potential candidates for immunomodulatory therapy. Prostase/KLK4 is a member of the kallikrein gene family shown to be highly restricted in expression to human prostate epithelium and regulated by androgenic hormones (Nelson et al., 1999b). Prostase/KLK4 shares 35% amino acid identity with PSA and 78% identity with the porcine enamel matrix serine proteinase 1, an enzyme involved in enamel matrix degradation and with a putative role in the disruption of intercellular junction adhesion (Nelson et al., 1999b). The tissue-specific expression profile of KLK4 suggests that this molecule is likely to be an excellent candidate Ag for the development of vaccine and immunotherapeutic agents against prostate cancer. It has recently been shown that $CD4^+$ T cells exist in the peripheral circulation of normal donors that recognize naturally processed epitopes derived from KLK4. Three peptide epitopes are identified that correspond to amino acids 155–169, 160–174, and 125–139 of KLK4. Furthermore, T cells specific for these epitopes exist in peripheral blood mononuclear cells (PBMC) from multiple normal males that express the relevant class II molecules. These preliminary studies support the further evaluation of whole gene-, protein-, or peptide-based prostase/KLK4 cancer vaccine strategies.

Mouse RTVP-1 (mRTVP-1; related to testes-specific, vespid, and pathogenesis proteins) gene, a direct target of p53 with proapoptotic activities in various cancer cell lines including prostate cancer, was identified by using differential display PCR and extensive promoter analysis (Ren et al., 2002). The mRTVP-1 protein has 255 amino acids and differs from the human RTVP-1 (hRTVP-1) (Rich et al., 1996) protein by two short in-frame deletions of two and nine amino acids. Overexpression of mRTVP-1 induced apoptosis in both murine and human prostate cancer cell lines. Deletion of the signal peptide from the N terminus of RTVP-1 reduced its apoptotic activities, suggesting that a secreted and soluble form of RTVP-1 may mediate, in part, its proapoptotic activities (Ren et al., 2002). Adenovirus-based mRTVP-1 (AdmRTVP-1) gene therapy was shown to significantly reduce primary tumor as well as lung metastasis in an orthotopic, metastatic mouse model of prostate cancer (Satoh et al., 2003) confirming its antiangiogenic activity. Interestingly, significant increased natural killer and cytotoxic T lymphocyte activities were also found in mouse-bearing tumors following AdmRTVP-1-treatment indicating that RTVP-1 serves as not only an antiangiogenic gene but also as a new target of immunotherapeutics for metastatic prostate cancer.

Dentritic cell (DC)-based tumor vaccine

DCs, the most potent antigen-presenting cells (APC), are involved in native T cell activation. Because the interaction between activated, antigen-loaded, myeloid-type DCs and T-cells is a critical event in eliciting a cellular immune response to tumor antigens and enhancing the survival of CTLs recruited to the tumor site by protecting these effector cells from tumor-induced apoptosis (Mailliard and Lotze, 2001), their use for the active immunotherapy of malignancies has been of considerable interest (Banchereau and Steinman, 1998). Studies in prostate cancer using monocyte-derived DCs pulsed with peptides derived from PSMA in combination with radiotherapy and hormonal therapy resulted in objective responses in 8 of 33 patients (Tjoa et al., 1998). A smaller study used CD34[+] derived DCs pulsed with a fusion protein of human GM-CSF and prostatic acid phosphatase led to falling levels of serum PSA in 3 of 13 patients (Burch et al., 2000). To date, no toxicity has been observed with DC vaccines apart from slight fever and painful lymph nodes. Antigen can be delivered to DCs in the form of MHC-restricted peptides, proteins, tumor-derived antigenic mixtures, or through transfection with genetic materials, each of which greatly influences the pathway and efficacy of T cell activation by DCs (Gilboa et al., 1998). In all of the above, mRNA-loaded DC vaccines represents a new and effective strategy to stimulate CTL responses since mRNA can be generated and characterized easier than protein, and have the advantage of expanding the scope of vaccination by presenting multiple epitopes for different MHC haplotypes to every cancer patient, independent of their genetic background. Indeed, experiments in mice have demonstrated the development of both protective and therapeutic antitumor responses by using mRNA-loaded DC vaccines (Ashley et al., 1997; Boczkowski et al., 1996; Heiser et al., 2000). Recently a phase I trial using autologous dendritic cells (DCs) transfected with mRNA encoding PSA (Heiser et al., 2002) was performed to evaluate its safety, feasibility, and efficacy to induce T cell responses against the self-protein PSA in patients with metastatic prostate cancer. The demonstration of vaccine safety, successful *in vivo* induction of PSA-specific immunity, and impact on surrogate clinical endpoints provides a scientific rationale for further clinical investigation of RNA-transfected DCs in the treatment of human cancer.

Immunomodulatory Gene Therapy

Patients with advanced prostate cancer exhibit alterations in the patterns of cytokine production that lead to decreased cellular immunity, evidenced by the down-regulation of many cytokines, such as TNF-α, interferons (IFNs), and IL-2 (Elsasser-Beile et al., 1993). Conversely, elevated levels of TH2 cytokines, such as IL-4 (Hrouda et al., 1998), can promote antibody-based immunity rather than cellular-based immunity. Other causes of impaired tumor detection by the immune system in prostate cancer patients include secretion of inhibitory substances such as IL-10, TGF-β (Stearns et al., 1999), abnormal T-lymphocyte signal transduction (Healy et al., 1998) and expression of Fas ligand (FasL), which may enable tumor cells to induce apoptosis in Fas-expressing tumor infiltrating lymphocytes (Hedlund et al., 1998; Liu et al., 1998).

Introduction of cytokine genes into tumor cells, an approach described as *ex vivo* gene therapy, allows the sustained local release of cytokines capable of enhancing the intensity and quality of the immune response to tumor. Preclinical studies have been shown that gene-modified tumor vaccines expressing specific cytokines, including IFN-γ, IL-2 (Vieweg et al., 1994) and GM-CSF (Sanda et al., 1994), induce T cell- specific responses that can result in antitumor effects. Based on these findings, evaluation of the clinical feasibility of these cytokines (Belldegrun et al., 2001) and GM-CSF (Simons and Mikhak, 1998) gene modified prostate cancer cell vaccines were undertaken. In contrast to *ex vivo* cancer vaccine, *in situ* gene-modified immunotherapy may have some practical and conceptual benefits from the simplicity of vector injection into a tumor and expression of cytokine genes directly within a population of cancer cells (Hitt and Gauldie, 2000). More recently, several viral vectors, including herpes simplex viruses (Parkinson et al., 2003), adenoviruses (Hull et al., 2000; Nasu et al., 1999), and canarypox viruses (Siemens et al., 2000) are being applied to cancer cytokine gene therapy to demonstrate its feasibility to treat prostate cancer through *in vivo* gene delivery.

It is now evident that complete T cell activation requires two signals. The first is provided by antigen-specific signals arising from interactions between the T cell receptor (TCR) and antigen/MHC. The second signal arises from antigen-independent interactions between the CD28 molecule on the T cell surface with the costimulatory B7 family of ligands (CD80 and CD86), commonly expressed on APC. Numerous studies have demonstrated that provision of these costimulatory B7 ligands to cancer cells from diverse tissue origins bypasses the requirement for exogenous APC help, culminating in potent and tumor-specific CD8$^+$ T cell activation (Chen et al., 1992; Townsend and Allison, 1993; Townsend et al., 1994). The CD28 homolog, CTLA-4, also binds to B7, but with an approximately 20-fold higher affinity than CD28 (Linsley et al., 1994). In contrast to the B7/CD28 interaction, however, the B7/CTLA-4 interaction delivers an inhibitory signal to T cells (Krummel and Allison, 1995). Therefore, the outcome of TCR signaling is dependent on the competing stimulatory and inhibitory interactions of B7 with CD28 and CTLA-4, respectively. *In vivo*, prostate cancer cells transduced to express the B7.1 ligand (Kwon et al., 1997) and antibody-mediated blockade of the T cell CTLA-4 (Kwon et al., 1999; Kwon et al., 1997) can augment host antitumor responses, as has been demonstrated in a transgenic TRAMP mouse model that closely parallel the biology and progression of human prostate cancer (Gingrich et al., 1996) suggesting that appropriate manipulation of T cell costimulatory and inhibitory signals may provide a fundamental and highly adaptable basis for prostate cancer immunotherapy.

In addition to immune stimulation, the issue of overcoming active immune suppression must also be considered when developing an immune-based strategy for cancer therapy, particularly with regard to secreted soluble factors known to down-regulate immune function and antitumor response. TGF-β (Letterio and Roberts, 1998), which has previously been shown to act in a critical inhibitory fashion on most cells of the immune system and is secreted by a wide variety of tumor types, is frequently associated with mechanisms of tumor escape from immunosurveillance. The potency of TGF-β. as an immunosuppressive cytokine makes it an attractive target as anticancer therapy. Shah *et al* (Shah et al., 2002) recently demonstrated that abrogation of TGF-β signaling in the immune compartment via retrovirus-mediated expression of a dominant-negative TGF-β type II receptor in transplanted BM-derived stem cells leads to the generation of mature leukocytes capable of increasing survival, reducing metastases in mice when animals were challenged with highly tumorigenic melanoma or prostate cancer cells. This finding suggests that an immunotheapy approach to induce TGF-β insensibility may be a potent anticancer therapy. However, because of the potency of TGF-β as an immunoregulatory cytokine critical for the maintenance of immune homeostasis, blockage of TGF-β signaling could potentially generate widespread autoimmunity and inflammation. Thus the safety of employing perturbations in the TGF-β signaling processes for cancer immunotherapeutics needs further investigation.

GENE THERAPY HUMAN CLINICAL TRIALS

The lethal phenotype of prostate cancer involves androgen-independent and bone metastatic lesions. Because of the well-known mortality, morbidity and skeletal complications including severe bone pain, pathologic fracture, spinal cord compression syndrome, cranial nerve foramena, and hypercalcemia commonly associated with hormone refractory prostate cancer bone metastasis (Franks, 1956; Harada et al., 1992; Jemal et al., 2003; Mintz and Smith, 1934), a large number of clinical trials have been implemented to assess clinical responsiveness of advanced prostate cancer to gene and drug therapy. In this section, we summarized in table form most of the gene therapeutic clinical trials conducted to treat localized and distant disseminated prostate cancer. Because of the rather limited number of clinical trials involving the treatment of metastatic cancers (Benjamin et al., 2001; Kubo et al., 2003), we will focus our attention on discussing first the use of gene therapy for localized prostate cancer, followed by gene therapy in the treatment of metastatic prostate cancer.

Numerous therapeutic approaches including clinical trials targeting metastases to soft tissues are ongoing and can be sub-categorized based on each molecular mechanism. Examples of gene therapy for the treatment of cancer metastasis to bone are rare and will be reviewed below, Two clinical trials of gene therapy application to bone are reported in the literature: one on the metastatic prostate cancer to bone and the other on the treatment of primary osteosarcoma in bone. A phase I dose-escalation clinical trial we conducted employed both patients with localized and metastatic hormone-refractory prostate cancer using Ad-OC-hsv-TK (Kubo et al., 2003), and the other trial is a phase I/II study of intravenous injections of Ad-OC-E1 (OCaP1) in patients with refractory osteosarcoma metastatic to lung (Benjamin et al., 2001). Because of the small number of reports regarding of gene therapy for bone metastatsis, we will review our trial for the treatment of prostate cancer bone metastasis in a separate section below. We began our review below first with gene therapy application to treat primarily localized prostate cancer and in patients with prostate cancer micro-metastasis.

Gene Therapy Clinical Trials for Prostate Cancer

A total of 46 gene therapy trials for prostate cancer were either completed or are being conducted presently in the United States (http://www.wiley.co.uk/genmed/clinical/, http://www4.od.nih.gov/oba/rac/clinicaltrial.htm). These clinical trials are summarized in Table 3. Therapeutic strategies of these trials can be categorized as immune-based gene therapy (25 trials), tumor suppressor-based corrective gene therapy (6 trials), genes directed toward the activation of pro-drugs via the transfer of enzymes to achieve "bystander" and cytoreductive effects on tumors (8 trials), and a conditional replicating-based adenoviral therapy (7 trials).

Table 3. Current clinical trials of prostate cancer gene therapy

Investigator/Location	Indication	Gene(s)	Phase	Route	Vector
A. Belldegrun UCLA	Primary or recurrent local	IL-2	I	Intratumoral	Lipofm (Leuvectin)
A. P. Chen National Naval Medical Center, Bethesda	Metastatic	PSA	I	Intradermoral	Pox
R. A. Figlin UCLA	Metastatic and local reccurrent	MUC-1/IL-2	I/II	IM	Pox
J. T. Holt Vanderbilt University, Nashville	Advanced	Antisense c-myc RNA	I	Intraprostatic	Retro
D.W. Kufe and J.P. Eder Dana Farber Cancer Institute, Boston	Advanced	PSA	I	Intradermal	Pox
D. F. Paulson Duke University Medical Center, Durham	Locally advanced or metastatic	IL-2	I	Intradermal	Cationic Liposome Complex
M. G. Sanda University of Michigan	Locally advanced T2-T3	PSA	I	Intradermal	Pox
P. T. Scardino Baylor College, Houston	Locally recurrent	HSV-TK	I/II	Intratumoral	Adeno
J. W. Simons Johns Hopkins, Baltimore	Metastatic	GM-CSF	I	SC	Retro
M. S. Steiner University of Tennessee		BRCA-1	I/II	Intratumoral	Retro
S. J. Hall Mount Sinai, New York	T1c, T2b&C	HSV-TK	I/II	Intratumoral	Adeno
A. Belldegrun UCLA	Locally advanced or recurrent	p53 (SCH58500)	I	Intratumoral	Adeno
C. J. Logothetis MD Anderson, Houston	Locally advanced	p53 (INGN201)	I	Intraprostatic	Adeno
J. W. Simons Johns Hopkins, Baltimore	Metastatic	GM-CSF	II	SC	Retro

(Continued on next page)

                    Gene Therapy for Prostate Cancer Bone Metastasis

(Table 3 continued)

D. Kadmon Baylor College, Houston	Clinically localized	HSV-TK	I	Intratumoral	Adeno
J. W. Simons Johns Hopkins, Baltimore	Locally recurrent	PSA	I	Intratumoral	Adeno (CN706)
L. W. Chung and T. A. Gardner University of Virginia	Metastatic or local recurrent	Osteocalcin-HSV-TK	I	Intratumoral	Adeno
Dana Farber Cancer Institute, Boston	Advanced	PSA	II	IM	Pox
E. J. Small Univ California San Francisco	Micro-metastatic	GM-CSF	I	SC	Retro
H. L. Kaufman Albert Einstein Cancer Center, New York	Advanced	PSA	I	Intraderm/ IM	Pox
J. Vieweg Duke University Medical Center, Durham	Advanced	PSA	I-II	IV	rna transfer
A. Belldegrun UCLA	local	IL-2	I-II	Intratum	lipofect (Leuvectin)
E. J. Small UCSF	Advanced	GM-CSF	II	SC	Retro
J. H. Kim Henry Ford Health System, Detroit	Local recurrent	CD+ HSV-TK	I-II	Intratum	Adeno
E. B. Butler Baylor College, Houston	T2-T3	HSV-TK	I/II	Intratum	Adenov
J. R. Gingrich University of Tennessee	Locally advanced	p16	I	Intratum	Adeno
M. K. Terris Palo Alto Vet. Adm. Stanford	Locally recurrent	PSA	I/II	Intratum	Adeno (CV787)
G. Wilding University of Wisconsin, Madison	Metastatic	PSA	I/II	IV	Adeno (CV787)
A. Belldegrun UCLA	Locally recurrent	IL-2	I/II	Intratum	Lipofect (Leuvectin)
B. Dahut National Naval Medical Center, Bethesda	Localized	PSA	II	Intraderm/ IM	Pox

(Continued on next page)

(Table 3 continued)

P. M. Arlen NCI, Bethesda	Micro-metastatic	PSA	II	Intraderm/IM	Pox
J. Vieweg Duke University Medical Center, Durham	Metastatic	Tumour RNA	I	IV	RNA transfer
A. Pollack MD Anderson	T1-T3	p53	II	Intraprostatic	Adeno
T. A. Gardner Indiana University	Metastatic or locally recurrent	OC-E1a	I	Intratum	Adeno
S. O. Freytag Henry Ford Health System	localized	CD/HSV-TK	I	Intratum	Adeno
D. M. Lubaroff University of Iowa	Metastatic	PSA	I	SC	Adeno
B. J. Miles Baylor College	Local recurrent	IL-12	I	Intratum	Adeno
T. L. DeWeese Johns Hopkins Oncology Center	Clinically localized	PSA	II	Intratum	Adeno (CV7606)
E. J. Small UCSF	Metastatic	PSA	II	IV	Adeno (CV787)
E. Dula West Coast Clinical Research	Metastatic	GM-CSF	I	SC	AAV
S. O. Freytag Henry Ford Health System	T2a-T4	E. coli CD / HSV-TK	I	Intratum	Adeno
H. Scher MSCKK	Relapsed	PSMA	I	IM	plasmid DNA
J. Corman VA Puget Sound Health Care System	Metastatic	GM-CSF	I/II	SC	AAV
A. J. Pantuck UCLA	Recurrent	MUC-1 / IL2	II	SC	Vaccina Virus
J. Vieweg Duke University Medical Center	Metastatic	Human Telomerase Reverse Transcriptase	I	Intradermal	RNA transfusion
J. Corman VA Puget Sound Health Care System	Locally recurrent	PSA	I / II	Intratum	Adeno (CG7060)

In the immune modulation approach, antitumor immune response is mediated by expressing interleukin-2 (IL-2) (n=6), granulocyte-macrophage-colony stimulating factor (GM-CSF) (n=6), PSA (n=9), tumor RNA (n=1), expressing IL-12 (n=1), PSMA (n=1), and human telomerase reverse transcriptase (n=1). Simons *et al* (Johns Hopkins) reported the induction of tumor-specific immunity after subcutaneous injection of GM-CSF transfected and irradiated autologous tumor cells in three out of eight vaccinated patients. Although no immunity to PSA was obtained, antibodies from the sera of three patients detected polypeptides in LNCaP, PC3 and normal prostate epithelial cells (Simons et al., 1999). Vaccinia virus expressing PSA elicits a PSA-specific IgM response (Hodge et al., 1995; Sanda et al., 1999). Cutaneous vaccinia-PSA vaccinations were without local complications and resulted in a specific T-cell response to peptide from PSA in a phase I clinical trial at Dana-Farber/Harvard Cancer Center (Eder et al., 2000). Of 33 recurrent prostate cancer patients treated with a recombinant vaccinia virus encoding human PSA (rV-PSA), 14 showed stable PSA levels for at least 6 months. Nine patients remained stable for 11-25 months; six of these remain progression free with stable PSA levels (Eder et al., 2000). At National Cancer Institute, a phase I clinical study of 42 patients with advanced metastatic prostate cancer was also conducted using rV-PSA (Gulley et al., 2002). Pantuck *et al* constructed a vaccinia virus expressing MUC1, a tumor antigen present on prostate, breast, lung, and other cancers, in combination with IL-2 (Pantuck et al., 2000; Pantuck et al., 2001). After intramuscular injection of this recombinant virus, PSA decline was observed in 1 of 15 patients, whereas in several patients white blood cell activity increased, as did expression of TNF-α and IFN-γ suggesting MUC1 gene expression coupled to local production of IL-2 can advance the stimulation of CTL response in patients. Belldegrun et al conducted a Phase I clinical trial for evaluating the safety and efficacy of delivering Leuvectin, a DNA-lipid complex encoding IL-2 gene intratumorally into patients with locally recurrent prostate cancer at UCLA (Belldegrun et al., 2001). In this trial, 57% of the enrolled patients showed transient decrease of PSA with no significant changes in American Urologic Association Symptom Scores during the entire course of treatment (Belldegrun et al., 2001). By using DC-mediated immunotherapy strategy, a study of phase II trial, involving infusions of autologous DC and two PSMA peptides, was recently completed and reported by Tjoa and colleaques (Tjoa et al., 1999). Thirty percent of the participants, including subjects with hormone-refractory metastastic disease, and those with suspected local recurrence of prostate cancer, were identified as clinical responders suggesting that DC-based cancer vaccines in the future may provide an additional avenue for advanced prostate cancer.

As corrective gene therapy, six clinical trials have been conducted using tumor suppressor genes. All these approaches aimed to replace defective or mutated genes related to tumorigenesis and tumor growth. Mutation of p53 gene is a late event in the progression of prostate cancer and is associated with advanced (metastatic) stage, loss of differentiation, and the transition from androgen-dependent to androgen-independent growth in experimental and clinical prostate cancer (Navone et al., 1993). Three clinical trials with adenovirus carrying wild-type p53 are in progress at the University of Texas M. D. Anderson Cancer Center and UCLA. Logothetis et al. have treated 30 patients with either locally advanced, had high Gleason scores or high PSA-expressing prostate cancers using wild-type p53 carried in an adenoviral vector and delivered by intraprostatic injection. Patients with a 25% reduction in tumor size or greater, assessed by ultrasound, were given repeat treatments. A total of 38 treatments were given, without significant side effects. TUNEL assay and assays for p53 on radical prostatectomy specimens and post-treatment tissue biopsies verified that p53 protein production can be induced even in tumors without p53 immunostaining at the onset of this study, and that apoptosis in tumor cells can be triggered (Pisters LL, 2001). Other than p53, the breast cancer gene (BRCA 1) and p16 are also used as tumor suppressors for corrective gene therapy. PTEN that inhibit the PI3-kinase growth pathway signal transduction and recently discovered tumor suppressor gene, pHyde, might be new candidates for corrective gene therapy based on the promising preclinical data (Davies et al., 2002; Steiner et al., 2000).

Suicide gene therapies involve the delivery of genes to cancer cells where the encoded enzymes locally convert inactive pro-drugs into active metabolites that lead to cell cycle arrest and cell death. This kind of gene directed enzyme pro-drug therapies enable more precise control of cell-kill than the therapies using tumor suppressor genes because the timing of pro-drug administration can be precisely determined to augment therapeutic efficacy. In addition, non-infected cells are also expected to be damaged by a "bystander" gene-induced therapeutic effects. The widely applied pro-drug-suicide gene systems are the herpes simplex virus thymidine kinase (HSV-TK)/ganciclovir (GCV) system and the *Escherichia coli* cytosine deaminase (CD)/5-fluorocytosine (5-FC) system. Five clinical trials using HSV-TK/GCV system and 3 trials using a fusion suicide gene system of CD/5-FC plus HSV-TK/GCV have been applied so far. A Phase I clinical trial of adenovirus-HSV-TK/GCV was conducted at Baylor College of Medicine for patients with local recurrence of prostate cancer after definitive irradiation therapy (Herman *et al.*, 1999). Of 18 patients enrolled, one patient at the highest dose level developed spontaneously reversible grade 4 thrombocytopenia and grade 3 hepatotoxicity (Herman et al., 1999). The safety of this therapy was further investigated in a multiple and repeated injection fashion, demonstrating mild and self-limiting side effects (Shalev *et al.*, 2000). The efficacy was documented in a report of an extended phase I/II study as follows; an initial cycle of HSV-TK/GCV gene therapy caused a significant prolongation of the mean serum PSA-doubling time from 15.9 to 42.5 months and in 28 of the injected patients (77.8%) there was a mean PSA reduction of 28% (Miles et al., 2001). These authors also demonstrated an interesting finding where positive correlation between the density of CD8$^+$ T cells in posttreatment biopsy specimens and the number of apoptotic cells was observed (Miles et al., 2001).

Henry Ford Health System (Detroit, MI) conducted a phase I study for locally recurrent prostate cancer using a unique vector of a replication-competent adenovirus delivering a CD/HSV-1 TK fusion gene (Ad5-CD/Tk*rep*) to tumors (Freytag et al., 2002). Ad5-CD/Tk*rep* was injected intraprostatically into 16 patients with local recurrent prostate cancer after definitive radiation therapy. Ninety-four percent of the adverse events observed were grade 1 or 2 in nature. Seven of 16 (44%) patients demonstrated a ≥25% decrease in serum PSA, and 3 of 16 (19%) patients demonstrated a ≥50% decrease in serum PSA. Two patients were negtative for adenocarcinoma at one year follow-up confirmed by sextant needle biopsy. Although Ad5-CD/TK*rep* viral DNA could be detected in blood as far out as day 76, no infectious adenovirus was detected in patient serum or urine (Freytag et al., 2002).

At the University of Virginia, we conducted a phase I clinical trial of adenovirus vector carrying osteocalcin promoter-driven hsv-TK in localized and metastatic hormone-refractory prostate cancer with the goal of co-targeting tumor and stroma. The details of this trial are described in a separate section below.

One of the major limitations of replication deficient viral-based vectors is the insufficient delivery of therapeutic genes to cancer cells. To enhance the transduction efficiency, replication competent viral vectors (capable of replicating in host cells that contain the complement factors that can drive the viral replication) were examined in several studies (Hsieh et al., 2002; Latham et al., 2000; Matsubara et al., 2001; Rodriguez et al., 1997; Walker et al., 1999). The early expressed adenoviral genes, *E1a* and *E1b*, are necessary in viral replication. E1a is known to bind the retinoblastoma (Rb) gene product, while E1b binds p53 (Braithwaite and Jenkins, 1989; Zantema et al., 1985). As Rb and p53 negatively regulate the cell cycle, binding or inhibition of Rb and p53 forces the cell to enter S phase of cell cycle, where the viral genome can be multiplied for self-replication. In 1997, Rodriguez *et al.* (Rodriguez et al., 1997), reported on the development of a replication-competent, E3-deleted, cytolytic Ad5 adenovirus called CN706 (subsequently renamed CV706), with replication that was restricted to PSA-producing cells. This restricted replication was achieved by the insertion of a minimal promoter-enhancer construct of the human PSA enhancer (*PSE*) 5' of E1A, 3' of the E1A promoter, resulting in PSA-regulated expression of E1A. This E1A regulation, in turn, resulted in the restriction of CV706 replication primarily to cells expressing PSA. Single, intratumoral, injections of CV706 into the PSA-producing human prostate cancer LNCaP xenograft model resulted in rapid regression of those established tumors with a concomitant decrement in serum PSA. These findings were translated into a Phase I clinical trial conducted at Johns Hopkins Hospital for the treatment of patients with locally recurrent prostate cancer after radiation therapy (DeWeese et al., 2001). In this study, CV706 was found to be safe and was not associated with irreversible grade 3 or any grade 4 toxicity. Posttreatment prostatic biopsies and detection of a delayed "peak" of circulating copies of virus provided evidence of intraprostatic replication of CV706. Biopsies after viral injection showed viral replication only in prostate epithelial cells. All five patients who achieved a $\geq 50\%$ reduction in PSA were treated with the highest two doses of CV706 (DeWeese et al., 2001).

Another improved replication-competent Ad vector, CV787, contains the E1a adenoviral gene under probasin promoter control and the E1b gene under PSA promoter control (Yu et al., 1999). This enables CV787 to get higher tumor specificity than CV706. CV787 is further added the Ad5 E3 region, eventually this virus get enhanced cytolytic effects compared with CN702 (Yu et al., 1999). A few clinical trials using CV787 adenovirus are ongoing for patients with not only local recurrence but also metastatic prostate cancer via intraveneous injection of this viral vector (see Table 3, UCSF/Mt. Zion Cancer Center, University of Wisconsin Comprehensive Cancer Center).

Phase I Dose Escalation Clinical Trial of Adenovirus Vector Carrying Osteocalcin Promoter-driven Herpes Simplex Virus Thymidine Kinase in Localized and Metastatic Hormone-Refractory Prostate Cancer

While men with early stage prostate cancer can be treated effectively by surgery, radiation and/or hormonal therapy, once the disease has become hormone-independent and progressed to lymph nodes and bone there is no available effective therapy to prolong the patient's survival. Osseous metastases are currently treated by external beam radiation therapy (Szostak and Kyprianou, 2000) or radiopharmaceuticals (Graham et al., 1999; Lee et al., 1996; Turner et al., 2001) which offer symptomatic palliation and prevent pathologic fracture, but are associated with myelosuppression in patients with osseous metastases. Although chemotherapy and second-line hormonal therapy have limited roles in the treatment of hormone-independent advanced prostate cancer, several new therapeutic combinations including bone-directed targeting have recently shown early promise (Tu et al., 2001). In addition, recent studies indicate that bisphosphonates (Heidenreich et al., 2001; Papapoulos et al., 2000) and endothelin-1 receptor antagonist (Nelson et al., 1999a; Stephenson, 2001) may have a role in the treatment of prostate cancer bone metastasis and associated complications. As the literature reveals, new alternative approaches for treating hormone-independent prostate cancer metastasis to bone and visceral organs are being urgently sought.

Osteocalcin (OC), a major noncollagenous bone matrix protein, is expressed prevalently in prostate cancer epithelial cells, adjacent fibromuscular stromal cells, and osteoblasts in locally recurrent prostate cancer and prostate cancer bone metastasis (Matsubara et al., 2001). Our pre-clinical models demonstrated the efficacy of a recombinant, replication-defective adenovirus, osteocalcin promoter-driven herpes-simplex-virus thymidine kinase (Ad-OC-hsv-TK) (Cheon et al., 1997; Gardner et al., 1998; Ko et al., 1996; Shirakawa et al., 1998) and a replication-competent Ad-OC-E1a (Matsubara et al., 2001) or Ad-hOC-E1 (Hsieh et al., 2002) adenovirus capable of co-targeting prostate tumor epithelium and supporting stromal cells, resulting in effective tumor regression in immune-compromised mice.

Based on these promising pre-clinical results, we constructed Ad-OC-hsv-TK to cotarget prostate cancer cells and their surrounding stromal cells. A phase I dose-escalating trial of intra-tumoral injection of Ad-OC-hsv-TK followed by oral valacyclovir (VAL) was conducted at the University of Virginia (Charlottesville, VA) in 11 men with hormone refractory metastatic or localized recurrent prostate cancer (2 local recurrent, 5 osseous metastasis, and 4 lymph node metastasis) to assess the potential toxicity of this therapy and to determine the usefulness of this vector for the palliation of androgen-independent prostate cancer metastasis (Kubo et al., 2003). This is the first clinical trial in which therapeutic adenoviruses are injected directly into prostate cancer lymph node and bone metastasis. Eleven men were treated with an escalating dose of Ad-OC-hsv-*TK*, 2.5×10^8 to $2.5 \times$

10^{10} plaque-forming units (pfu) (5×10^{9} to 5×10^{11} viral particles) on Days 1 and 8, followed by oral valacyclovir (VAL, 1 gram twice daily for 21 days).

Results show that (1) all patients tolerated this therapy with no serious adverse events; (2) local cell death was observed in treated lesions in seven patients (63.6%) as assessed by terminal deoxynucleotidyl transferase mediated dUTP nick end labeling (TUNEL) assay, and histomorphological change (mediation of fibrosis) was detected in all posttreated specimens; (3) one patient showed stabilization of the treated lesion for 317 days with no alternative therapy. Of the two patients who complained of tumor-associated symptoms before the treatment, one patient with bone pain had resolution of pain, although significant remission of treated lesions was not observed by image examination; (4) CD8-positive T cells were predominant compared with CD4-positive T cells, B cells (L26 positive), and natural killer cells (CD56 positive) in posttreated tissue specimens; (5) levels of HSV *TK* gene transduction correlated well with coxsackie-adenovirus receptor expression but less well with the titers of adenovirus injected; and (6) intrinsic OC expression and the efficiency of hsv TK gene transduction affected the levels of hsv TK protein expression in clinical specimens. Our data suggest that this form of gene therapy requires further development for the treatment of androgen-independent prostate cancer metastasis although histopathological and immunohistochemical evidence of apoptosis was observed in the specimens treated. Further studies including the development of improved viral delivery, via the use of replication-competent Ad vectors, will enhance the efficacy of this form of gene therapy.

FUTURE GENE THERAPY PROSPECTIVE

One of the most challenging problems facing prostate cancer treatment is to develop a rational and effective therapy to repress the development and progression of multiple bone and visceral lesions in high-risk prostate cancer patients with the hope of extending their survival and improve their overall quality of life. This strategy, if implement successfully, is expected to achieve not only short-term palliation in symptoms but also the long-term benefit by reducing mortality, morbidity and skeletal complications associated with advanced prostate cancer. Most of gene therapy for prostate cancer today including our clinical trial show acceptable toxicity, high degree of specificity and some local therapeutic effects as evidenced by biochemical, histomorphologic and clinical evaluations. Unfortunately, overall results from gene therapy trials showed that most of the clinical responses recorded were transient in nature and limited in scope. The challenge remains was how to develop a gene therapy strategy so that long-lasting responses and complete remission of prostate cancer bone and visceral metastases are possible. We believe the following areas of improvement are essential before gene therapy will be widely adopted as an integral part of cancer therapy for the treatment of localized and metastatic prostate cancer:

1. Improved delivery of target genes to cancer cells: This will require further development of improved vectors and delivery systems so that a large number of tumor cells can express efficiently the desired transgene for longer duration. Since the lethality from cancer is contributed largely by metastasis, delivery of transgene to metastatic tumor cells outside of the prostate gland is likely to be achieved more efficiently by systemic rather than intratumoral route. Thus effort must be directed at the development of vectors that could be injected or taken orally with high level of transgene expression by all cancer cells, or alternatively all cancer cells including the non-transduced cells be affected by the transgene via either direct or indirect mechanisms such as the "bystander" effect. In case if immunogene therapy is applied, tumor cell-bearing antigens or vaccines can be applied successfully by subcutaneous inoculation method. To improve further transgene expression in cancer but not normal host vital organs, strategies are needed to improve transcriptional and transductional targeting of cancer cells as illustrated above in this chapter;

2. Reduced immunogenicity of the viral and non-viral vectors for continued and long-term application: Efficiency of transgene delivery and expression in target cells is dependent upon the concentration of the vector in plasma or tissue and its accumulated time intervals of cell and tissue contact during transgene delivery. Viral vectors, such as Ad and vaccinia viruses employing in most of current clinical applications are considered as highly immunogenic agents. Thus strategies must be sought to design viral and non-viral vectors which are non-immunogenic so that they can be given continuously, bypassing host immune responses to vectors or target genes, with increased accumulation of transgene in target cancer cells. Alternatively, different viral vectors and their variants may be applied sequentially to evade host immune response in an effort to improve transgene delivery to target cells.

3. Improved specificity of transgene delivery to and expression in cancer and adjacent stromal cells: It is becoming increasing clear that cancer-microenvironment interaction could determine ultimately the malignant progression and survival of cancer cells. While the basic premise is to eradicate cancer cells without damaging the normal host organs, targeting

cancer cells is understandable necessary but alone may be insufficient to eradicate the growth of both primary and metastatic prostate cancers permanently. Cancer is an organ comprising of both cancer and cancer-adjacent cells, such as prostate and bone stroma located within cancer-associated microenvironment. Thus to achieve the best possible therapeutic response of cancer growth in the host, both cancer and its microenvironment can be selected as potential therapeutic targets. This concept is supported and appreciated through the understanding of the biology of cancer-stroma interactions which contribute to enhance cancer growth and survival. Moreover, it is well documented that neovasculature originated from the stroma is required to support the continued cancer growth and dissemination. The "vicious cycle" between cancer and stroma represents not only cancer cell responsive to the "inductive cue" emancipated from the stroma, but also the realization of the plasticity of cancer and stromal cells in the microenvironment which could undergo permanent genotypic and phenotypic alterations, mediated by factors produced by cancer cells as well as cells within tumor-associated microenvironment. Thus, to achieve the most effective and optimal targeting of the tumors, cotargeting cancer and stroma with gene therapy either applies alone or in combination with other treatment modalities could generate profound therapeutic benefits to patients with prostate cancer metastasis.

4. Improved efficacy of cancer-specific therapeutic genes targeting at lethal phenotypes of prostate cancer: Among prostate cancer variants, there are high-, intermediate- and low-risk subtype. To improve the survival of high-risk prostate cancer patients, more potent and selective therapeutic gene(s) must be developed targeting at prostate cancer bone and visceral metastases. It is likely that such therapeutic genes can be successfully developed only after carefully examine and validate critical molecular pathways relevant to the development of lethal phenotypes of prostate cancer as manifested by increased cell proliferation, survival under androgen-deprived conditions, resistance to chemotherapy and radiation therapy and failure to commit to terminal differentiation and apoptotic death. New cancer-specific therapeutic genes may be discovered through the investigation of the molecular determinants that enabling androgen-independent prostate cancer cells to survive under hormone-deprived condition. The design of viral vectors with the ability of expressing transgene in both androgen receptor (AR-positive as well as –negative cells, irrespective of their basal AR and cell signaling status. Better predictive methods, molecular sensing technologies, animal models and basic understanding of the molecular pathways leading to cancer cell growth control are essential ingredients for the development of new and

more effective therapeutic genes targeting prostate cancer growth and metastasis; and

5. Combinatory targeting strategies must be designed using gene therapy in combination with surgery, hormone therapy, chemotherapy, and/or radiation therapy: Based on the published literature on the development of therapeutic strategies for the treatment of prostate cancer and other forms of malignancies, it is likely that gene therapy will need to be applied together with other forms of therapeutic modalities before it can reach its peak activity with the potential of "curing" patients with localized and disseminated prostate cancer. Understanding mechanistically how gene therapy will work in concert with other therapeutic modalities, such as surgery, hormone, radiation and chemotherapy, to achieve synergism could affect profoundly the clinical outcome and ultimately the survival of patients.

In summary, this article summarized current literatures on the pre-clinical and clinical investigations of gene therapy for prostate cancer with special emphasis on prostate cancer bone metastasis. We predict rapid progresses will be made in the design of vectors, therapeutic genes and deliver system as our understanding accelerated in recent years in the areas of prostate cancer biology and development of better animal models mimicking clinical prostate cancer and metastasis. Facing with 30,000 prostate cancer death per year and patients are suffered from fear of pains, skeletal complications and hopelessness prospect of survival, it becomes an urgent need to speed-up discoveries in the area of gene therapy for the treatment of prostate cancer bone metastasis.

REFERENCES

Adachi, Y., Reynolds, P. N., Yamamoto, M., Grizzle, W. E., Overturf, K., Matsubara, S., Muramatsu, T. and Curiel, D. T. (2000): Midkine promoter-based adenoviral vector gene delivery for pediatric solid tumors. *Cancer Research* **60**, 4305-10.

Anderson, W. F. (1998): Human gene therapy. *Nature* **392**, 25-30.

Aprikian, A. G., Cordon-Cardo, C., Fair, W. R., Zhang, Z. F., Bazinet, M., Hamdy, S. M. and Reuter, V. E. (1994): Neuroendocrine differentiation in metastatic prostatic adenocarcinoma. *Journal of Urology* **151**, 914-9.

Asano, M., Yukita, A., Matsumoto, T., Kondo, S. and Suzuki, H. (1995): Inhibition of tumor growth and metastasis by an immunoneutralizing monoclonal antibody to human vascular endothelial growth factor/vascular permeability factor121. *Cancer Research* **55**, 5296-301.

Ashley, D. M., Faiola, B., Nair, S., Hale, L. P., Bigner, D. D. and Gilboa, E. (1997): Bone marrow-generated dendritic cells pulsed with tumor extracts or tumor RNA induce antitumor immunity against central nervous system tumors. *Journal of Experimental Medicine* **186**, 1177-82.

Aumuller, G. (1989): Morphologic and regulatory aspects of prostatic function. *Anat Embryol (Berl)* **179**, 519-31.

Bailey, S. M. and Hart, I. R. (1997): Nitroreductase activation of CB1954--an alternative 'suicide' gene system. *Gene Therapy* **4**, 80-1.

Bailey, S. M., Knox, R. J., Hobbs, S. M., Jenkins, T. C., Mauger, A. B., Melton, R. G., Burke, P. J., Connors, T. A. and Hart, I. R. (1996): Investigation of alternative prodrugs for use with E. coli nitroreductase in 'suicide gene' approaches to cancer therapy. *Gene Therapy* **3**, 1143-50.

Bakker, A. B., Schreurs, M. W., de Boer, A. J., Kawakami, Y., Rosenberg, S. A., Adema, G. J. and Figdor, C. G. (1994): Melanocyte lineage-specific antigen gp100 is recognized by melanoma-derived tumor-infiltrating lymphocytes. *Journal of Experimental Medicine* **179**, 1005-9.

Banchereau, J. and Steinman, R. M. (1998): Dendritic cells and the control of immunity. *Nature* **392**, 245-52.

Barnett, B. G., Tillman, B. W., Curiel, D. T. and Douglas, J. T. (2002): Dual targeting of adenoviral vectors at the levels of transduction and transcription enhances the specificity of gene expression in cancer cells. *Molecular Ther* **6**, 377-85.

Becker, C. M., Farnebo, F. A., Iordanescu, I., Behonick, D. J., Shih, M. C., Dunning, P., Christofferson, R., Mulligan, R. C., Taylor, G. A., Kuo, C. J. and Zetter, B. R. (2002): Gene therapy of prostate cancer with the soluble vascular endothelial growth factor receptor flk1. *Cancer Biol Ther* **1**, 548-53.

Behrend, E. I., Craig, A. M., Wilson, S. M., Denhardt, D. T. and Chambers, A. F. (1995): Expression of antisense osteopontin RNA in metastatic mouse fibroblasts is associated with reduced malignancy. *Ann N Y Acad Sci* **760**, 299-301.

Belldegrun, A., Tso, C. L., Zisman, A., Naitoh, J., Said, J., Pantuck, A. J., Hinkel, A., deKernion, J. and Figlin, R. (2001): Interleukin 2 gene therapy for prostate cancer: phase I clinical trial and basic biology. *Human Gene Therapy* **12**, 883-92.

Benjamin, R., Helman, L., Meyers, P. and Reaman, G. (2001): A phase I/II dose escalation and activity study of intravenous injections of OCaP1 for subjects with refractory osteosarcoma metastatic to lung. *Human Gene Therapy* **12**, 1591-3.

Bergelson, J. M., Cunningham, J. A., Droguett, G., Kurt-Jones, E. A., Krithivas, A., Hong, J. S., Horwitz, M. S., Crowell, R. L. and Finberg, R. W. (1997): Isolation of a common receptor for Coxsackie B viruses and adenoviruses 2 and 5. *Science* **275**, 1320-3.

Bilbao, G., Feng, M., Rancourt, C., Jackson, W. H., Jr. and Curiel, D. T. (1997): Adenoviral/retroviral vector chimeras: a novel strategy to achieve high-efficiency stable transduction in vivo. *Faseb J* **11**, 624-34.

Boczkowski, D., Nair, S. K., Snyder, D. and Gilboa, E. (1996): Dendritic cells pulsed with RNA are potent antigen-presenting cells in vitro and in vivo. *Journal of Experimental Medicine* **184**, 465-72.

Braithwaite, A. W. and Jenkins, J. R. (1989): Ability of p53 and the adenovirus E1b 58-kilodalton protein to form a complex is determined by p53. *Journal of Virology* **63**, 1792-9.

Brichard, V., Van Pel, A., Wolfel, T., Wolfel, C., De Plaen, E., Lethe, B., Coulie, P. and Boon, T. (1993): The tyrosinase gene codes for an antigen recognized by autologous cytolytic T lymphocytes on HLA-A2 melanomas. *Journal of Experimental Medicine* **178**, 489-95.

Brown, J. M., Corey, E., Lee, Z. D., True, L. D., Yun, T. J., Tondravi, M. and Vessella, R. L. (2001): Osteoprotegerin and rank ligand expression in prostate cancer. *Urology* **57**, 611-6.

Burch, P. A., Breen, J. K., Buckner, J. C., Gastineau, D. A., Kaur, J. A., Laus, R. L., Padley, D. J., Peshwa, M. V., Pitot, H. C., Richardson, R. L., Smits, B. J., Sopapan, P., Strang, G., Valone, F. H. and Vuk-Pavlovic, S. (2000): Priming tissue-specific cellular immunity in a phase I trial of autologous dendritic cells for prostate cancer. *Clinical Cancer Research* **6**, 2175-82.

Calmels, T. P., Mattot, V., Wernert, N., Vandenbunder, B. and Stehelin, D. (1995): Invasive tumors induce c-ets1 transcription factor expression in adjacent stroma. *Biol Cell* **84**, 53-61.

Camps, J. L., Chang, S. M., Hsu, T. C., Freeman, M. R., Hong, S. J., Zhau, H. E., von Eschenbach, A. C. and Chung, L. W. (1990): Fibroblast-mediated acceleration of human epithelial tumor growth in vivo. *Proceedings of the National Acadamy of Sciences U S A* **87**, 75-9.

Caplen, N. J., Higginbotham, J. N., Scheel, J. R., Vahanian, N., Yoshida, Y., Hamada, H., Blaese, R. M. and Ramsey, W. J. (1999): Adeno-retroviral chimeric viruses as in vivo transducing agents. *Gene Therapy* **6**, 454-9.

Chen, L., Ashe, S., Brady, W. A., Hellstrom, I., Hellstrom, K. E., Ledbetter, J. A., McGowan, P. and Linsley, P. S. (1992): Costimulation of antitumor immunity by the B7 counterreceptor for the T lymphocyte molecules CD28 and CTLA-4. *Cell* **71**, 1093-102.

Chen, L., Waxman, D. J., Chen, D. and Kufe, D. W. (1996): Sensitization of human breast cancer cells to cyclophosphamide and ifosfamide by transfer of a liver cytochrome P450 gene. *Cancer Research* **56**, 1331-40.

Chen, L., Yu, L. J. and Waxman, D. J. (1997): Potentiation of cytochrome P450/cyclophosphamide-based cancer gene therapy by coexpression of the P450 reductase gene. *Cancer Research* **57**, 4830-7.

Chen, S. H., Shine, H. D., Goodman, J. C., Grossman, R. G. and Woo, S. L. (1994): Gene therapy for brain tumors: regression of experimental gliomas by adenovirus-mediated gene transfer in vivo. *Proceedings of the National Acadamy of Sciences U S A* **91**, 3054-7.

Cheon, J., Ko, S. C., Gardner, T. A., Shirakawa, T., Gotoh, A., Kao, C. and Chung, L. W. (1997): Chemogene therapy: osteocalcin promoter-based suicide gene therapy in combination with methotrexate in a murine osteosarcoma model. *Cancer Gene Therapy* **4**, 359-65.

Chung, L. W. and Auble, K. (1988): Characterization of fetal urogenital sinus-induced prostatic hyperplasia in the mouse: time course, hormonal requirement, age dependency and responsiveness of various adult organs to growth induction by fetal urogenital sinus tissues. *Biol Reprod* **39**, 50-7.

Chung, L. W., Chang, S. M., Bell, C., Zhau, H. E., Ro, J. Y. and von Eschenbach, A. C. (1989): Co-inoculation of tumorigenic rat prostate mesenchymal cells with non-tumorigenic epithelial cells results in the development of carcinosarcoma in syngeneic and athymic animals. *International Journal of Cancer* **43**, 1179-87.

Chung, L. W., Kao, C., Sikes, R. A. and Zhau, H. E. (1997): Human prostate cancer progression models and therapeutic intervention. *Hinyokika Kiyo* **43**, 815-20.

Chung, L. W., Matsuura, J. and Runner, M. N. (1984): Tissue interactions and prostatic growth. I. Induction of adult mouse prostatic hyperplasia by fetal urogenital sinus implants. *Biol Reprod* **31**, 155-63.

Coleman, R. E., Houston, S., James, I., Rodger, A., Rubens, R. D., Leonard, R. C. and Ford, J. (1992): Preliminary results of the use of urinary excretion of pyridinium crosslinks for monitoring metastatic bone disease. *British Journal of Cancer* **65**, 766-8.

Conget, P. A. and Minguell, J. J. (2000): Adenoviral-mediated gene transfer into ex vivo expanded human bone marrow mesenchymal progenitor cells. *Experimental Hematology* **28**, 382-90.

Cooper, C. R., Chay, C. H. and Pienta, K. J. (2002): The role of alpha(v)beta(3) in prostate cancer progression. *Neoplasia* **4**, 191-4.

Cooper, C. R., McLean, L., Walsh, M., Taylor, J., Hayasaka, S., Bhatia, J. and Pienta, K. J. (2000): Preferential adhesion of prostate cancer cells to bone is mediated by binding to bone marrow endothelial cells as compared to extracellular matrix components in vitro. *Clinical Cancer Research* **6**, 4839-47.

Corey, E., Brown, L. G., Quinn, J. E., Poot, M., Roudier, M. P., Higano, C. S. and Vessella, R. L. (2003): Zoledronic Acid exhibits inhibitory effects on osteoblastic and osteolytic metastases of prostate cancer. *Clinical Cancer Research* **9**, 295-306.

Coussens, L. M. and Werb, Z. (2002): Inflammation and cancer. *Nature* **420**, 860-7.

Curatolo, C., Ludovico, G. M., Correale, M., Pagliarulo, A., Abbate, I., Cirrillo Marucco, E. and Barletta, A. (1992): Advanced prostate cancer follow-up with prostate-specific antigen, prostatic acid phosphatase, osteocalcin and bone isoenzyme of alkaline phosphatase. *European Urology* **21**, 105-7.

Curiel, D. T. (1999): Strategies to adapt adenoviral vectors for targeted delivery. *Ann N Y Acad Sci* **886**, 158-71.

Dannull, J., Diener, P. A., Prikler, L., Furstenberger, G., Cerny, T., Schmid, U., Ackermann, D. K. and Groettrup, M. (2000): Prostate stem cell antigen is a promising candidate for immunotherapy of advanced prostate cancer. *Cancer Research* **60**, 5522-8.

Davies, M. A., Kim, S. J., Parikh, N. U., Dong, Z., Bucana, C. D. and Gallick, G. E. (2002): Adenoviral-mediated expression of MMAC/PTEN inhibits proliferation and metastasis of human prostate cancer cells. *Clinical Cancer Research* **8**, 1904-14.

Delannoy-Courdent, A., Mattot, V., Fafeur, V., Fauquette, W., Pollet, I., Calmels, T., Vercamer, C., Boilly, B., Vandenbunder, B. and Desbiens, X. (1998): The expression of an Ets1 transcription factor lacking its activation domain decreases uPA proteolytic activity and cell motility and impairs normal tubulogenesis and cancerous scattering in mammary epithelial cells. *J Cell Sci* **111** (Pt 11), 1521-34.

DeWeese, T. L., van der Poel, H., Li, S., Mikhak, B., Drew, R., Goemann, M., Hamper, U., DeJong, R., Detorie, N., Rodriguez, R., Haulk, T., DeMarzo, A. M., Piantadosi, S., Yu, D. C., Chen, Y., Henderson, D. R., Carducci, M. A., Nelson, W. G. and Simons, J. W. (2001): A phase I trial of CV706, a replication-competent, PSA selective oncolytic adenovirus, for the treatment of locally recurrent prostate cancer following radiation therapy. *Cancer Research* **61**, 7464-72.

Dong, J. Y., Fan, P. D. and Frizzell, R. A. (1996): Quantitative analysis of the packaging capacity of recombinant adeno-associated virus. *Human Gene Therapy* **7**, 2101-12.

Dong, Z., Greene, G., Pettaway, C., Dinney, C. P., Eue, I., Lu, W., Bucana, C. D., Balbay, M. D., Bielenberg, D. and Fidler, I. J. (1999): Suppression of angiogenesis, tumorigenicity and metastasis by human prostate cancer cells engineered to produce interferon-beta. *Cancer Research* **59**, 872-9.

Eastham, J. A., Chen, S. H., Sehgal, I., Yang, G., Timme, T. L., Hall, S. J., Woo, S. L. and Thompson, T. C. (1996): Prostate cancer gene therapy: herpes simplex virus thymidine kinase gene transduction followed by ganciclovir in mouse and human prostate cancer models. *Human Gene Therapy* **7**, 515-23.

Eder, J. P., Kantoff, P. W., Roper, K., Xu, G. X., Bubley, G. J., Boyden, J., Gritz, L., Mazzara, G., Oh, W. K., Arlen, P., Tsang, K. Y., Panicali, D., Schlom, J. and Kufe, D. W. (2000): A phase I trial of a recombinant vaccinia virus expressing prostate-specific antigen in advanced prostate cancer. *Clinical Cancer Research* **6**, 1632-8.

Edlund, M., Miyamoto, T., Sikes, R. A., Ogle, R., Laurie, G. W., Farach-Carson, M. C., Otey, C. A., Zhau, H. E. and Chung, L. W. (2001): Integrin expression and usage by prostate cancer cell lines on laminin substrata. *Cell Growth Differ* **12**, 99-107.

Elenbaas, B. and Weinberg, R. A. (2001): Heterotypic signaling between epithelial tumor cells and fibroblasts in carcinoma formation. *Experimental Cell Research* **264**, 169-84.

Elsasser-Beile, U., von Kleist, S., Fischer, R., Martin, M., Wetterauer, U., Gallati, H. and Monting, J. S. (1993): Impaired cytokine production in whole blood cell cultures of patients with urological carcinomas. *J Cancer Res Clin Oncol* **119**, 430-3.

Felding-Habermann, B., O'Toole, T. E., Smith, J. W., Fransvea, E., Ruggeri, Z. M., Ginsberg, M. H., Hughes, P. E., Pampori, N., Shattil, S. J., Saven, A. and Mueller, B. M. (2001): Integrin activation controls metastasis in human breast cancer. *Proceedings of the National Acadamy of Sciences U S A* **98**, 1853-8.

Feng, M., Jackson, W. H., Jr., Goldman, C. K., Rancourt, C., Wang, M., Dusing, S. K., Siegal, G. and Curiel, D. T. (1997): Stable in vivo gene transduction via a novel adenoviral/retroviral chimeric vector. *Nat Biotechnol* **15**, 866-70.

Folkman, J. (1971): Tumor angiogenesis: therapeutic implications. *New England Journal of Medicine* **285**, 1182-6.

Folkman, J. (2001): A new family of mediators of tumor angiogenesis. *Cancer Investigation* **19**, 754-5.

Fong, L., Brockstedt, D., Benike, C., Breen, J. K., Strang, G., Ruegg, C. L. and Engleman, E. G. (2001): Dendritic cell-based xenoantigen vaccination for prostate cancer immunotherapy. *Journal of Immunology* **167**, 7150-6.

Fonseca, M. J., Storm, G., Hennink, W. E., Gerritsen, W. R. and Haisma, H. J. (1999): Cationic polymeric gene delivery of beta-glucuronidase for doxorubicin prodrug therapy. *J Gene Med* **1**, 407-14.

Franks, L. M. (1956): The spread of prostate cancer. *J Pathol Bacteriol* **72**, 603-11.

Franks, L. M., Riddle, P. N., Carbonell, A. W. and Gey, G. O. (1970): A comparative study of the ultrastructure and lack of growth capacity of adult human prostate epithelium mechanically separated from its stroma. *Journal of Pathology* **100**, 113-9.

Freytag, S. O., Khil, M., Stricker, H., Peabody, J., Menon, M., DePeralta-Venturina, M., Nafziger, D., Pegg, J., Paielli, D., Brown, S., Barton, K., Lu, M., Aguilar-Cordova, E. and Kim, J. H. (2002): Phase I study of replication-competent adenovirus-mediated double suicide gene therapy for the treatment of locally recurrent prostate cancer. *Cancer Research* **62**, 4968-76.

Friedlos, F., Davies, L., Scanlon, I., Ogilvie, L. M., Martin, J., Stribbling, S. M., Spooner, R. A., Niculescu-Duvaz, I., Marais, R. and Springer, C. J. (2002): Three new prodrugs for suicide gene therapy using carboxypeptidase G2 elicit bystander efficacy in two xenograft models. *Cancer Research* **62**, 1724-9.

Gardner, T. A., Ko, S. C., Kao, C., Shirakawa, T., Cheon, J., Gotoh, A., Wu, T. T., Sikes, R. A., Zhau, H. E., Cui, Q., Balian, G. and Chung, L. W. K. (1998): Exploiting stromal-epithelial interaction for model development and new strategies of gene therapy for prostate cancer and osteosarcoma metastases. *Gene Ther Mol Biol* **2**, 41-58.

Gerber, H. P., McMurtrey, A., Kowalski, J., Yan, M., Keyt, B. A., Dixit, V. and Ferrara, N. (1998): Vascular endothelial growth factor regulates endothelial cell survival through the phosphatidylinositol 3'-kinase/Akt signal transduction pathway. Requirement for Flk-1/KDR activation. *Journal of Biological Chemistry* **273**, 30336-43.

Gilboa, E., Nair, S. K. and Lyerly, H. K. (1998): Immunotherapy of cancer with dendritic-cell-based vaccines. *Cancer Immunol Immunother* **46**, 82-7.

Gingrich, J. R., Barrios, R. J., Morton, R. A., Boyce, B. F., DeMayo, F. J., Finegold, M. J., Angelopoulou, R., Rosen, J. M. and Greenberg, N. M. (1996): Metastatic prostate cancer in a transgenic mouse. *Cancer Research* **56**, 4096-102.

Glaspy, J. A. (2002): Therapeutic options in the management of renal cell carcinoma. *Semin Oncol* **29**, 41-6.

Gleave, M., Hsieh, J. T., Gao, C. A., von Eschenbach, A. C. and Chung, L. W. (1991): Acceleration of human prostate cancer growth in vivo by factors produced by prostate and bone fibroblasts. *Cancer Research* **51**, 3753-61.

Gleave, M. E., Hsieh, J. T., von Eschenbach, A. C. and Chung, L. W. (1992): Prostate and bone fibroblasts induce human prostate cancer growth in vivo: implications for bidirectional tumor-stromal cell interaction in prostate carcinoma growth and metastasis. *Journal of Urology* **147**, 1151-9.

Goldman, C. K., Kendall, R. L., Cabrera, G., Soroceanu, L., Heike, Y., Gillespie, G. Y., Siegal, G. P., Mao, X., Bett, A. J., Huckle, W. R., Thomas, K. A. and Curiel, D. T. (1998): Paracrine expression of a native soluble vascular endothelial growth factor receptor inhibits tumor growth, metastasis and mortality rate. *Proceedings of the National Acadamy of Sciences U S A* **95**, 8795-800.

Goncalves, M. A., van der Velde, I., Janssen, J. M., Maassen, B. T., Heemskerk, E. H., Opstelten, D. J., Knaan-Shanzer, S., Valerio, D. and de Vries, A. A. (2002): Efficient generation and amplification of high-capacity adeno-associated virus/adenovirus hybrid vectors. *Journal of Virology* **76**, 10734-44.

Graham, M. C., Scher, H. I., Liu, G. B., Yeh, S. D., Curley, T., Daghighian, F., Goldsmith, S. J. and Larson, S. M. (1999): Rhenium-186-labeled hydroxyethylidene diphosphonate dosimetry and dosing guidelines for the palliation of skeletal metastases from androgen-independent prostate cancer. *Clinical Cancer Research* **5**, 1307-18.

Gu, Z., Thomas, G., Yamashiro, J., Shintaku, I. P., Dorey, F., Raitano, A., Witte, O. N., Said, J. W., Loda, M. and Reiter, R. E. (2000): Prostate stem cell antigen (PSCA expression increases with high gleason score, advanced stage and bone metastasis in prostate cancer. *Oncogene* **19**, 1288-96.

Guise, T. A., Yin, J. J. and Mohammad, K. S. (2003): Role of endothelin-1 in osteoblastic bone metastases. *Cancer* **97**, 779-84.

Gulley, J., Chen, A. P., Dahut, W., Arlen, P. M., Bastian, A., Steinberg, S. M., Tsang, K., Panicali, D., Poole, D., Schlom, J. and Michael Hamilton, J. (2002): Phase I study of a vaccine using recombinant vaccinia virus expressing PSA (rV-PSA) in patients with metastatic androgen-independent prostate cancer. *Prostate* **53**, 109-17.

Harada, M., Iida, M., Yamaguchi, M. and Shida, K. (1992): Analysis of bone metastasis of prostatic adenocarcinoma in 137 autopsy cases, pp. 137-82. In Kerr and Yamanaka (Eds): Prostate cancer and bone metastasis, Plenum Press, New York.

Harui, A., Suzuki, S., Kochanek, S. and Mitani, K. (1999): Frequency and stability of chromosomal integration of adenovirus vectors. *Journal of Virology* **73**, 6141-6.

Hayashi, N., Cunha, G. R. and Parker, M. (1993): Permissive and instructive induction of adult rodent prostatic epithelium by heterotypic urogenital sinus mesenchyme. *Epithelial Cell Biology* **2**, 66-78.

Healy, C. G., Simons, J. W., Carducci, M. A., DeWeese, T. L., Bartkowski, M., Tong, K. P. and Bolton, W. E. (1998): Impaired expression and function of signal-transducing zeta chains in peripheral T cells and natural killer cells in patients with prostate cancer. *Cytometry* **32**, 109-19.

Hedlund, T. E., Duke, R. C., Schleicher, M. S. and Miller, G. J. (1998): Fas-mediated apoptosis in seven human prostate cancer cell lines: correlation with tumor stage. *Prostate* **36**, 92-101.

Heidenreich, A., Hofmann, R. and Engelmann, U. H. (2001): The use of bisphosphonate for the palliative treatment of painful bone metastasis due to hormone refractory prostate cancer. *Journal of Urology* **165**, 136-40.

Heine, D., Muller, R. and Brusselbach, S. (2001): Cell surface display of a lysosomal enzyme for extracellular gene- directed enzyme prodrug therapy. *Gene Therapy* **8**, 1005-10.

Heiser, A., Coleman, D., Dannull, J., Yancey, D., Maurice, M. A., Lallas, C. D., Dahm, P., Niedzwiecki, D., Gilboa, E. and Vieweg, J. (2002): Autologous dendritic cells transfected with prostate-specific antigen RNA stimulate CTL responses against metastatic prostate tumors. *Journal of Clinical Investigation* **109**, 409-17.

Heiser, A., Dahm, P., Yancey, D. R., Maurice, M. A., Boczkowski, D., Nair, S. K., Gilboa, E. and Vieweg, J. (2000): Human dendritic cells transfected with RNA encoding prostate-specific antigen stimulate prostate-specific CTL responses in vitro. *Journal of Immunology* **164**, 5508-14.

Herman, J. R., Adler, H. L., Aguilar-Cordova, E., Rojas-Martinez, A., Woo, S., Timme, T. L., Wheeler, T. M., Thompson, T. C. and Scardino, P. T. (1999): In situ gene therapy for adenocarcinoma of the prostate: a phase I clinical trial. *Human Gene Therapy* **10**, 1239-49.

Hitt, M. M. and Gauldie, J. (2000): Gene vectors for cytokine expression in vivo. *Curr Pharm Des* **6**, 613-32.

Hodge, J. W., Schlom, J., Donohue, S. J., Tomaszewski, J. E., Wheeler, C. W., Levine, B. S., Gritz, L., Panicali, D. and Kantor, J. A. (1995): A recombinant vaccinia virus expressing human prostate-specific antigen (PSA): safety and immunogenicity in a non-human primate. *International Journal of Cancer* **63**, 231-7.

Honn, K. V. and Tang, D. G. (1992): Adhesion molecules and tumor cell interaction with endothelium and subendothelial matrix. *Cancer Metastasis Rev* **11**, 353-75.

Hrouda, D., Baban, B., Dunsmuir, W. D., Kirby, R. S. and Dalgleish, A. G. (1998): Immunotherapy of advanced prostate cancer: a phase I/II trial using Mycobacterium vaccae (SRL172). *British Journal of Urology* **82**, 568-73.

Hsieh, C. L., Yang, L., Miao, L., Yeung, F., Kao, C., Yang, H., Zhau, H. E. and Chung, L. W. (2002): A novel targeting modality to enhance adenoviral replication by vitamin D (3) in androgen-independent human prostate cancer cells and tumors. *Cancer Research* **62**, 3084-92.

Huber, B. E., Austin, E. A., Good, S. S., Knick, V. C., Tibbels, S. and Richards, C. A. (1993): In vivo antitumor activity of 5-fluorocytosine on human colorectal carcinoma cells genetically modified to express cytosine deaminase. *Cancer Research* **53**, 4619-26.

Huber, B. E., Austin, E. A., Richards, C. A., Davis, S. T. and Good, S. S. (1994): Metabolism of 5-fluorocytosine to 5-fluorouracil in human colorectal tumor cells transduced with the cytosine deaminase gene: significant antitumor effects when only a small percentage of tumor cells express cytosine deaminase. *Proceedings of the National Acadamy of Sciences U S A* **91**, 8302-6.

Hubert, R. S., Vivanco, I., Chen, E., Rastegar, S., Leong, K., Mitchell, S. C., Madraswala, R., Zhou, Y., Kuo, J., Raitano, A. B., Jakobovits, A., Saffran, D. C. and Afar, D. E. (1999): STEAP: a prostate-specific cell-surface antigen highly expressed in human prostate tumors. *Proceedings of the National Acadamy of Sciences U S A* **96**, 14523-8.

Hull, G. W., McCurdy, M. A., Nasu, Y., Bangma, C. H., Yang, G., Shimura, S., Lee, H. M., Wang, J., Albani, J., Ebara, S., Sato, T., Timme, T. L. and Thompson, T. C. (2000): Prostate cancer gene therapy: comparison of adenovirus-mediated expression of interleukin 12 with interleukin 12 plus B7-1 for in situ gene therapy and gene-modified, cell-based vaccines. *Clinical Cancer Research* **6**, 4101-9.

Hyytinen, E. R., Thalmann, G. N., Zhau, H. E., Karhu, R., Kallioniemi, O. P., Chung, L. W. and Visakorpi, T. (1997): Genetic changes associated with the acquisition of androgen-independent growth, tumorigenicity and metastatic potential in a prostate cancer model. *British Journal of Cancer* **75**, 190-5.

Ingber, D. E. (2002): Cancer as a disease of epithelial-mesenchymal interactions and extracellular matrix regulation. *Differentiation* **70**, 547-60.

Jackson, M. W., Roberts, J. S., Heckford, S. E., Ricciardelli, C., Stahl, J., Choong, C., Horsfall, D. J. and Tilley, W. D. (2002): A potential autocrine role for vascular endothelial growth factor in prostate cancer. *Cancer Research* **62**, 854-9.

Jacob, K., Webber, M., Benayahu, D. and Kleinman, H. K. (1999): Osteonectin promotes prostate cancer cell migration and invasion: a possible mechanism for metastasis to bone. *Cancer Research* **59**, 4453-7.

Jemal, A., Murray, T., Samuels, A., Ghafoor, A., Ward, E. and Thun, M. J. (2003): Cancer statistics, 2003. *CA Cancer J Clin* **53**, 5-26.

Johansson, N., Ahonen, M. and Kahari, V. M. (2000): Matrix metalloproteinases in tumor invasion. *Cell Mol Life Sci* **57**, 5-15.

Kanai, F. (2001): Transcriptional targeted gene therapy for hepatocellular carcinoma by adenovirus vector. *Molecular Biotechnology* **18**, 243-50.

Kaplan, J. M., Armentano, D., Sparer, T. E., Wynn, S. G., Peterson, P. A., Wadsworth, S. C., Couture, K. K., Pennington, S. E., St George, J. A., Gooding, L. R. and Smith, A. E. (1997): Characterization of factors involved in modulating persistence of transgene expression from recombinant adenovirus in the mouse lung. *Human Gene Therapy* **8**, 45-56.

Kavanaugh, D. Y. and Carbone, D. P. (1996): Immunologic dysfunction in cancer. *Hematol Oncol Clin North Am* **10**, 927-51.

Kawakami, Y., Eliyahu, S., Delgado, C. H., Robbins, P. F., Rivoltini, L., Topalian, S. L., Miki, T. and Rosenberg, S. A. (1994): Cloning of the gene coding for a shared human melanoma antigen recognized by autologous T cells infiltrating into tumor. *Proceedings of the National Acadamy of Sciences U S A* **91**, 3515-9.

Keck, P. J., Hauser, S. D., Krivi, G., Sanzo, K., Warren, T., Feder, J. and Connolly, D. T. (1989): Vascular permeability factor, an endothelial cell mitogen related to PDGF. *Science* **246**, 1309-12.

Kerr, J. S., Slee, A. M. and Mousa, S. A. (2000): Small molecule alpha(v) integrin antagonists: novel anticancer agents. *Expert Opin Investig Drugs* **9**, 1271-9.

Kim, K. J., Li, B., Winer, J., Armanini, M., Gillett, N., Phillips, H. S. and Ferrara, N. (1993): Inhibition of vascular endothelial growth factor-induced angiogenesis suppresses tumour growth in vivo. *Nature* **362**, 841-4.

Kim, K. R., Yoshizaki, T., Miyamori, H., Hasegawa, K., Horikawa, T., Furukawa, M., Harada, S., Seiki, M. and Sato, H. (2000): Transformation of Madin-Darby canine kidney (MDCK) epithelial cells by Epstein-Barr virus latent membrane protein 1 (LMP1) induces expression of Ets1 and invasive growth. *Oncogene* **19**, 1764-71.

Kitange, G., Kishikawa, M., Nakayama, T., Naito, S., Iseki, M. and Shibata, S. (1999a): Expression of the Ets-1 proto-oncogene correlates with malignant potential in human astrocytic tumors. *Mod Pathol* **12**, 618-26.

Kitange, G., Shibata, S., Tokunaga, Y., Yagi, N., Yasunaga, A., Kishikawa, M. and Naito, S. (1999b): Ets-1 transcription factor-mediated urokinase-type plasminogen activator expression and invasion in glioma cells stimulated by serum and basic fibroblast growth factors. *Laboratory Investigation* **79**, 407-16.

Kleeff, J., Fukahi, K., Lopez, M. E., Friess, H., Buchler, M. W., Sosnowski, B. A. and Korc, M. (2002): Targeting of suicide gene delivery in pancreatic cancer cells via FGF receptors. *Cancer Gene Therapy* **9**, 522-32.

Ko, S. C., Cheon, J., Kao, C., Gotoh, A., Shirakawa, T., Sikes, R. A., Karsenty, G. and Chung, L. W. (1996): Osteocalcin promoter-based toxic gene therapy for the treatment of osteosarcoma in experimental models. *Cancer Research* **56**, 4614-9.

Koeneman, K. S., Kao, C., Ko, S. C., Yang, L., Wada, Y., Kallmes, D. F., Gillenwater, J. Y., Zhau, H. E., Chung, L. W. and Gardner, T. A. (2000): Osteocalcin-directed gene therapy for prostate-cancer bone metastasis. *World Journal of Urology* **18**, 102-10.

Koeneman, K. S., Yeung, F. and Chung, L. W. (1999): Osteomimetic properties of prostate cancer cells: a hypothesis supporting the predilection of prostate cancer metastasis and growth in the bone environment. *Prostate* **39**, 246-61.

Koistinen, P., Pulli, T., Uitto, V. J., Nissinen, L., Hyypia, T. and Heino, J. (1999): Depletion of alphaV integrins from osteosarcoma cells by intracellular antibody expression induces bone differentiation marker genes and suppresses gelatinase (MMP-2) synthesis. *Matrix Biology* **18**, 239-51.

Krasnykh, V. N., Mikheeva, G. V., Douglas, J. T. and Curiel, D. T. (1996): Generation of recombinant adenovirus vectors with modified fibers for altering viral tropism. *Journal of Virology* **70**, 6839-46.

Krummel, M. F. and Allison, J. P. (1995): CD28 and CTLA-4 have opposing effects on the response of T cells to stimulation. *Journal of Experimental Medicine* **182**, 459-65.

Kubo, H., Gardner, T. A., Wada, Y., Koeneman, K. S., Gotoh, A., Yang, L., Kao, C., Lim, S. D., Amin, M. B., Yang, H., Black, M. E., Matsubara, S., Nakagawa, M., Gillenwater, J. Y., Zhau, H. E. and Chung, L. W. (2003): Phase I dose escalation clinical trial of adenovirus vector carrying osteocalcin promoter-driven herpes simplex virus thymidine kinase in localized and metastatic hormone-refractory prostate cancer. *Human Gene Therapy* **14**, 227-41.

Kumar, R. and Fidler, I. J. (1998): Angiogenic molecules and cancer metastasis. *In Vivo* **12**, 27-34.

Kwon, E. D., Foster, B. A., Hurwitz, A. A., Madias, C., Allison, J. P., Greenberg, N. M. and Burg, M. B. (1999): Elimination of residual metastatic prostate cancer after surgery and adjunctive cytotoxic T lymphocyte-associated antigen 4 (CTLA-4) blockade immunotherapy. *Proceedings of the National Acadamy of Sciences U S A* **96**, 15074-9.

Kwon, E. D., Hurwitz, A. A., Foster, B. A., Madias, C., Feldhaus, A. L., Greenberg, N. M., Burg, M. B. and Allison, J. P. (1997): Manipulation of T cell costimulatory and inhibitory signals for immunotherapy of prostate cancer. *Proceedings of the National Acadamy of Sciences U S A* **94**, 8099-103.

Lapidot, T. and Kollet, O. (2002): The essential roles of the chemokine SDF-1 and its receptor CXCR4 in human stem cell homing and repopulation of transplanted immune-deficient NOD/SCID and NOD/SCID/B2m(null) mice. *Leukemia* **16**, 1992-2003.

Latham, J. P., Searle, P. F., Mautner, V. and James, N. D. (2000): Prostate-specific antigen promoter/enhancer driven gene therapy for prostate cancer: construction and testing of a tissue-specific adenovirus vector. *Cancer Research* **60**, 334-41.

Lee, C. K., Aeppli, D. M., Unger, J., Boudreau, R. J. and Levitt, S. H. (1996): Strontium-89 chloride (Metastron) for palliative treatment of bony metastases. The University of Minnesota experience. *American Journal of Clinical Oncology* **19**, 102-7.

Lee, S. J., Kim, H. S., Yu, R., Lee, K., Gardner, T. A., Jung, C., Jeng, M. H., Yeung, F., Cheng, L. and Kao, C. (2002): Novel prostate-specific promoter derived from PSA and PSMA enhancers. *Molecular Therapy* **6**, 415-21.

Lee, Y., Schwarz, E., Davies, M., Jo, M., Gates, J., Wu, J., Zhang, X. and Lieberman, J. R. (2003): Differences in the cytokine profiles associated with prostate cancer cell induced osteoblastic and osteolytic lesions in bone. *Journal of Orthopaedic Research* **21**, 62-72.

Lee, Y. J., Galoforo, S. S., Battle, P., Lee, H., Corry, P. M. and Jessup, J. M. (2001): Replicating adenoviral vector-mediated transfer of a heat-inducible double suicide gene for gene therapy. *Cancer Gene Therapy* **8**, 397-404.

Lenschow, D. J. and Bluestone, J. A. (1993): T cell co-stimulation and in vivo tolerance. *Current Opinions in Immunology* **5**, 747-52.

Letterio, J. J. and Roberts, A. B. (1998): Regulation of immune responses by TGF-beta. *Annu Rev Immunol* **16**, 137-61.

Li, Y., Pong, R. C., Bergelson, J. M., Hall, M. C., Sagalowsky, A. I., Tseng, C. P., Wang, Z. and Hsieh, J. T. (1999): Loss of adenoviral receptor expression in human bladder cancer cells: a potential impact on the efficacy of gene therapy. *Cancer Research* **59**, 325-30.

Liapis, H., Flath, A. and Kitazawa, S. (1996): Integrin alpha V beta 3 expression by bone-residing breast cancer metastases. *Diagnostic Molecular Pathology* **5**, 127-35.

Lin, D. L., Tarnowski, C. P., Zhang, J., Dai, J., Rohn, E., Patel, A. H., Morris, M. D. and Keller, E. T. (2001): Bone metastatic LNCaP-derivative C4-2B prostate cancer cell line mineralizes in vitro. *Prostate* **47**, 212-21.

Link, C. J., Jr., Levy, J. P., McCann, L. Z. and Moorman, D. W. (1997): Gene therapy for colon cancer with the herpes simplex thymidine kinase gene. *Journal of Surgical Oncology* **64**, 289-94.

Linsley, P. S., Greene, J. L., Brady, W., Bajorath, J., Ledbetter, J. A. and Peach, R. (1994): Human B7-1 (CD80) and B7-2 (CD86) bind with similar avidities but distinct kinetics to CD28 and CTLA-4 receptors. *Immunity* **1**, 793-801.

Liotta, L. A. and Kohn, E. C. (2001): The microenvironment of the tumour-host interface. *Nature* **411**, 375-9.

Lissbrant, I. F., Stattin, P., Damber, J. E. and Bergh, A. (1997): Vascular density is a predictor of cancer-specific survival in prostatic carcinoma. *Prostate* **33**, 38-45.

Liu, Q. Y., Rubin, M. A., Omene, C., Lederman, S. and Stein, C. A. (1998): Fas ligand is constitutively secreted by prostate cancer cells in vitro. *Clinical Cancer Research* **4**, 1803-11.

Mailliard, R. B. and Lotze, M. T. (2001): Dendritic cells prolong tumor-specific T-cell survival and effector function after interaction with tumor targets. *Clinical Cancer Research* **7**, 980s-988s.

Matsubara, S., Wada, Y., Gardner, T. A., Egawa, M., Park, M. S., Hsieh, C. L., Zhau, H. E., Kao, C., Kamidono, S., Gillenwater, J. Y. and Chung, L. W. (2001): A conditional replication-competent adenoviral vector, Ad-OC-E1a, to cotarget prostate cancer and bone stroma in an experimental model of androgen-independent prostate cancer bone metastasis. *Cancer Research* **61**, 6012-9.

McNeal, J. (1990): Pathology of benign prostatic hyperplasia. Insight into etiology. *Urol Clin North Am* **17**, 477-86.

Miles, B. J., Shalev, M., Aguilar-Cordova, E., Timme, T. L., Lee, H. M., Yang, G., Adler, H. L., Kernen, K., Pramudji, C. K., Satoh, T., Gdor, Y., Ren, C., Ayala, G., Wheeler, T. M., Butler, E. B., Kadmon, D. and Thompson, T. C. (2001): Prostate-specific antigen response and systemic T cell activation after in situ gene therapy in prostate cancer patients failing radiotherapy. *Human Gene Therapy* **12**, 1955-67.

Millauer, B., Longhi, M. P., Plate, K. H., Shawver, L. K., Risau, W., Ullrich, A. and Strawn, L. M. (1996): Dominant-negative inhibition of Flk-1 suppresses the growth of many tumor types in vivo. *Cancer Research* **56**, 1615-20.

Miller, G. J., Runner, M. N. and Chung, L. W. (1985): Tissue interactions and prostatic growth: II. Morphological and biochemical characterization of adult mouse prostatic hyperplasia induced by fetal urogenital sinus implants. *Prostate* **6**, 241-53.

Mintz, E. R. and Smith, G. G. (1934): Autopsy findings in 100 cases of prostate cancer. *New England Journal of Medicine* **211**, 479-87.

Mitani, K., Graham, F. L., Caskey, C. T. and Kochanek, S. (1995): Rescue, propagation and partial purification of a helper virus-dependent adenovirus vector. *Proceedings of the National Acadamy of Sciences U S A* **92**, 3854-8.

Miyagi, T., Hori, O., Koshida, K., Egawa, M., Kato, H., Kitagawa, Y., Ozawa, K., Ogawa, S. and Namiki, M. (2002): Antitumor effect of reduction of 150-kDa oxygen-regulated protein expression on human prostate cancer cells. *International Journal of Urology* **9**, 577-85.

Mocellin, S., Wang, E. and Marincola, F. M. (2001): Cytokines and immune response in the tumor microenvironment. *Journal of Immunotherapy* **24**, 392-407.

Monsky, W. L., Mouta Carreira, C., Tsuzuki, Y., Gohongi, T., Fukumura, D. and Jain, R. K. (2002): Role of host microenvironment in angiogenesis and microvascular functions in human breast cancer xenografts: mammary fat pad versus cranial tumors. *Clinical Cancer Research* **8**, 1008-13.

Morsy, M. A. and Caskey, C. T. (1999): Expanded-capacity adenoviral vectors--the helper-dependent vectors. *Mol Med Today* **5**, 18-24.

Muller, A., Homey, B., Soto, H., Ge, N., Catron, D., Buchanan, M. E., McClanahan, T., Murphy, E., Yuan, W., Wagner, S. N., Barrera, J. L., Mohar, A., Verastegui, E. and Zlotnik, A. (2001): Involvement of chemokine receptors in breast cancer metastasis. *Nature* **410**, 50-6.

Mundy, G. R. (1997): Mechanisms of bone metastasis. *Cancer* **80**, 1546-56.

Murakami, T., Maki, W., Cardones, A. R., Fang, H., Tun Kyi, A., Nestle, F. O. and Hwang, S. T. (2002): Expression of CXC chemokine receptor-4 enhances the pulmonary metastatic potential of murine B16 melanoma cells. *Cancer Research* **62**, 7328-34.

Murphy, G., Tjoa, B., Ragde, H., Kenny, G. and Boynton, A. (1996): Phase I clinical trial: T-cell therapy for prostate cancer using autologous dendritic cells pulsed with HLA-A0201-specific peptides from prostate-specific membrane antigen. *Prostate* **29**, 371-80.

Naito, S., Shimizu, K., Nakashima, M., Nakayama, T., Ito, T., Ito, M., Yamashita, S. and Sekine, I. (2000): Overexpression of Ets-1 transcription factor in angiosarcoma of the skin. *Pathol Res Pract* **196**, 103-9.

Nakayama, T., Ito, M., Ohtsuru, A., Naito, S., Nakashima, M., Fagin, J. A., Yamashita, S. and Sekine, I. (1996): Expression of the Ets-1 proto-oncogene in human gastric carcinoma: correlation with tumor invasion. *American Journal of Pathology* **149**, 1931-9.

Nakayama, T., Ito, M., Ohtsuru, A., Naito, S. and Sekine, I. (2001): Expression of the ets-1 proto-oncogene in human colorectal carcinoma. *Mod Pathol* **14**, 415-22.

Nasu, Y., Bangma, C. H., Hull, G. W., Lee, H. M., Hu, J., Wang, J., McCurdy, M. A., Shimura, S., Yang, G., Timme, T. L. and Thompson, T. C. (1999): Adenovirus-mediated interleukin-12 gene therapy for prostate cancer: suppression of orthotopic tumor growth and pre-established lung metastases in an orthotopic model. *Gene Therapy* **6**, 338-49.

Navone, N. M., Troncoso, P., Pisters, L. L., Goodrow, T. L., Palmer, J. L., Nichols, W. W., von Eschenbach, A. C. and Conti, C. J. (1993): p53 protein accumulation and gene mutation in the progression of human prostate carcinoma. *Journal of the National Cancer Institute* **85**, 1657-69.

Nelson, J. B., Nguyen, S. H., Wu-Wong, J. R., Opgenorth, T. J., Dixon, D. B., Chung, L. W. and Inoue, N. (1999a): New bone formation in an osteoblastic tumor model is increased by endothelin-1 overexpression and decreased by endothelin A receptor blockade. *Urology* **53**, 1063-9.

Nelson, P. S., Gan, L., Ferguson, C., Moss, P., Gelinas, R., Hood, L. and Wang, K. (1999b): Molecular cloning and characterization of prostase, an androgen-regulated serine protease with prostate-restricted expression. *Proceedings of the National Acadamy of Sciences U S A* **96**, 3114-9.

Nemeth, J. A., Yousif, R., Herzog, M., Che, M., Upadhyay, J., Shekarriz, B., Bhagat, S., Mullins, C., Fridman, R. and Cher, M. L. (2002): Matrix metalloproteinase activity, bone matrix turnover and tumor cell proliferation in prostate cancer bone metastasis. *Journal of the National Cancer Institute* **94**, 17-25.

Nettelbeck, D. M., Jerome, V. and Muller, R. (2000): Gene therapy: designer promoters for tumour targeting. *Trends Genet* **16**, 174-81.

Nishihara, E., Nagayama, Y., Mawatari, F., Tanaka, K., Namba, H., Niwa, M. and Yamashita, S. (1997): Retrovirus-mediated herpes simplex virus thymidine kinase gene transduction renders human thyroid carcinoma cell lines sensitive to ganciclovir and radiation in vitro and in vivo. *Endocrinology* **138**, 4577-83.

Nishizaki, M., Fujiwara, T., Tanida, T., Hizuta, A., Nishimori, H., Tokino, T., Nakamura, Y., Bouvet, M., Roth, J. A. and Tanaka, N. (1999): Recombinant adenovirus expressing wild-type p53 is antiangiogenic: a proposed mechanism for bystander effect. *Clinical Cancer Research* **5**, 1015-23.

Nossal, G. J. (1994): Negative selection of lymphocytes. *Cell* **76**, 229-39.

Oettgen, P., Finger, E., Sun, Z., Akbarali, Y., Thamrongsak, U., Boltax, J., Grall, F., Dube, A., Weiss, A., Brown, L., Quinn, G., Kas, K., Endress, G., Kunsch, C. and Libermann, T. A. (2000): PDEF, a novel prostate epithelium-specific ets transcription factor, interacts with the androgen receptor and activates prostate-specific antigen gene expression. *Journal of Biological Chemistry* **275**, 1216-25.

Okegawa, T., Li, Y., Pong, R. C., Bergelson, J. M., Zhou, J. and Hsieh, J. T. (2000): The dual impact of coxsackie and adenovirus receptor expression on human prostate cancer gene therapy. *Cancer Research* **60**, 5031-6.

Olumi, A. F., Dazin, P. and Tlsty, T. D. (1998): A novel coculture technique demonstrates that normal human prostatic fibroblasts contribute to tumor formation of LNCaP cells by retarding cell death. *Cancer Research* **58**, 4525-30.

Olumi, A. F., Grossfeld, G. D., Hayward, S. W., Carroll, P. R., Tlsty, T. D. and Cunha, G. R. (1999): Carcinoma-associated fibroblasts direct tumor progression of initiated human prostatic epithelium. *Cancer Research* **59**, 5002-11.

Ozaki, I., Mizuta, T., Zhao, G., Yotsumoto, H., Hara, T., Kajihara, S., Hisatomi, A., Sakai, T. and Yamamoto, K. (2000): Involvement of the Ets-1 gene in overexpression of matrilysin in human hepatocellular carcinoma. *Cancer Research* **60**, 6519-25.

Pantuck, A. J., Zisman, A. and Belldegrun, A. S. (2000): Gene therapy for prostate cancer at the University of California, Los Angeles: preliminary results and future directions. *World Journal of Urology* **18**, 143-7.

Pantuck, A. J., Zisman, A., Henderson, D., Wilson, D., Schreiber, A. and Belldegrun, A. (2001): New biologicals for prostate cancer prevention: Genes, vaccines and immune-based interventions. *Urology* **57**, 95-9.

Papapoulos, S. E., Hamdy, N. A. and van der Pluijm, G. (2000): Bisphosphonates in the management of prostate carcinoma metastatic to the skeleton. *Cancer* **88**, 3047-53.

Parkinson, R. J., Mian, S., Bishop, M. C., Gray, T., Li, G., McArdle, S. E., Ali, S. and Rees, R. C. (2003): Disabled infectious single cycle herpes simplex virus (DISC-HSV) is a candidate vector system for gene delivery/expression of GM-CSF in human prostate cancer therapy. *Prostate* **56**, 65-73.

Parmiani, G., Castelli, C., Dalerba, P., Mortarini, R., Rivoltini, L., Marincola, F. M. and Anichini, A. (2002): Cancer immunotherapy with peptide-based vaccines: what have we achieved? Where are we going? *Journal of the National Cancer Institute* **94**, 805-18.

Pathak, S., Nemeth, M. A., Multani, A. S., Thalmann, G. N., von Eschenbach, A. C. and Chung, L. W. (1997): Can cancer cells transform normal host cells into malignant cells? *British Journal of Cancer* **76**, 1134-8.

Pisters LL, M. T., Troncoso P, Brisbay S, Hossan E, Pettaway C, Wood C, Evans R, Steiner M, Merritt J, Logothetis C. (2001): Intraprostatic Ad-p53 gene therapy induces apoptosis in locally advanced adenocarcinoma of the prostate. *Proceedings of the American Society of Clinical Oncology*, pp. 175a [abstract 699].

Quaranta, V. (2002): Motility cues in the tumor microenvironment. Differentiation **70**, 590-8.

Reiter, R. E., Gu, Z., Watabe, T., Thomas, G., Szigeti, K., Davis, E., Wahl, M., Nisitani, S., Yamashiro, J., Le Beau, M. M., Loda, M. and Witte, O. N. (1998): Prostate stem cell antigen: a cell surface marker overexpressed in prostate cancer. *Proceedings of the National Acadamy of Sciences U S A* **95**, 1735-40.

Ren, C., Li, L., Goltsov, A. A., Timme, T. L., Tahir, S. A., Wang, J., Garza, L., Chinault, A. C. and Thompson, T. C. (2002): mRTVP-1, a novel p53 target gene with proapoptotic activities. *Molecular Cellular Biology* **22**, 3345-57.

Rhee, H. W., Zhau, H. E., Pathak, S., Multani, A. S., Pennanen, S., Visakorpi, T. and Chung, L. W. (2001): Permanent phenotypic and genotypic changes of prostate cancer cells cultured in a three-dimensional rotating-wall vessel. *In Vitro Cell Dev Biol Anim* **37**, 127-40.

Rich, T., Chen, P., Furman, F., Huynh, N. and Israel, M. A. (1996): RTVP-1, a novel human gene with sequence similarity to genes of diverse species, is expressed in tumor cell lines of glial but not neuronal origin. *Gene* **180**, 125-30.

Rodriguez, R., Schuur, E. R., Lim, H. Y., Henderson, G. A., Simons, J. W. and Henderson, D. R. (1997): Prostate attenuated replication competent adenovirus (ARCA) CN706: a selective cytotoxic for prostate-specific antigen-positive prostate cancer cells. *Cancer Research* **57**, 2559-63.

Rogulski, K. R., Wing, M. S., Paielli, D. L., Gilbert, J. D., Kim, J. H. and Freytag, S. O. (2000): Double suicide gene therapy augments the antitumor activity of a replication-competent lytic adenovirus through enhanced cytotoxicity and radiosensitization. *Human Gene Therapy* **11**, 67-76.

Roland, S. (1958): Calsium studies in ten cases of ost4eoblasti prostatic metastasis. *Journal of Urology* **79**, 339-42.

Ronnov-Jessen, L., Petersen, O. W., Koteliansky, V. E. and Bissell, M. J. (1995): The origin of the myofibroblasts in breast cancer. Recapitulation of tumor environment in culture unravels diversity and implicates converted fibroblasts and recruited smooth muscle cells. *Journal of Clinical Investigation* **95**, 859-73.

Rosolen, A., Frascella, E., di Francesco, C., Todesco, A., Petrone, M., Mehtali, M., Zacchello, F., Zanesco, L. and Scarpa, M. (1998): In vitro and in vivo antitumor effects of retrovirus-mediated herpes simplex thymidine kinase gene-transfer in human medulloblastoma. *Gene Ther* **5**, 113-20.

Ross, S., Spencer, S. D., Holcomb, I., Tan, C., Hongo, J., Devaux, B., Rangell, L., Keller, G. A., Schow, P., Steeves, R. M., Lutz, R. J., Frantz, G., Hillan, K., Peale, F., Tobin, P., Eberhard, D., Rubin, M. A., Lasky, L. A. and Koeppen, H. (2002): Prostate stem cell antigen as therapy target: tissue expression and in vivo efficacy of an immunoconjugate. *Cancer Research* **62**, 2546-53.

Saffran, D. C., Raitano, A. B., Hubert, R. S., Witte, O. N., Reiter, R. E. and Jakobovits, A. (2001): Anti-PSCA mAbs inhibit tumor growth and metastasis formation and prolong the survival of mice bearing human prostate cancer xenografts. *Proceedings of the National Acadamy of Sciences U S A* **98**, 2658-63.

Salgaller, M. L., Lodge, P. A., McLean, J. G., Tjoa, B. A., Loftus, D. J., Ragde, H., Kenny, G. M., Rogers, M., Boynton, A. L. and Murphy, G. P. (1998a): Report of immune monitoring of prostate cancer patients undergoing T-cell therapy using dendritic cells pulsed with HLA-A2-specific peptides from prostate-specific membrane antigen (PSMA. *Prostate* **35**, 144-51.

Salgaller, M. L., Tjoa, B. A., Lodge, P. A., Ragde, H., Kenny, G., Boynton, A. and Murphy, G. P. (1998b): Dendritic cell-based immunotherapy of prostate cancer. *Crit Rev Immunol* **18**, 109-19.

Sanda, M. G., Ayyagari, S. R., Jaffee, E. M., Epstein, J. I., Clift, S. L., Cohen, L. K., Dranoff, G., Pardoll, D. M., Mulligan, R. C. and Simons, J. W. (1994): Demonstration of a rational strategy for human prostate cancer gene therapy. *Journal of Urology* **151**, 622-8.

Sanda, M. G., Smith, D. C., Charles, L. G., Hwang, C., Pienta, K. J., Schlom, J., Milenic, D., Panicali, D. and Montie, J. E. (1999): Recombinant vaccinia-PSA (PROSTVAC) can induce a prostate-specific immune response in androgen-modulated human prostate cancer. *Urology* **53**, 260-6.

Satoh, T., Timme, T. L., Saika, T., Ebara, S., Yang, G., Wang, J., Ren, C., Kusaka, N., Mouraviev, V. and Thompson, T. C. (2003): Adenoviral Vector-Mediated mRTVP-1 Gene Therapy for Prostate Cancer. *Human Gene Therapy* **14**, 91-101.

Schoggins, J. W., Gall, J. G. and Falck-Pedersen, E. (2003): Subgroup B and f fiber chimeras eliminate normal adenovirus type 5 vector transduction in vitro and in vivo. *Journal of Virology* **77**, 1039-48.

Sementchenko, V. I. and Watson, D. K. (2000): Ets target genes: past, present and future. *Oncogene* **19**, 6533-48.

Shah, A. H., Tabayoyong, W. B., Kundu, S. D., Kim, S. J., Van Parijs, L., Liu, V. C., Kwon, E., Greenberg, N. M. and Lee, C. (2002): Suppression of tumor metastasis by blockade of transforming growth factor beta signaling in bone marrow cells through a retroviral-mediated gene therapy in mice. *Cancer Research* **62**, 7135-8.

Shao, R., Xia, W. and Hung, M. C. (2000): Inhibition of angiogenesis and induction of apoptosis are involved in E1A-mediated bystander effect and tumor suppression. *Cancer Research* **60**, 3123-6.

Shekhar, M. P., Pauley, R. and Heppner, G. (2003): Host microenvironment in breast cancer development: extracellular matrix-stromal cell contribution to neoplastic phenotype of epithelial cells in the breast. *Breast Cancer Research* **5**, 130-5.

Shirakawa, T., Ko, S. C., Gardner, T. A., Cheon, J., Miyamoto, T., Gotoh, A., Chung, L. W. and Kao, C. (1998): In vivo suppression of osteosarcoma pulmonary metastasis with intravenous osteocalcin promoter-based toxic gene therapy. *Cancer Gene Therapy* **5**, 274-80.

Siemens, D. R., Austin, J. C., Hedican, S. P., Tartaglia, J. and Ratliff, T. L. (2000): Viral vector delivery in solid-state vehicles: gene expression in a murine prostate cancer model. *Journal of the National Cancer Institute* **92**, 403-12.

Simons, J. W. and Mikhak, B. (1998): Ex-vivo gene therapy using cytokine-transduced tumor vaccines: molecular and clinical pharmacology. *Semin Oncol* **25**, 661-76.

Simons, J. W., Mikhak, B., Chang, J. F., DeMarzo, A. M., Carducci, M. A., Lim, M., Weber, C. E., Baccala, A. A., Goemann, M. A., Clift, S. M. ando, D. G., Levitsky, H. I., Cohen, L. K., Sanda, M. G., Mulligan, R. C., Partin, A. W., Carter, H. B., Piantadosi, S., Marshall, F. F. and Nelson, W. G. (1999): Induction of immunity to prostate cancer antigens: results of a clinical trial of vaccination with irradiated autologous prostate tumor cells engineered to secrete granulocyte-macrophage colony-stimulating factor using ex vivo gene transfer. *Cancer Research* **59**, 5160-8.

Singh, S., Barrett, J., Sakata, K., Tozer, R. G. and Singh, G. (2002): ETS proteins and MMPs: partners in invasion and metastasis. *Curr Drug Targets* **3**, 359-67.

Sotomayor, E. M., Borrello, I. and Levitsky, H. I. (1996): Tolerance and cancer: a critical issue in tumor immunology. *Crit Rev Oncog* **7**, 433-56.

Stearns, M. E., Garcia, F. U., Fudge, K., Rhim, J. and Wang, M. (1999): Role of interleukin 10 and transforming growth factor beta1 in the angiogenesis and metastasis of human prostate primary tumor lines from orthotopic implants in severe combined immunodeficiency mice. *Clinical Cancer Research* **5**, 711-20.

Steiner, M. S., Zhang, X., Wang, Y. and Lu, Y. (2000): Growth inhibition of prostate cancer by an adenovirus expressing a novel tumor suppressor gene, pHyde. *Cancer Research* **60**, 4419-25.

Stephenson, J. (2001): Experimental prostate cancer drugs slow disease progression. *Journal of the American Medical Association* **286**, 34.

Stribbling, S. M., Friedlos, F., Martin, J., Davies, L., Spooner, R. A., Marais, R. and Springer, C. J. (2000): Regressions of established breast carcinoma xenografts by carboxypeptidase G2 suicide gene therapy and the prodrug CMDA are due to a bystander effect. *Human Gene Therapy* **11**, 285-92.

Su, L., Mukherjee, A. B. and Mukherjee, B. B. (1995): Expression of antisense osteopontin RNA inhibits tumor promoter-induced neoplastic transformation of mouse JB6 epidermal cells. *Oncogene* **10**, 2163-9.

Sung, S. Y. and Chung, L. W. (2002): Prostate tumor-stroma interaction: molecular mechanisms and opportunities for therapeutic targeting. *Differentiation* **70**, 506-21.

Sweeney, P., Karashima, T., Kim, S. J., Kedar, D., Mian, B., Huang, S., Baker, C., Fan, Z., Hicklin, D. J., Pettaway, C. A. and Dinney, C. P. (2002): Anti-vascular endothelial growth factor receptor 2 antibody reduces tumorigenicity and metastasis in orthotopic prostate cancer xenografts via induction of endothelial cell apoptosis and reduction of endothelial cell matrix metalloproteinase type 9 production. *Clinical Cancer Research* **8**, 2714-24.

Szostak, M. J. and Kyprianou, N. (2000): Radiation-induced apoptosis: predictive and therapeutic significance in radiotherapy of prostate cancer (review). *Oncology Report* **7**, 699-706.

Taichman, R. S., Cooper, C., Keller, E. T., Pienta, K. J., Taichman, N. S. and McCauley, L. K. (2002): Use of the stromal cell-derived factor-1/CXCR4 pathway in prostate cancer metastasis to bone. *Cancer Research* **62**, 1832-7.

Thalmann, G. N., Anezinis, P. E., Chang, S. M., Zhau, H. E., Kim, E. E., Hopwood, V. L., Pathak, S., von Eschenbach, A. C. and Chung, L. W. (1994): Androgen-independent cancer progression and bone metastasis in the LNCaP model of human prostate cancer. *Cancer Research* **54**, 2577-81.

Thalmann, G. N., Sikes, R. A., Devoll, R. E., Kiefer, J. A., Markwalder, R., Klima, I., Farach-Carson, C. M., Studer, U. E. and Chung, L. W. (1999): Osteopontin: possible role in prostate cancer progression. *Clincial Cancer Research* **5**, 2271-7.

Thalmann, G. N., Sikes, R. A., Wu, T. T., Degeorges, A., Chang, S. M., Ozen, M., Pathak, S. and Chung, L. W. (2000): LNCaP progression model of human prostate cancer: androgen-independence and osseous metastasis. *Prostate* **44**, 91-103 Jul 1;44(2).

Tjoa, B. A., Erickson, S. J., Bowes, V. A., Ragde, H., Kenny, G. M., Cobb, O. E., Ireton, R. C., Troychak, M. J., Boynton, A. L. and Murphy, G. P. (1997): Follow-up evaluation of prostate cancer patients infused with autologous dendritic cells pulsed with PSMA peptides. *Prostate* **32**, 272-8.

Tjoa, B. A., Simmons, S. J., Bowes, V. A., Ragde, H., Rogers, M., Elgamal, A., Kenny, G. M., Cobb, O. E., Ireton, R. C., Troychak, M. J., Salgaller, M. L., Boynton, A. L. and Murphy, G. P. (1998): Evaluation of phase I/II clinical trials in prostate cancer with dendritic cells and PSMA peptides. *Prostate* **36**, 39-44.

Tjoa, B. A., Simmons, S. J., Elgamal, A., Rogers, M., Ragde, H., Kenny, G. M., Troychak, M. J., Boynton, A. L. and Murphy, G. P. (1999): Follow-up evaluation of a phase II prostate cancer vaccine trial. *Prostate* **40**, 125-9.

Tomko, R. P., Xu, R. and Philipson, L. (1997): HCAR and MCAR: the human and mouse cellular receptors for subgroup C adenoviruses and group B coxsackieviruses. *Proceedings of the National Acadamy of Sciences U S A* **94**, 3352-6.

Topf, N., Worgall, S., Hackett, N. R. and Crystal, R. G. (1998): Regional 'pro-drug' gene therapy: intravenous administration of an adenoviral vector expressing the E. coli cytosine deaminase gene and systemic administration of 5-fluorocytosine suppresses growth of hepatic metastasis of colon carcinoma. *Gene Therapy* **5**, 507-13.

Torrent, C., Jullien, C., Klatzmann, D., Perricaudet, M. and Yeh, P. (2000): Transgene amplification and persistence after delivery of retroviral vector and packaging functions with E1/E4-deleted adenoviruses. *Cancer Gene Therapy* **7**, 1135-44.

Townsend, S. E. and Allison, J. P. (1993): Tumor rejection after direct costimulation of CD8+ T cells by B7-transfected melanoma cells. *Science* **259**, 368-70.

Townsend, S. E., Su, F. W., Atherton, J. M. and Allison, J. P. (1994): Specificity and longevity of antitumor immune responses induced by B7-transfected tumors. *Cancer Research* **54**, 6477-83.

Tu, S. M., Millikan, R. E., Mengistu, B., Delpassand, E. S., Amato, R. J., Pagliaro, L. C., Daliani, D., Papandreou, C. N., Smith, T. L., Kim, J., Podoloff, D. A. and Logothetis, C. J.

(2001): Bone-targeted therapy for advanced androgen-independent carcinoma of the prostate: a randomised phase II trial. *Lancet* **357**, 336-41.

Turner, S. L., Gruenewald, S., Spry, N. and Gebski, V. (2001): Less pain does equal better quality of life following strontium-89 therapy for metastatic prostate cancer. *British Journal of Cancer* **84**, 297-302.

Tuxhorn, J. A., Ayala, G. E. and Rowley, D. R. (2001): Reactive stroma in prostate cancer progression. *Journal of Urology* **166**, 2472-83.

Tuxhorn, J. A., Ayala, G. E., Smith, M. J., Smith, V. C., Dang, T. D. and Rowley, D. R. (2002): Reactive stroma in human prostate cancer: induction of myofibroblast phenotype and extracellular matrix remodeling. *Clinical Cancer Research* **8**, 2912-23.

van der Poel, H. G., Molenaar, B., van Beusechem, V. W., Haisma, H. J., Rodriguez, R., Curiel, D. T. and Gerritsen, W. R. (2002): Epidermal growth factor receptor targeting of replication competent adenovirus enhances cytotoxicity in bladder cancer. *Journal of Urology* **168**, 266-72.

Varani, J., Dame, M. K., Wojno, K., Schuger, L. and Johnson, K. J. (1999): Characteristics of nonmalignant and malignant human prostate in organ culture. *Laboratory Investigation* **79**, 723-31.

Varner, J. A. and Cheresh, D. A. (1996): Integrins and cancer. *Current Opinions in Cell Biology* **8**, 724-30.

Vieweg, J., Rosenthal, F. M., Bannerji, R., Heston, W. D., Fair, W. R., Gansbacher, B. and Gilboa, E. (1994): Immunotherapy of prostate cancer in the Dunning rat model: use of cytokine gene modified tumor vaccines. *Cancer Research* **54**, 1760-5.

Walker, J. R., McGeagh, K. G., Sundaresan, P., Jorgensen, T. J., Rabkin, S. D. and Martuza, R. L. (1999): Local and systemic therapy of human prostate adenocarcinoma with the conditionally replicating herpes simplex virus vector G207. *Human Gene Therapy* **10**, 2237-43.

Waltregny, D., Bellahcene, A., Van Riet, I., Fisher, L. W., Young, M., Fernandez, P., Dewe, W., de Leval, J. and Castronovo, V. (1998): Prognostic value of bone sialoprotein expression in clinically localized human prostate cancer. *Journal of the National Cancer Institute* **90**, 1000-8.

Wang, J. M., Deng, X., Gong, W. and Su, S. (1998): Chemokines and their role in tumor growth and metastasis. *Journal of Immunological Methods* **220**, 1-17.

Wang, R. F., Robbins, P. F., Kawakami, Y., Kang, X. Q. and Rosenberg, S. A. (1995): Identification of a gene encoding a melanoma tumor antigen recognized by HLA-A31-restricted tumor-infiltrating lymphocytes. *Journal of Experimental Medicine* **181**, 799-804.

Waxman, D. J., Chen, L., Hecht, J. E. and Jounaidi, Y. (1999): Cytochrome P450-based cancer gene therapy: recent advances and future prospects. Drug Metab Rev **31**, 503-22.

Weber, G. F. (2001): The metastasis gene osteopontin: a candidate target for cancer therapy. *Biochim Biophys Acta* **1552**, 61-85.

Wei, M. X., Tamiya, T., Hurford, R. K., Jr., Boviatsis, E. J., Tepper, R. I. and Chiocca, E. A. (1995): Enhancement of interleukin-4-mediated tumor regression in athymic mice by in situ retroviral gene transfer. *Human Gene Therapy* **6**, 437-43.

Wernert, N. (1997): The multiple roles of tumour stroma. *Virchows Arch* **430**, 433-43.

Wesseling, J. G., Bosma, P. J., Krasnykh, V., Kashentseva, E. A., Blackwell, J. L., Reynolds, P. N., Li, H., Parameshwar, M., Vickers, S. M., Jaffee, E. M., Huibregtse, K., Curiel, D. T. and Dmitriev, I. (2001): Improved gene transfer efficiency to primary and established human pancreatic carcinoma target cells via epidermal growth factor receptor and integrin-targeted adenoviral vectors. *Gene Therapy* **8**, 969-76.

Weyel, D., Sedlacek, H. H., Muller, R. and Brusselbach, S. (2000): Secreted human beta-glucuronidase: a novel tool for gene-directed enzyme prodrug therapy. *Gene Therapy* 7, 224-31.

Wickham, T. J. (2000): Targeting adenovirus. *Gene Therapy* 7, 110-4.

Wickham, T. J., Mathias, P., Cheresh, D. A. and Nemerow, G. R. (1993): Integrins alpha v beta 3 and alpha v beta 5 promote adenovirus internalization but not virus attachment. *Cell* 73, 309-19.

Wickham, T. J., Segal, D. M., Roelvink, P. W., Carrion, M. E., Lizonova, A., Lee, G. M. and Kovesdi, I. (1996): Targeted adenovirus gene transfer to endothelial and smooth muscle cells by using bispecific antibodies. *Journal of Virology* 70, 6831-8.

Wildner, O., Morris, J. C., Vahanian, N. N., Ford, H., Jr., Ramsey, W. J. and Blaese, R. M. (1999): Adenoviral vectors capable of replication improve the efficacy of HSVtk/GCV suicide gene therapy of cancer. *Gene Therapy* 6, 57-62.

Wojtowicz-Praga, S. (1997): Reversal of tumor-induced immunosuppression: a new approach to cancer therapy. *Journal of Immunotherapy* 20, 165-77.

Wong, Y. C. and Wang, Y. Z. (2000): Growth factors and epithelial-stromal interactions in prostate cancer development. *Int Rev Cytol* 199, 65-116.

Wu, H. C., Hsieh, J. T., Gleave, M. E., Brown, N. M., Pathak, S. and Chung, L. W. (1994): Derivation of androgen-independent human LNCaP prostatic cancer cell sublines: role of bone stromal cells. *International Journal of Cancer* 57, 406-12.

Wu, L., Matherly, J., Smallwood, A., Adams, J. Y., Billick, E., Belldegrun, A. and Carey, M. (2001): Chimeric PSA enhancers exhibit augmented activity in prostate cancer gene therapy vectors. *Gene Therapy* 8, 1416-26.

Wu, T. T., Sikes, R. A., Cui, Q., Thalmann, G. N., Kao, C., Murphy, C. F., Yang, H., Zhau, H. E., Balian, G. and Chung, L. W. (1998): Establishing human prostate cancer cell xenografts in bone: induction of osteoblastic reaction by prostate-specific antigen-producing tumors in athymic and SCID/bg mice using LNCaP and lineage-derived metastatic sublines. *International Journal of Cancer* 77, 887-94.

Xu, J., Kalos, M., Stolk, J. A., Zasloff, E. J., Zhang, X., Houghton, R. L., Filho, A. M., Nolasco, M., Badaro, R. and Reed, S. G. (2001): Identification and characterization of prostein, a novel prostate-specific protein. *Cancer Research* 61, 1563-8.

Xu, J., Stolk, J. A., Zhang, X., Silva, S. J., Houghton, R. L., Matsumura, M., Vedvick, T. S., Leslie, K. B., Badaro, R. and Reed, S. G. (2000): Identification of differentially expressed genes in human prostate cancer using subtraction and microarray. *Cancer Research* 60, 1677-82.

Yamamoto, M., Alemany, R., Adachi, Y., Grizzle, W. E. and Curiel, D. T. (2001): Characterization of the cyclooxygenase-2 promoter in an adenoviral vector and its application for the mitigation of toxicity in suicide gene therapy of gastrointestinal cancers. *Molecular Therapy* 3, 385-94.

Yang, Y., Jooss, K. U., Su, Q., Ertl, H. C. and Wilson, J. M. (1996): Immune responses to viral antigens versus transgene product in the elimination of recombinant adenovirus-infected hepatocytes in vivo. *Gene Therapy* 3, 137-44.

Yeung, F. and Chung, L. W. (2002): Molecular basis of co-targeting prostate tumor and stroma. *J Cell Biochem Suppl* 38, 65-72.

Yeung, F., Law, W. K., Yeh, C. H., Westendorf, J. J., Zhang, Y., Wang, R., Kao, C. and Chung, L. W. (2002): Regulation of human osteocalcin promoter in hormone-independent human prostate cancer cells. *Journal of Biological Chemistry* 277, 2468-76.

Yu, D. C., Chen, Y., Seng, M., Dilley, J. and Henderson, D. R. (1999): The addition of adenovirus type 5 region E3 enables calydon virus 787 to eliminate distant prostate tumor xenografts. *Cancer Research* **59**, 4200-3.

Zabner, J., Freimuth, P., Puga, A., Fabrega, A. and Welsh, M. J. (1997): Lack of high affinity fiber receptor activity explains the resistance of ciliated airway epithelia to adenovirus infection. *Journal of Clinical Investigation* **100**, 1144-9.

Zantema, A., Schrier, P. I., Davis-Olivier, A., van Laar, T., Vaessen, R. T. and van der, E. A. (1985): Adenovirus serotype determines association and localization of the large E1B tumor antigen with cellular tumor antigen p53 in transformed cells. *Molecular Cellular Biology* **5**, 3084-91.

Zhang, J., Dai, J., Qi, Y., Lin, D. L., Smith, P., Strayhorn, C., Mizokami, A., Fu, Z., Westman, J. and Keller, E. T. (2001): Osteoprotegerin inhibits prostate cancer-induced osteoclastogenesis and prevents prostate tumor growth in the bone. *Journal of Clinical Investigation* **107**, 1235-44.

Zhang, L. Q., Mei, Y. F. and Wadell, G. (2003): Human adenovirus serotypes 4 and 11 show higher binding affinity and infectivity for endothelial and carcinoma cell lines than serotype 5. *Journal of General Virology* **84**, 687-95.

Chapter 12

CANCER CELLS HOMING TO BONE: THE SIGNIFICANCE OF CHEMOTAXIS AND CELL ADHESION

Carlton R. Cooper[1], Robert A. Sikes[1], Brian E. Nicholson[2], Yan-Xi Sun[3], Kenneth J. Pienta[4] and Russell S. Taichman[3]

[1]*Department of Biological Sciences, University of Delaware, Newark DE,* [2]*Department of Urology, University of Virginia Health System, Charlottesville, VA;* [3]*Periodontics/ Prevention/Geriatrics, University of Michigan, Ann Arbor, MI; and* [4]*Departments of Internal Medicine and Surgery, University of Michgian, Ann Arbor, MI*

INTRODUCTION

Cancer cell metastasis is a complex process involving several well-characterized steps. To metastasize successfully, tumor cells must first detach from a primary mass, enter the blood circulation or lymphatics. Subsequently, tumors must home to a particular organ, adhere to the endothelium lining the capillaries of that organ, exit the circulation where they must adhere to organ-specific extra-cellular matrix (ECM) components to begin new growth in an foreign environment (Geldof, 1997). Although the metastatic pattern of some cancers may be explained by anatomy, such as the pattern of efferent venous and lymphatic drainage, anatomy does not account for the metastatic pattern of all cancers (Nicolson *et al.*, 1984). This suggests that other factors contribute significantly to the metastatic fate of cancer cells.

Both breast and prostate cancer cells preferentially metastasize to bone, causing intense pain, spinal cord compression, and pathological fractures (Rubens, 1998). Indeed, more than 80% of prostate cancer patients will have bone lesions at autopsy (Jacobs, 1983) and more than 90% of these will be osteoblastic (Koutsilieris, 1995). Prostate cancer homing to the lumbar spine specifically has been reported to be mediated by the connection of the periprostatic venous vessel to the vertebral venous plexus. Batson, using human cadavers and experimental animals, demonstrated that when a dye was injected into the deep dorsal vein of the penis, it reached the vertebral venous plexus of the lumbar spine via the prostatic venous plexus (Batson, 1940). In animal studies, some of the dye entered the caval vein, but the application of abdominal pressure resulted in the dye passing into the vertebral venous system, later termed the Batson's plexus (Geldof, 1997). These observations together suggested that under increased abdominal pressure, prostate cancer cells reach the lumbar spine by retrograde blood flow in the Batson's plexus.

Batson's plexus may explain prostate cancer metastasis to the lumbar spine, but it does not explain prostate cancer metastasis to other bony sites or breast cancer metastasis to the bone. Nor can the metastatic preference be explained by blood volume as bone is a less vascular organ than the liver and lungs (Orr *et al.*, 1993; Yoneda, 1998). Therefore, other mechanisms must be involved in the homing of cancer cells to bone. Cell chemotaxis and adhesion are steps in the metastatic cascade and these steps may contribute to a cancer cell's ability to preferentially target the bone marrow. This chapter will discuss the possible roles of chemotaxis and cell adhesion in the preferential metastasis of tumors to bone, with an emphasis on breast and prostate cancers. Attention will be given to chemotactic molecules and receptors, cell adhesion molecules (CAMs), cell-to-cell interactions, and cell-to-ECM interactions that are involved.

CANCER CELL CHEMOTAXIS

A cancer cell homing to a particular organ may be determined by the mechanical trapping in the microvasculature of the first organ encountered, the volume of blood entering an organ, or by following a concentration gradient of organ-specific chemotactic molecules (Yoneda, 1998). The relatively low volume of blood supplied to the bone (5-10% of the cardiac output) when compared to the significantly greater volume supplied to other organs, such as the lung and liver, targeted by breast and prostate cancer cells, is an unsatisfying explanation for why these cancers' preferentially metastasize to bone (Orr *et al.*, 1993; Yoneda, 1998). Thus, bone-derived chemotactic factors may contribute to the bone marrow homing of breast and prostate cancer cells and their ability to establish bony metastases. During bone remodeling, many potential chemoattractants for cancer cells are synthesized and/or released. Previous investigations have detailed that collagen I peptides, components of bone marrow fibroblast-conditioned media, transforming growth factor-beta (TGF-β), insulin-like growth factors (IGF) I and II, osteonectin and others may all serve as chemoattractants for tumors (Asosingh *et al.*, 2000; Cooper *et al.*, 2000).

Recently stromal-derived factor-1 (SDF-1 or CXCL12) and its receptor, CXCR4 are critical molecules that participate in hematopoietic stem cell homing (Kim and Broxmeyer, 1999; Aiuti *et al*, 1999a). Gene knockout investigations of both the receptor and the ligand demonstrate that normal fetal liver hematopoiesis occurs in homozygous animals, but marrow engraftment by hematopoietic cells does not occur (Aiuti *et al*, 1999b; Nagasawa *et al*, 1996;Peled *et al*, 1999). In addition, CXCR4 expression levels correlate with the ability of human progenitors to engraftment into the marrow in nude mice, and blockade of CXCR4 prevents engraftment into the bone marrow (Peled *et al*, 1999). Most germane to this chapter are data that demonstrate that tumor progression may be associated with alterations in CXCR4 levels.

Müller *et al.* recently reported that CXCR4 and CXCL12 are central players in regulating metastasis by demonstrating that normal breast tissues express little CXCR4, whereas breast neoplasms express high levels of CXCR4 (Muller *et al*, 2001). Furthermore, antibody to CXCR4 blocked the metastatic spread of the tumors to the lung and lymph nodes. Protein extracts from the extracellular matrices derived from normal human lung, liver, skin and muscle, and conditioned media from human primary bone-marrow and lymph-node stromal cells were also evaluated for their chemotactic activity on breast cancer cells. The data demonstrated that protein extracts of lung, liver and conditioned media from human bone-marrow or lymph-node stromal cells induced chemotactic responses in breast cancer cells, indicating that extracts derived from these organs contain chemotactic factors. The chemotactic activity was significantly reduced in the presence of anti-CXCR4 antibodies. In contrast, protein extracts from organs, such as the skin or muscle tissue colonized less frequently by breast cancer cells, exhibited weak overall chemoattractive properties for breast cancer cells, and the weak migratory responses were not affected by anti-CXCR4 antibodies. Similarly, CXCR4 mRNA levels are elevated in glioblastoma multiforme in regions of angiogenesis and degeneration, but deceased in areas of rapid cell proliferation and may be a general characteristic of neuroblastoma cells that supports their preferential metastasis into the bone marrow (Geminder *et al*, 2001). Results consistent with these have also been reported for human melanoma cell lines and melanoma cells that had macroscopically infiltrated draining lymph nodes (Robledo *et al*, 2001), neuroblastomas (Geminder *et al.*, 2001), pancreatic and renal carcinomas (Gerritsen *et al*, 2002;Koshiba *et al*, 2000). These results are also consistent with those of Zeelenberg *et al.* who transfected CXCL12 who fused to a KDEL sequence into mouse T cell hybridoma TAM2D2. The CXCL12-KDEL fusion protein was retained in the endoplasmic reticulum by the KDEL-receptor, and bound to CXCR4 which was therefore also retained. This prevented the metastasis of the cell line to many different tissues (Zeelenberg *et al*, 2001). Yet CXCR4 is clearly not a generalized feature of all carcinomas. Several digestive tract cancers including colon, esophageal, gastric and premalignant liver disease (hepatitis C viral infected livers) do not alter their expression of the receptor. Moreover, CXCR4 expression may even be reduced in hepatocellular carcinomas (Mitra *et al*, 1999). These investigations suggest that CXCR4 may play an important role in neoplastic events including the development metastasis of a wide variety of solid tumors including prostate carcinomas (Muller *et al*, 2001;2002).

Prostate cancer cells also appear to migrate in response to a CXCL12 gradient (Taichman *et al.*, 2002). We recently reported that PC-3 (derived from a bone metastasis), LNCaP (lymph node metastasis), and C4-2B cell lines (a subline of LNCaP derived from a bone metastasis in a mouse model) and DU 145 (derived from a brain metastasis) expressed the CXCR4 transcript. Western blot analysis demonstrated that PC-3, DU145, and C4-2B expressed CXCR4 protein, with cell lines derived from bone metastases having a higher expression. The CXCR4 receptor was determined to be active in PC-3 cells based on CXCL12 stimulation of ERK-1/ERK-2 pathways. Finally, it was shown that CXCL12 stimulated the transendothelial migration of prostate cancer through a monolayer of human bone endothelial (HBME) cells, and the invasion of prostate cancer cells through collagen type I, a major protein in bone ECM, and matrigel. In preliminary experiments (Sikes et al, unpublished observations) testing the effects of IL-8 and CXCL12 (50 ng/ml) on the adhesion of LNCaP and LNCaP C4-2B cells to HBME, we found that LNCaP cells responded with a reproducible increase in attachment using IL-8 while CXCL12 had no effect. LNCaP C4-2, a bone metastatic variant of the LNCaP parental cells responded with an increased attachment to HBME cells in response to CXCL12 ($\geq 15\%$) while IL-8 was actually inhibitory to a similar extent. These observations suggest that CXCL12/CXCR4 may contribute to prostate cancer's preferential metastasis to the skeleton. More recently, we have demonstrated using high-density tissue microarrays constructed from clinical samples obtained from a cohort of over 600 patients that CXCR4 protein expression is significantly elevated in localized and metastatic cancers (Sun *et al*, 2003)(Sun *et al*, submitted). At the RNA level, human PCa tumors also express CXCR4 and message, but overall, they were not significantly different, suggesting post-transcriptional regulation of the receptor plays a major role in regulating protein expression. Similar observations were made for CXCL12 message, but in this case more CXCL12 message was expressed by metastastic lesions as compared to normal tissues (Sun *et al*, 2003). Using PCa cell lines, it was possible to verify that PCa cells express CXCL12 mRNA, regulate expression of the message in response to ligand, and secrete biologically active protein (Unpublished observations). Furthermore, neutralizing antibody to CXCL12 decreased the proliferation of LNCaP C4-2B metastastic tumor cells (Sun *et al*, 2003). A similar dependence for growth by prostate cancers was recently observed *in vivo* for PC3 cells over-expressing the CXCR4 receptor (Derash-Yahana *et al*, 2003).

PROSTATE CANCER-ENDOTHELIUM INTERACTION: DOCKING AND LOCKING

Cancer cell adhesion to organ microvascular endothelial cells is a critical step in the bone metastatic cascade because it determines the site of metastasis and is necessary for cancer cell extravasation (Pauli *et al.*, 1988; Jahroudi *et al.*, 1995; Voura *et al.*, 1998). A recent study demonstrated that the adhesion of cancer cells to the endothelium initiated cancer cell proliferation within the vessel prior to extravasation (Al-Mehdi *et al.*, 2000). Studies from our laboratory demonstrated that the prostate cancer cells preferentially adhered to immortalized human bone marrow endothelial (HBME) cells when compared to immortalized human umbilical vein endothelial cells (HUVEC), immortalized human aortic endothelial cells (HAEC-I), and immortalized human dermal microvascular endothelial cells (HDMVEC) (Lehr *et al.*, 1998; Cooper *et al.*, 2000). These observations were confirmed in another investigation that demonstrated PC-3 cells preferentially adhered to a primary culture of HBME cells as compared to primary cultures of HUVECs and lung microvascular endothelial cells Hs888Lu (Scott *et al.*, 2001). Together, these studies suggest a role for prostate cancer-endothelial interaction in prostate cancer metastasis to bone.

Tumor cell binding to the microvascular endothelium involves two distinct steps described in the docking and locking hypothesis (Honn *et al.*, 1992). The initial docking of the tumor cell to the endothelium is mediated by lectins. Integrins are responsible for the subsequent locking of the tumor cell to the endothelium. Both lectins and integrins have been implicated in

PC-3 cell adhesion to HBME cells. PC-3 cells, treated with galactose-rich modified citrus pectin, an antibody to galectin-3, and arginine-glycine-aspartic (RGD) peptides, reduced their ability to bind HBME cell monolayers *in vitro* (Lehr *et al.*, 1998). The effects of modified citrus pectin and galectin-3 polyclonal antibody suggest the involvement of lectin, while the RGD peptide effect suggests integrin involvement. Other investigations suggest that beta-1 integrins, CD44 isoforms, hyaluronan pericellular matrix, and a type C cell surface lectin, expressed on the surface of PC-3 cells, may also mediate PC-3-HBME adhesion (Kierszenbaum *et al.*, 2000; Scott *et al.*, 2001; Simpson *et al.*, 2001). Glinsky and colleagues demonstrated that Thomsen-Friedenreich (T) antigen, a simple mucin-type disaccharide, expressed on most cancer cells, including breast and prostate, contributed to cancer cell-HBME adhesion (Glinsky *et al.*, 2001). It was first demonstrated that both MDA-MB-435 breast cancer cells and DU-145 prostate cancer cells expressed T antigen on their surfaces, and subsequently it was showed that their adhesion to HUVEC and HBME were T antigen-dependent. The tumor cell-endothelial adhesion mediated by T antigen could be disrupted by synthetic compounds that either mimicked or masked the carbohydrate structure, implicating T antigen as a useful target for the development of anti-adhesive cancer therapeutics.

Hyaluronan (HA) is a ubiquitous high molecular weight glycosaminoglycan component of extracellular and cell-associated matrices. The production of HA correlates with cancer progression and corresponds to dedifferentiation of prostate cancer (Simpson *et al.*, 2001; Simpson *et al.*, 2002). Simpson and colleagues demonstrated that HA pericellular matrix was present on PC-3 cells and it's subline PC-3 M-LN4, which has enhanced metastatic potential in mice and homes to bone upon intracardial injection (Simpson *et al.*, 2001). HA pericellular matrix was not observed on DU145 and LNCaP. These observations correspond to the greater percent binding of PC-3 and PC-3M-LN4 to HBME cells, called BMEC-1 cells, as compared to DU145 and LNCaP cells. Interestingly, the adhesion of PC-3 and PC-3M-LN4 to HBME cells was HA-dependent, but adhesion to HUVEC and human bone stromal cells (BMSC) were HA-independent. Although DU145 and LNCaP cells adhered poorly to HBME cells in this study, the minor adhesion that was detected was HA-independent. The presence of HA in PC-3 and PC-3M-LN4 was mediated by a higher expression of HA synthetase (HAS), a transmembrane enzyme that catalyzes the biosynthesis of HA. When HAS2 and HAS3 expression was reduced in PC-3M-LN4 cells by antisense technology, noticeable reductions in their binding to HBME cells was observed (Simpson *et al.*, 2002). Moreover, transfection of LNCaP cells with HAS2 or the HAS3 isoform conferred an increased ability to bind HBME cells. These data indicate that the elevated expression of HAS and the subsequent HA surface retention on prostate cancer cells may contribute to their ability to bind bone-marrow endothelium, thereby preferentially colonizing the skeleton.

Cortactin, a cortical actin-associated protein that is a prominent substrate of the protein, tyrosine kinase Src, may be important for breast cancer cell adhesion to HBME cells and transendothelial migration (Li *et al.*, 2001). MDA-MB-231 breast cancer cells over-expressing cortactin were evaluated for their abilities to bind HBME cell monolayers and to transverse HBME cell monolayers. Cortactin enhanced the adhesive affinity of MDA-MB-231 for HBME cells by 62% and enhanced transendothelial cell migration by 72% (Li *et al.*, 2001). MDA-MB-231 cells over-expressing a mutant cortactin deficient in tyrosine phosphorylation adhesion to HBME cell monolayers was 45% less than controls, and their transendothelial cell migration was 40% less than controls(Li *et al.*, 2001). Thus cortactin may contribute to breast cancer metastasis to bone by increasing the adhesion of breast cancer cells to bone-marrow endothelium and the invasion of breast cancer cells into bone tissues.

Further examination of PCa cell lines have demonstrated that that beta-1 integrins expressed on HBME cells may not mediate PC-3 cell adhesion (Cooper *et al.*, 2000). An other integrin candidate molecule that may be important in metastasis is the $\alpha_v\beta_3$ integrin - reported to mediate the adhesion of PC-3 and DU145 cells to cytokine-activated HUVEC monolayers (Romanov *et al.*, 1999). We recently characterized $\alpha_v\beta_3$ expression in a variety of prostate cancer cells and determined that of the cells that were tested, $\alpha_v\beta_3$ expression on PC-3 cells was the highest. The role of $\alpha_v\beta_3$ in PC-3-HBME adhesion was then examined by treating PC-3 cells with LM609, a well-characterized $\alpha_v\beta_3$ blocking antibody, prior to performing adhesion assays on HBME. LM609 treatment did not alter the adhesion of PC-3 cells to HBME cell monolayers, suggesting that $\alpha_v\beta_3$ expressed on PC-3 cells does not mediate preferential adhesion (manuscript in press). Although HBME cells also express $\alpha_v\beta_3$, its role in the PC-3-HBME interaction is more difficult to evaluate as the treatment of HBME cells with LM609 causes their detachment from the plastic substratum. Presently, CAMs involved in PC-3-HBME interaction that are specifically expressed on HBME cell surfaces have yet to be identified and characterized.

As will be discussed in a later section, the LNCaP lineage related cell lines have markedly different usage of integrin heterodimers that may be involved in docking or locking to marrow endothelial cells. We have directly tested the adhesion of LNCaP and C4-2 cell adhesion to osteoblasts or HBME cells *in vitro* (Sikes et al., Submitted). Interestingly, despite the more malignant phenotype of C4-2 cells *in vivo* the overall adhesion to osteoblasts or HBME cells was essentially identical (data not presented). In fact, when compared to P69, a T-antigen transformed poorly tumorigenic prostate epithelial cell line, the tumor cell lines actually adhered much less. Therefore, under these conditions we observed an inverse correlation between the tumorigenic behavior of a cell and its adhesive potential. When the invasion of an HBME lawn was compared across the same cell series, the transmigration of the cell lines was directly proportional to their tumorigenic and metastatic potential (data not presented). These findings would therefore dispute the locking and docking hypothesis as a perhaps a statistical argument and that the only cells that establish themselves are those that have the potential to, or can be induced via paracrine interactions to migrate/extravasate. The usage of different integrin pairs, functional reassortment of $\alpha_v\beta_3$, and perhaps the ligand-independent utilization/signaling of integrins used extensively in LNCaP, e.g. $\alpha_6\beta_4$, are responsible for the enhanced migration of C4-2 cells through the marrow endothelium. These intriguing results however do not take into account the potential effects of modulating factors derived from the marrow stroma, and thus require further experimental validation in the future.

PROSTATE CANCER-ENDOTHELIUM INTERACTION: MODULATING FACTORS

The expression of CAMs on endothelial cells, as well as on cancer cells, is not static but is dynamic and strictly controlled by factors such as growth factors (GFs), cytokines, and the composition of the extracellular matrix (ECM) (Pauli *et al.*, 1988; Augustin-Voss *et al.*, 1991; Haraldsen *et al.*, 1996; Kostenuik *et al.*, 1997; Khatib *et al.*, 1999). Some CAMs involved in "docking and locking" a cancer cell to the microvascular endothelium are typically not produced by endothelial cells until stimulated by a cytokine (Taichman *et al.*, 1991; Haraldsen *et al.*, 1996). Although several studies suggest that preferential adhesion of circulating prostate cancer cells to bone marrow endothelium partly contributes to the metastatic pattern observed in advanced prostate cancer, it is important to consider that these adhesion studies were done in the absence of naturally occurring soluble factors. These soluble factors, which could be GFs, cytokines, and extra-cellular matrix components, may alter the expression of the CAMs involved. Therefore, the effects of these modulating factors on CAM expression should be considered when trying to identify CAMs involved in cancer cell-endothelial cell interaction. This consideration is especially vital to the study of PCa adhesion to HBME cells due to the plethora of growth factors and cytokines in the bone marrow (Mohan *et al.*, 1991).

For these reasons we also investigated how PCa cell adhesion to HBME cell monolayers is affected by growing HBME cells on soluble ECM components extracted from kidney, bone, and placenta (Cooper *et al.*, 2000). The growth of HBME cells on bone, kidney, and placenta ECM proteins significantly increased their ability to bind PC-3 cells, independent of the ECM protein concentrations. Bone matrix components were expected to selectively enhance PC-3 cell adhesion to HBME cells; however, similar results with kidney and placenta ECM components were demonstrated. These results suggest that the expression of CAMs involved in PC-3-HBME cell interaction is also regulated by soluble components of the bone matrix.

In another study, we determined the effects of tumor necrosis factor-alpha (TNF-α), transforming growth factor-beta (TGF-β), and dihydrotestosterone (DHT) on PC-3-HBME interaction (Cooper *et al.*, 2002). Both TNF-α and TGF-β regulate CAM expression on endothelial cells and TGF-β also regulates CAM expression on PC-3 cells (Haraldsen *et al.*, 1996; Cohen *et al.*, 1997; Festuccia *et al.*, 1999). DHT enhances the effect of TNF-α on HUVEC monolayers and may contribute to the effect of TNF-α on HBME cell monolayers (McCrohon *et al.*, 1999). The treatment of HBME cells with TGF-β prior to performing adhesion assays significantly reduced PC-3 cell adhesion in a dose-dependent fashion. However, the treatment of PC-3 cells with TGF-β did not alter the PC-3-HBME adhesion. TNF-α alone, or in combination with DHT, did not demonstrate a measurable effect in these adhesion assays (Cooper *et al.*, 2002).

In a recent study, we determined the effect of CXCL12 on prostate cancer cell adhesion to HBME cell monolayers (Taichman *et al.*, 2002). C4-2B and PC-3 cells were pretreated with CXCL12, ranging from 0 to 200 ng/ml for 30 min. at 37°C prior to performing adhesion assays. The data demonstrated that CXCL12 significantly increased the adhesion of both PC-3 and C4-2B cells to HBME cell monolayers in a concentration-dependent manner.

The effects of bone ECM components and TGF-β on HBME cell growth was not determined in the above studies, so it is possible that altered HBME cell growth, mediated by both of these soluble bone factors, could alter PC-

3-HBME cell interaction (Cooper *et al.*, 2000; Cooper *et al.*, 2002). To characterize the effects that bone ECM components and TGF-β have on the growth of HBME cells in our adhesion assay model system, HBME cells were grown on bone ECM components for 24 hours or treated with TGF-β for 24 hours and growth rates were determined. The data demonstrated that neither bone ECM components nor TGF-β significantly altered the growth of HBME cells in our adhesion assays (Cooper *et al.*, in press). These results suggest that the enhanced adhesion of PC-3 cells to HBME cell monolayers mediated by bone ECM components and the reduced adhesion of PC-3 cells to HBME cell monolayers mediated by TGF-β are due to these soluble factors' ability to regulate CAM expression on HBME cells.

Besides TGF-β and ECM components, the bone microenvironment contains other cytokines that could conceivably modulate prostate cancer cell interaction with the bone marrow endothelium. One family of cytokines is the bone morphogenetic proteins (BMP), which is a group of proteins belonging to the extended TGF-β family (Mohan *et al.*, 1991). These proteins, including BMP 1 to 7, induce cartilage and bone formation and have been reported to regulate integrin expression and subsequently, cell adhesion (Nissinen *et al.*, 1997; Koeneman *et al.*, 1999). Normal human prostate and neoplastic human prostate cell lines express BMPs with BMP-4 being the most prevalent (Harris *et al.*, 1994 ; Koeneman *et al.*, 1999). Although BMP expression by prostate cancer cell lines is reported to contribute specifically to the osteoblastic nature of bone lesions mediated by prostate cancer cells, their role in prostate cancer adhesion to bone marrow endothelium has not been explored. We demonstrated in a previous study that TGF-β had a significant effect on PC-3 adhesion to HBME cell monolayers (Cooper *et al.*, 2002). Because BMPs belong to the extended TGF-β family, it is possible that these cytokines, like TGF-β, can alter PC-3-HBME interaction as well.

The potential role of BMPs in PC-3-HBME interaction was determined by treating HBME cell monolayers with BMP 4, -5, and -6 or by treating PC-3 cells with the same for approximately 24 hours prior to performing the adhesion assays (Cooper *et al.*, in press). The treatment of HBME cell monolayers with BMP- 4, -5, and -6 at several concentrations did not significantly alter PC-3-HBME adhesion or the growth of HBME cells. BMP-4 treatment of PC-3 cells significantly increased their ability to bind HBME cell monolayers in a dose-dependent fashion. Interestingly, BMP-5 and -6 treatments of PC-3 cells failed to alter their interaction with HBME cell monolayers (data not shown). This study strongly suggests that distinct BMPs have varying effects on prostate cancer cell adhesion to bone endothelium and that BMP-4 specifically may increase prostate cancer cell adhesion to the bone endothelium.

Once the prostate cancer cell has "locked" on to the bone-marrow endothelium, it must extravasate through the endothelial barrier into the underlying bone microenvironment. The expression of the thrombin receptor, protease activated receptor (PAR1), may contribute to prostate cancer's transendothelial migration and invasion into the bone matrix (Chay *et al.*, 2002). We demonstrated that PAR1 expression in prostate cancer tissue was elevated when compared to normal tissue. Interestingly, PAR1 expression was further increased in those cell lines derived from bone metastases (PC-3 and VCaP) compared to those derived from soft-tissue metastases (LNCaP, DuCaP, and Du145) (Chay *et al.*, 2002). The activation of PAR1 by thrombin contributes to cancer cell motility as well as the secretion of matrix metalloproteinases (MMPs) and vascular endothelial growth factor (VEGF). PAR1 activation also alters the cell cytoskeleton that allows movement through the endothelial monolayer. Furthermore, it was demonstrated that prostate cancer adhesion to a HBME cell monolayer caused endothelial retraction *in vitro* (Cooper *et al.*, in press, Cancer 2003). The exact function of PAR1 expression and thrombin in prostate cancer's metastasis has yet to be determined; however, these data suggest that PAR1 enhanced-expression on bone-derived prostate cancer cells may be important in targeting these cells to the bone.

PROSTATE CANCER CELL-BONE ECM INTERACTION

Following transendothelial migration, breast and prostate cancer cells attach to specific components of the bone ECM (Zheng *et al.*, 1999; Byzova *et al.*, 2000; Cooper *et al.*, 2000; Kiefer *et al.*, 2001; Cooper *et al.*, 2002). The bone ECM is primarily composed of collagen type I (>95%) (Kiefer *et al.*, 2001). Previous studies reported that PC-3 cells adhered strongly to collagen type I and that this adhesion was increased in the presence of TGF-β (10 ng/ml), found in high levels in the bone microenvironment (Kostenuik *et al.*, 1997). This adhesion was mediated by integrins alpha3-beta1 and alpha2-beta1, and TGF-β treatment increased cell adhesion to collagen type I by increasing alpha2-beta1 expression on PC-3 cells (Kostenuik *et al.*, 1996; Kostenuik *et al.*, 1997; Festuccia *et al.*, 1999; Kiefer *et al.*, 2001). Kiefer and Farach-Carson (Kiefer *et al.*, 2001) demonstrated that PC-3 cell adhesion to collagen type I stimulated an increase in cyclin D1 expression followed by an increase in cell division. Inhibitor studies implicated the activation of phosphatidylinositol 3-kinase (PI3K), map kinase (MAPK) and p70S6 kinase in the collagen-mediated effect on PC-3 cells.

The bone ECM also consists of non-collagenous molecules such as bone sialoprotein (BSP), osteopontin, vitronectin, fibronectin, osteocalcin, thrombospondin, and osteonectin (Kiefer *et al.*, 2001). Studies have demonstrated that prostate and breast cancer cells adhere to several of these non-collagenous ECM proteins, including BSP, osteopontin, vitronectin, and fibronectin. One fascinating observation is that $\alpha_V\beta_3$, expressed on breast and prostate cancer cells, is a natural receptor for many of the non-collagenous ECM proteins (Byzova *et al.*, 2000; Zheng *et al.*, 2000; Cooper *et al.*, 2002; Pecheur *et al.*, 2002). Previously, we have shown that the LNCaP cell line, which does not utilize $\alpha_V\beta_3$ heterodimers to bind osteopontin, laminin and vitronectin, progressed to C4-2, where there was a marked utilization of $\alpha_V\beta_3$ to bind these substrates as shown by inhibitory antibody competition (Edlund *et al.*, 2001). Not only did $\alpha_V\beta_3$ expression mediate the adhesion of C4-2 cells to laminin, vitronectin and osteopontin but it also mediated cell migration on these substrates. Additional integrins being utilized by C4-2 but not LNCaP to bind noncollagenous proteins of the bone were α_3 and β_1. Although, β_1 was shown not to be responsible for PC-3 cell invasion, it may still play a role in C4-2 cell migration/invasion. These data strongly implicate the role of integrins in the transmigration of C4-2 cells into the marrow stroma in addition to having a direct effect on the binding to marrow endothelial cells. These data indicate that most of these functions are directed by $\alpha_6\beta_4$ in LNCaP and suggest that a functional reassortment of integrins has occurs coincident with the acquisition of additional metastatic traits by C4-2.

Similar observations were made for the PC-3 cell line where receptor engagement after binding to osteopontin and vitronectin led to increased tyrosine phosphorylation of focal adhesion kinase (FAK), a signaling molecule activated by integrins and able to regulate cell migration (Zheng *et al.*, 1999). FAK activation resulted in the activation of the PI3K/Akt pathway followed by prostate cancer cell adhesion and migration on osteopontin and vitronectin (Zheng *et al.*, 2000; Cooper *et al.*, 2002).

Breast cancer cell adhesion to cortical bone is also $\alpha_V\beta_3$ dependent (Pecheur *et al.*, 2002). Pechuer and colleagues demonstrated that breast cancer cell line B02, a bone-homing subline of MDA-MB-231, constitutively over-expressed $\alpha_V\beta_3$ and caused osteolytic lesions in mice (Pecheur *et al.*, 2002). Adhesion studies revealed that B02 adhesion to cortical bone and BSP was significantly greater than in the parental cell line, and this adhesion was significantly reduced in the presence of anti-$\alpha_V\beta_3$

antibody LM609, demonstrating that this gain in adhesion was $\alpha_v\beta_3$ - dependent.

ANTI-ADHESIVE CANCER THERAPY

Once breast and prostate cancer cells have metastasized to the bone, these cancers are often refractory to available anticancer therapies, resulting in 39,600 female deaths and 30,200 male deaths in the United States, respectively (Keller *et al.*, 2001; Kiefer *et al.*, 2001; Yoneda *et al.*, 2001; Jemal *et al.*, 2002). Therefore, preventing or reducing the ability of these cancer cells to metastasize to the bone is a worthwhile goal to pursue that may yield significant clinical benefit. It has been reported here that cancer cell adhesion to bone-marrow endothelium and bone ECM components are required steps in the development of bone metastasis. The identification of the CAMs involved in these interactions will hopefully lead to the development of molecules that can block the function of these CAMs, implementing anti-adhesive cancer therapy (Chay *et al.*, 2002). The adhesion of breast and prostate cancer cells to HBME cell monolayers can be disrupted with synthetic compounds that bind to T-antigen expressed on the cancer cells, *in vitro* (Glinsky *et al.*, 2001). Another study demonstrated that modified citrus pectin can reduce PC-3 cell adhesion to HBME cell monolayers (Glinsky *et al.*, 2001). DeRoock and colleagues (DeRoock *et al.*, 2001) demonstrated that synthetic peptides inhibit the adhesion of DU145 to ECM proteins, including fibronectin, laminin1 and 5, and collagen IV. Bisphosphonates, commonly used to treat osteolytic bone disease by binding strongly to bone mineral and inhibiting bone resorption, has been shown to specifically inhibit breast (MDA-MB-231) and prostate cancer (PC-3) cells' ability to adhere to unmineralized and mineralized bone ECM (Boissier *et al.*, 1997). These studies strongly indicate that compounds that disrupt cell adhesion may have immense potential as anti-adhesive cancer therapeutics designed to prevent bone metastases in patients with early stage breast or prostate cancer.

CONCLUSIONS

Although the metastasis of specific types of cancer cells to the bone is likely to be mediated by a variety of chemotactic factors and CAMs, a few common themes have emerged from recent investigations. CXCL12 appears to be a common chemoattractant for breast, neuroblastoma, and prostate cancers and others, suggesting it may target other types of cancer cells to the bone as well. The Thomsen-Friedenreich (T) antigen, a lectin, and $\alpha_V\beta_3$, an integrin, are likely to participate in both breast and prostate cancer cell adhesion to bone-marrow endothelium and components of the bone ECM, respectively. It is conceivable that these CAMs, and perhaps others may be also involved in the ability of other types of cancer cells to interact with and colonize the bone. If the above is applicable to most cancers that metastasize to the bone, then designing therapies that block the activities of these molecules is a worthy pursuit that may yield significant clinical benefit.

ACKNOWLEDGMENTS

Some of the work reported herein was supported by several funding sources: an American Foundation for Urologic Diseases (AFUD) 1999 award (C.R.C) sponsored by AstraZeneca Pharmaceuticals, the cell culture core (R.A.S., Core Director) PO1 CA76465-01A2 (Weber, MJ-PI), the DOD prostate cancer research program grants DAMD-17-00-1-0049 (R.A.S),DAMD17-02-1-0100 (R.S.T), post-graduate training grant for Urologic Fellows 1 K12 DK02633-01 (B.E.N.), the SPORE grant at the University of Michigan Comprehensive Cancer Center Ref # P50 Ca 69568 (K.J.P.), AR46024 (R.S.T.), Comprehensive Cancer Grant Ref # CA 46592 (K.J.P), CaPCURE (K.J.P), and the National Institute of Dental and Craniofacial, DE13701 (R.ST).

REFERENCES

Aiuti, A., Webb, I. J., Bleul, C., Springer, T. and Gutierrez-Ramos, J. C. (1997) The chemokine SDF-1 is a chemoattractant for human CD34+ hematopoietic progenitor cells and provides a new mechanism to explain the mobilization of CD34+ progenitors to peripheral blood. *Journal of Experimental Medicine* **185**, 111-120.

Aiuti, A., Tavian, M., Cipponi, A., Ficara, F., Zappone, E., Hoxie, J., Peault, B. and Bordignon, C. (1999) Expression of CXCR4, the receptor for stromal cell-derived factor-1 on fetal and adult human lympho-hematopoietic progenitors. *European Journal of Immunology*, **29**, 1823-1831

Al-Mehdi, A. B., Tozawa, K., Fisher, A. B., Shientag, L., Lee, A. and Mushel, R. J. (2000) Intravascular origin of metastasis from the proliferation of endothelium-attached tumor cells: a new model of metastasis. *Nature Medicine* **6**, 100-102.

Asosingh, K., Gunthert, U., Bakkus, M. H., Raeve, H. D., Goes, E., I, I. V. R., Camp, B. V. and Vanderkerken, K. (2000) In vivo induction of insulin-like growth factor-I receptor and CD44v6 confers homing and adhesion to murine multiple myeloma cells. *Cancer Research* **60**, 3096-3104.

Augustin-Voss, H. G., Johnson, R. C. and Pauli, B. U. (1991) Modulation of endothelial cell surface glycoconjugate expression by organ-derived biomatrices. *Experimental Cell Research* **192**, 346-351.

Batson, O. V. (1940) The function of the vertebral veins and their role in the spread of metastases. *Annals of Surgery* **112**, 138-149.

Boissier, S., Magnetto, S., Frappart, L., Cuzin, B., Ebetino, F. H., Delmas, P. D. and Clezardin, P. (1997) Bisphosphonates inhibit prostate and breast carcinoma cell adhesion to unmineralized and mineralized bone extracellular matrices. *Cancer Research* **57**, 3890-3904.

Byzova, T. V., Kim, W., Midura, R. J. and Plow, E. F. (2000) Activation of integrin αvB3 regulates cell adhesion and migration on bone sialoprotein. *Experimental Cell Research* **254**, 299-308.

Chay, C. H., Cooper, C. R., Gendernalik, J. D., Dhanasekaran, S. M., Chinnaiyan, A. M., Rubin, M., Schmaier, A. H. and Pienta, K. J. (2002) A functional thrombin receptor (PAR1) is expressed on bone-derived prostate cancer cell lines. *Urology* **60**, 760-765.

Chay, C. H., Cooper, C. R., Hellerstedt, B. A. and Pienta, K. J. (2002) Antimetastatic drugs in prostate cancer. *Clinical Prostate Cancer* **1**, 14-19.

Cohen, M. C., Bereta, M. and Bereta, J. (1997) Effect of cytokines on tumour cell-endothelial interactions. *Indian Journal of. Biochemistry and Biophysic* **1-2**, 199-204.

Cooper, C. R., Bhatia, J. K., Muenchen, H. J., McLean, L., Hayasaka, S., Taylor, J., Poncza, P. J. and Pienta, K. J. (2002) The regulation of prostate cancer cell adesion to human bone marrow endothelial cell monolayers by androgen dihydrotesterone and cytokines. *Clinical and Experimental Metastasis* **19**, 25-33.

Cooper, C. R., Chay, C. H. and Pienta, K. J. (2002) The role of αvβ3 in prostate cancer progression. *Neoplasia* **4**, 1-4.

Cooper, C. R., McLean, L., Mucci, N. R., Poncza, P. and Pienta, K. J. (2000) Prostate cancer cell adhesion to quiescent endothelial cells is not mediated by beta-1 integrin subunit. *Anticancer Research* **20**, 4159-4162.

Cooper, C. R., Mclean, L., Walsh, M., Taylor, J., Hayasaka, S., Bhatia, J. and Pienta, K. J. (2000) Preferential adhesion to prostate cancer cells to bone is mediated by binding to bone marrow endothelial cells as compared to extracellular matrix components in vitro. *Clinical Cancer Research* **6**, 4839-4847.

Cooper, C. R. and Pienta, K. J. (2000) Cell adhesion and chemotaxis in prostate cancer metastasis to bone: a minireview. *Prostate Cancer and Prostatic Disease* **3**, 6-12.

Derash-Yahana, M., Pikarsky, E., Karplus, R., Kasem, S., Pal, B., Zeira, E., Abramovitch, R., Galun, E. and Pelid, A. (2003) High expression levels of CXCR4 are associated with human prostate growth, vascularization and metastasis. (Abstract).Keystone Symposia: Chemokines and Chemokine Receptors., 77.

DeRoock, I. B., Pennington, M. E., Sroka, T. C., Lam, K. S., Bowden, G. T., Bair, E. L. and Cress, A. E. (2001) Synthetic peptides inhibit adhesion of human tumor cells to extracellular matrix proteins. *Cancer Research* **61**, 3308-3313.

Edlund, M., Miyamoto, T., Sikes, R. A., Ogle, R., Laurie, G. W., Farach-Carson, M. C., Otey, C. A., Zhau, H. E. and Chung, L. W. K. (2001) Integrin expression and usage by prostate cancer cell lines on laminin substrata. *Cell Growth and Differentiation* **12**, 99-107.

Festuccia, C., Bologna, M., Gravina, G. L., Guerra, F., Angelucci, A., Villonava, I., Millimaggi, D. and Teti, A. (1999) Osteoblast conditioned media contained TGF-beta1 and modulat the migration of prostate tumor cells and their interactions with extracellular matrix components. *International Journal of Cancer* **81**, 395-403.

Geldof, A. A. (1997) Models for cancer skeletal metastasis:a reappraisal of Batson's Plexus. *Anticancer Research* **17**, 1535-1540.

Geminder, H., Sagi-Assif, O., Goldberg, L., Meshel, T., Rechavi, G., Witz, I. P. and Ben-Baruch, A. (2001) A possible role for CXCR4 and its ligand, the CXC Chemokine Stromal

Cell-derived Factor-1, in the development of bone marrow metastases in neuroblastoma. *Journal of Immunology* **167**, 4747-4757.

Gerritsen, M.E., Peale, F.V., Jr. and Wu, T. (2002) Gene expression profiling in silico: relative expression of candidate angiogenesis associated genes in renal cell carcinomas. *Experimental Nephrology*, **10**, 114-119.

Glinsky, V. V., Glinsky, G. V., Rittenhouse-Olson, K., Huflejt, M. E., Glinskii, O. V., Deutscher, S. L. and Quinn, T. P. (2001) The role of Thomsen-Friedenreich antigen in adhesion of human breast and prostate cancer cells to the endothelium. *Cancer Research* **61**, 4851-4857.

Guise, TA. How Metastases Home to Bone: The Attraction of Chemokines July 2002 Commentary on: Taichman RS, Cooper C, Keller ET, Pienta KJ, Taichman NS, McCauley LK. Use of the stromal cell-derived factor-1/CXCR4 pathway in prostate cancer metastasis to bone. Cancer Res. 2002 Mar 15;62(6):1832-7.   2002. Internet Communication

Haraldsen, G., Kvale, D., Lien, B., Farstad, I. N. and Brandtzaeg, P. (1996) Cytokine-regulated expression of E-selectin, intercellular adhesion molecule-1 (ICAM-1), and vascular cell adhesion molecule-1 (VCAM-1) in human microvascular endothelial cells. *Journal of Immunology* **156**, 2558-2565.

Harris, S. E., Harris, M. A., Mahy, P., Wozney, J., Feng, J. Q. and Mundy, G. R. (1994) Expression of bone morphogenetic protein messenger RNAs by normal rat and human prostate and prostate cancer cells. *The Prostate* **24**, 204-211.

Honn, K. V. and Tang, D. G. (1992) Adhesion molecules and tumor cell interaction with endothelium and subendothelial matrix. Cancer and Metastasis Reviews. **11**, 353-75.

Jacobs, S. C. (1983) Spread of prostatic cancer to bone. *Urology* **21**, 337-344.

Jahroudi, N. and Greenberger, J. S. (1995) The role of endothelial cells in tumor invasion and metastasis. *Journal of Neuro-Oncology* **23**, 99-108.

Jemal, A., Thomas, A., Murray, T. and Thun, M. (2002) Cancer Statistics, 2002. *CA Cancer J Clin* **52**, 23-47.

Keller, E. T., Zhang, J.R., Cooper, C. C., Smith, P., McCauley, L. K., Pienta, K. J. and Taichman, R. (2001) Prostate carcinoma skeletal metastases: cross-talk between tumor and bone. *Cancer and Metastasis Review* **20**, 333-49.

Khatib, A. M., Kontogiannea, M., Fallavollita, L., Jamison, B., Meterissian, S. and Brodt, P. (1999) Rapid induction of cytokine and E-selectin expression in the liver in response to metastatic tumor cells. *Cancer Research* **59**, 1356-1361.

Kiefer, J. A. and Farach-Carson, M. C. (2001) Type I collagen-mediated proliferation of PC3 prostate carcinoma cell line: implications for enhanced growth in the bone microenvironment. *Matrix Biology* **20**, 429-437.

Kierszenbaum, A. L., Rivkin, E., Chang, P. L., Tres, L. L. and Olsson, C. A. (2000) Galactosyl receptor, a cell surface C-type lectin of normal and tumoral prostate epithelial cells with binding affinity to endothelial cells. *The Prostate* **43**, 175-183.

Kim, C.H. and Broxmeyer, H.E. (1999) SLC/exodus2/6Ckine/TCA4 induces chemotaxis of hematopoietic progenitor cells: differential activity of ligands of CCR7, CXCR3, or CXCR4 in chemotaxis vs. suppression of progenitor proliferation. *Journal of Leukocyte Biology*, **66**, 455-461.

Koeneman, K. S., Yeung, F. and Chung, L. W. K. (1999) Osteomimetic properties of prostate cancer cells: A hypothesis supporting the predilection of prostate cancer metastasis and growth in the bone environment. *The Prostate* **39**, 246-261.

Koshiba, T., Hosotani, R., Miyamoto, Y., Ida, J., Tsuji, S., Nakajima, S., Kawaguchi, M., Kobayashi, H., Doi, R., Hori, T., Fujii, N. and Imamura, M. (2000) Expression of stromal cell-derived factor 1 and CXCR4 ligand receptor system in pancreatic cancer: a possible role for tumor progression. *Clinical Cancer Research*, 6, 3530-3535.

Kostenuik, P. J., Sanchez-Sweatman, O., Orr, F. W. and Singh, G. (1996) Bone cell matrix promotes the adhesion of human prostatic carcinoma cells via the alpha 2 beta 1 integrin. *Clinical and Experimental Metastasis* 14, 19-26.

Kostenuik, P. J., Singh, G. and Orr, F. W. (1997) Transforming growth factor-beta upregulates the integrin-mediated adhesion of human prostatic carcinoma cells to type I collagen. *Clinical and Experimental Metastasis* 15, 41-52.

Koutsilieris, M. (1995) Skeletal metastases in advanced prostate cancer: cell biology and therapy. *Critical reviews inOncology/Hematology* 18, 51-64.

Lehr, J. E. and Pienta, K. J. (1998) Preferential adhesion of prostate cancer cells to a human bone marrow endothelial cell line. *Journal of the National Cancer Institute* 90, 118-123.

Li, Y., Tondravi, M., Liu, J., Smith, E., Haudenschild, C. C., Kaczmarek, M. and Zhan, X. (2001) Cortactin potentiates bone metastasis of breast cancer cells. *Cancer Research* 61, 6906-6911.

McCrohon, J. A., Jessup, W., Handelsman, D. J. and Celermajer, D. S. (1999) Androgren exposure increases human monocyte adhesion to vascular endothelium and endothelial cell expression of vascular cell adhesion molecule-1. *Circulation* 99, 2317-2322.

Mitra, P., Shibuta, K., Mathai, J., Shimoda, K., Banner, B.F., Mori, M. and Barnard, G.F. (1999) CXCR4 mRNA expression in colon, esophageal and gastric cancers and hepatitis C infected liver. *International Journal of Oncology*, 14, 917-925.

Mohan, S. and Baylink, D. J. (1991) Bone growth factors. *Clinical Orthopaedics and Related Rresearch* 263, 30-48.

Muller, A., Homey, B., Soto, H., Ge, N., Catron, D., Buchanan, M. E., McClanahan, T., Murphy, E., W.Yuan, Wagner, S. N., Barrera, J. L., Mohar, A., Verastegui, E. and Zlotnik, A. (2001) Involvement of chemokine receptors in breast cancer metastasis. *Nature* 410, 50-56.

Nagasawa, T., Hirota, S., Tachibana, K., Takakura, N., Nishikawa, Kitamura, Y., Yoshida, N., Kikutani, H. and Kishimoto, T. (1996) Defects of B-cell lymphopoiesis and bone-marrow myelopoiesis in mice lacking the CXC chemokine PBSF/SDF-1. *Nature*, 382, 635-638.

Nicolson, G. L., Irimura, T., Nakajima, M. and Estrada, J. (1984). Metastatic cell attachment to and invasion of vascular endothelium and its underlying basal lamina using endothelial cell monolayers. <u>Cancer invasion and metastasis: biologic and therapeutic aspects</u>. Nicolson G. L. and Milas L. New York, Raven Press: 145-167.

Nissinen, L., Pirila, L. and Heino, J. (1997) Bone morphogenetic protein-2 is a regulator fo cell adhesion. *Experimental Cell Research* 230, 377-385.

Orr, F. W., Kostenuik, P., Sanchez-Sweatman, O. H. and Singh, G. (1993) Mechanisms involved in the metastasis of cancer to bone. *Breast Cancer Research and Treatment* 25, 151-163.

Pauli, B. U. and Lee, C.-L. (1988) Organ preference of metastasis: The role of organ-specifically modulated endothelial cells. *Laboratory Investigation* 58, 379-387.

Pecheur, I., Peyruchaud, O., Serre, C. M., Guglielmi, J., Voland, C., Bourre, F., Margue, C., Cohen-Solal, M., Buffet, A., Kieffer, N. and Clezardin, P. (2002) Integrin alpha(v)beta3 expression confers on tumor cells a greater propensity to metastasize to bone. *The FASEB Journal* 16, 1266-1268.

Peled, A., Petit, I., Kollet, O., Magid, M., Ponomaryov, T., Byk, Nagler, A., Ben-Hur, H., Many, A., Shultz, L., Lider, O., Alon, R., Zipori, D. and Lapidot, T. (1999) Dependence of human stem cell engraftment and repopulation of NOD/SCID mice on CXCR4. *Science*, **283**, 845-848.

Robledo, M.M., Bartolome, R.A., Longo, N., Rodriguez-Frade, J.M., Mellado, M., Longo, I., van, M.G., Sanchez-Mateos, P. and Teixido, J. (2001) Expression of functional chemokine receptors CXCR3 and CXCR4 on human melanoma cells. *Journal of Biological Chemistry*, **276**, 45098-45105.

Romanov, V. I. and Goligorsky, M. S. (1999) RGD-recognizing integrins mediate interactions of human prostate carcinoma cells with endothilial cells in vitro. The Prostate **39**, 108-118.

Rubens, R. D. (1998) Bone Metastases- The clinical problem. *European Journal of Cancer* **34**, 210-213.

Scott, L., Clarke, N., George, N., Shanks, J., Testa, N. and Lang, S. (2001) Interactions of human prostatic epithelial cells with bone marrow endothelium: binding and invasion. *British Journal of Cancer* **84**, 1417-1423.

Simpson, M. A., Reiland, J., Burger, S. R., Furch, L. T., Spicer, A. P., Theodore R. Oegema, J. and McCarthy, J. B. (2001) Hyaluronan synthase elevation in metastatic prostate carcinoma cells correlates with hyaluronan surface retention, a prerequisite for rapid adhesion to bone marrow endothelial cells. *Journal of Biological Chemistry* **276**, 17949-17957.

Simpson, M. A., Wilson, C. M., Furcht, L. T., Spicer, A. P., Theodore R. Oegema, J. and McCarthy, J. B. (2002) Manipulation of hyaluronan synthase expression in prostate adenocarcinoma cells alters pericellular matrix retention and adhesion to bone marrow endothelial cells. *Journal of Biology Chemistry* **277**, 10050-10057.

Sun, Y.-X., Wang, J., Shelburne, C.E., Lopatin, D.E., Chinnaiyan, A.M., Rubin, M.A., Pienta, K.J. and Taichman, R.S. (2003) The Expression of CXCR4 and CXCL12 (SDF-1) in Human Prostate Cancers (PCa) In Vivo. *Journal of Cell Biochemistry.*, **Submitted**.

Taichman, D. B., Cybulsky, M. I., Djaffar, I., Longenecker, B. M., Teixido, J., Rice, G. E., Aruffo, A. and Bevilacqua, M. P. (1991) Tumor cell surface alpha 4 beta 1 integrin mediates adhesion to vascular endothelium: demonstration of an interaction with the N-terminal domains of INCAM-110/VCAM-1. *Cell Regulation* 5, 347-355.

Taichman, R. S., Cooper, C., Keller, E. T., Pienta, K. J., Taichman, N. S. and McCauley, L. K. (2002) Use of the stromal cell-derived factor-1/CXCR4 pathway in prostate cancer metastasis to bone. *Cancer Research* **62**, 1832-1837.

Voura, E. B., Sandig, M. and Siu, C.-H. (1998) Cell-cell interactions during transendothelial migration of tumor cells. Microscopy Research and Technique **43**, 265-275.

Yoneda, T. (1998) Cellular and molecular mechanisms of breast and prostate cancer metastasis to bone. *European Journal of Cancer* **34**, 240-245.

Yoneda, T., Williams, P. J., Hiraga, T., Niewolna, M. and Nishimura, R. (2001) A bone-seeking clone exhibits different biological properties from the MDA-MB-231 parental human breast cancer cells and a brain-seeking clone in vivo and in vitro. *Journal of Bone and Mineral Research* **16**, 1486-1495.

Zeelenberg, I.S., Ruuls-Van Stalle, L. and Roos, E. (2001) Retention of CXCR4 in the endoplasmic reticulum blocks dissemination of a T cell hybridoma. *Journal of Clinical Investigation*, **108**, 269-277.

Zheng, D.-Q., Woodard, A. S., Fornaro, M., Tallini, G. and Languino, L. R. (1999) Prostatic carcinoma cell migration via $\alpha_v\beta_3$ integrin is modulated by a focal adhesion kinase pathway. *Cancer Research* **59**, 1655-1664.

Zheng, D.-Q., Woodard, A. S., Tallini, G. and Languino, L. R. (2000) Substrate specificity of αvβ3 integrin-mediated cell migration and phosphatidylinositol 3-kinase/AKT pathway activation. *Journal of Biological Chemistry* **275**, 24565-24574.

Chapter 13

HISTOLOGICAL, IMMUNOPHENOTYPIC AND HISTOMORPHOMETRIC CHARACTERIZATION OF PROSTATE CANCER BONE METASTASES

Martine P. Roudier[1], Eva Corey[1], Lawrence D. True[2], Celestia S. Hiagno[3], Susan M. Ott[4], and Robert L. Vessella[1,5]

[1]*Department of Urology, University of Washington Medical Center, Seattle,, WA;*
[2]*Department of Pathology, University of Washington Medical Center, Seattle WA;*
[3]*Department of Medicine (Oncology) University of Washington Medical Center, Seattle, WA;*
[4]*Department of Medicine (Metabolism), University of Washington Medical Center, Seattle, WA;* [5]*VA Puget Sound Health Care System, Research Service, Seattle, WA*

INTRODUCTION

Carcinoma of the prostate (CaP) is the most common malignancy in older men in the United States. In 2002, more than 200,000 cases of CaP were diagnosed and an estimated 32,000 Americans died of this cancer (Jemal et al., 2002). Most of the devastating effects of prostate cancer can be attributed to its tendency to metastasize to bone. At the time of clinical presentation, 8% of Caucasian-Americans and 14% of African-Americans already have bone metastasis (Coffey, 1993; Whitmore, 1990), and bone metastases will develop in the majority of patients with recurrent hormone-independent CaP. Bone metastases are a major cause of morbidity in patients with advanced CaP; major clinical features of bone metastases are intractable bone pain, fracture, spinal cord compression and eventually wasting and death. While the biology of the primary tumor has been intensively studied, the special aspects of CaP bone metastases that lead to abnormal bone growth not ordinarily seen in any other cancers are not extensively documented in the literature. In this chapter, we review the detection of CaP metastases, the predilection of CaP to spread to bone, the main phenotypic features of CaP in bone, and the characterization of the histological "osteoblastic" bone response. We conclude with a brief description of our osteoblastic xenograft model and comparison of this model to clinical bone metastases.

DISTRIBUTION OF CAP BONE METASTASES

Scintigraphy

In the past, the detection of bone metastases was accomplished using plain X-ray film radiography. However, the sensitivity of this technique is limited, since an increase of approximately 50% in bone mineral density is required to detect osteoblastic lesions (Paulson, 1980). Today, bone scintigraphy using Technetium^{99} methylene diophosphonate (Tc^{99}MDP) has supplanted X-ray radiography as a more sensitive tool in detecting metastases; it may detect bone metastases up to 18 months earlier than radiography (Galasko, 1969). Other advantages of bone scintigraphy include its convenience, efficiency in evaluating the entire skeleton, follow-up evaluations, and its inter-institutional reproducibility. The latter advantage is especially important in monitoring the effectiveness of different therapeutic modalities, *i.e.*, external beam radiation therapy and hormonal therapy. Although bone scintigraphy has high sensitivity in the diagnosis of bone metastasis, its specificity is limited when there is concurrent trauma, or degenerative or inflammatory diseases, or when only one scintigraphic abnormality is present (Jacobson et al., 1990; Paulson, 1980). Furthermore, Tc^{99}MDP bone scintigraphy has low sensitivity in detecting pure bone marrow involvement that is not associated with a bone response (Gulenchyn et al., 1987). In cases where the bone scintigraphy result is equivocal, additional imaging modalities such as X-ray plain film, magnetic resonance imaging (MRI) and/or ^{11}C-acetate positron emission tomography (PET)-imaging may help in making an accurate diagnosis (Oyama et al., 2002).

Another method of detecting osseous and non-osseous CaP metastases by scintigraphy relies on the targeting of tumor foci using radio-labeled monoclonal antibodies that are immunoreactive with an antigen expressed by the tumor cells. This approach is referred to as radioimmunoscintigraphy. For the imaging and detection of CaP metastases, the most success has come from the targeting of prostate specific membrane antigen (PSMA; see discussion on PSMA to follow) (Yao et al, 2002). One anti-PSMA imaging agent (ProstaScint, Cytogen, Princeton, NJ) is FDA approved for the imaging of CaP metastases in non-osseous tissues, although published studies also document the detection of bone metastases (Elgamal et al, 1998).

Bisphosphonates as scanning agents

The most commonly used agent for bone scintigraphy is Technetium[99] methylene diophosphonate. Although a current synonym for diophosphonate is "bisphosphonate" (BisP), the older term is used when these agents are coupled to a gamma-emitting radioisotope. These compounds are useful bone-scanning agents because of their high affinity for hydroxyapatite. BisP are preferentially delivered to sites of increased bone formation (Galasko, 1986). Uptake of BisP occurs during the mineralization phase of bone formation because the BisP moiety of the tracer adheres to newly formed bone crystals (McCarthy, 1997). Some lesions not associated with bone formation cannot be visualized by bone scintigraphy. For example, myeloma, lymphoma, leukemia, or highly anaplastic metastases, and metastases of long duration where the osteoblastic response is no longer active are difficult to detect by bone scintigraphy (Galasko, 1975; Galasko, 1977).

Bisphosphonates as therapeutic agents

In addition to their use as scanning agents, BisPs are also used for the treatment of diseases in which osteoclastic resorption is increased, such as Paget's disease, post-menopausal osteoporosis, hypercalcemia of malignancy, bone metastases due to solid tumors, and multiple myeloma. BisPs prevent, minimize, or delay skeletal morbidity secondary to osteoclast-tumor interactions. Various BisPs are available, with anti-resorptive potencies that vary from 1 to 1,000,000 fold: etidronate, clodronate, tiludronate, pamidronate, alendronate, risendronate, ibandronate and zoledronic acid. Recent studies have shown that these BisPs have distinct patterns of deposition in the bone. Pamidronate accumulates selectively in metaphyseal bone, diaphyseal periosteum and endosteum (Fitton et al., 1991). Etidronate binds to both bone-forming and bone-resorbing surfaces. The more potent alendronate binds preferentially to resorbing surfaces (Masarachia et al., 1996). Since all BisPs have a long half-life in bone (over 10 years), it is possible that long-term BisPs treatment saturates bone and interferes with the ability of a single dose of Tc[99]MDP to permit visualization of bone metastases.

Long term treatment and scintigraphy

Only a few studies have addressed the effect of BisP therapy on bone scintigraphy. Five studies have confirmed the usefulness of bone scintigraphy during short-term BisP treatment (Carrasquillo et al., 2001; Macro et al., 1995; Pecherstorfer et al., 1993; Ryan et al., 1992; Sandler et al., 1991). Macro reported that when a single pamidronate infusion was used in 6 patients with bone metastases and 5 patients with Paget's disease presenting with life-threatening hypercalcemia, the number and activity of bone metastases were unchanged from baseline when a second bone scintigraphy was performed 24 hours after pamidronate infusion (Macro et al., 1995). Also, Pecherstrorfer et al. reported that when clodronate was given for 3 weeks (300 mg per day by infusion) to women with breast cancer bone metastases, the sensitivity of scintigraphy using $Tc^{99}MDP$ in detecting bone metastases was not altered by administration of clodronate (Pecherstorfer et al., 1993). In contrast, two studies have shown adverse effects of BisP administration on the sensitivity of $Tc^{99}MDP$ scintigraphy. Watt et al. reported profound alterations in the distribution of the scanning agent after administration of etidronate at the time of injection of $Tc^{99}MDP$ (Watt et al., 1981) in an animal model. Similarly, Krasnow et al. reported a false-negative bone scintigraph due to etidronate therapy in a patient with CaP (Krasnow et al., 1988). In this report, the patient, with known CaP bone metastases, showed extensive soft tissue tracer accumulation but only minimal bone uptake after three months of treatment with etidronate.

Zoledronic acid, one of the most potent of the BisPs, has recently received FDA approval for treatment of CaP bone metastases. The first randomized placebo-controlled clinical trial using zoledronic acid for treatment of men with hormone-refractory CaP and osteoblastic bone metastases demonstrated that skeletal-related events were reduced and delayed by BisP therapy (Saad et al., 2002).

Therefore, in an effort to address the issue of whether BisP treatment affects the detection of CaP bone metastasis by scintigraphy, we performed a site-by-site comparison of 33 $Tc^{99}MDP$ bone scans and histological findings of 188 autopsy bone biopsies obtained from 11 CaP patients, five of whom were treated with pamidronate for up to 13 months (Roudier et al. 2003a). Concordance was observed in 86% of samples from patients who did not receive pamidronate, and in 82% of samples from pamidronate-treated patients. Scintigraphy false negatives (13%) were observed in four situations: (1) absence of bone change in the metastatic areas (12 sites, Figure 1); (2) osteonecrosis (therapeutic or tumor-related) at 5 sites; (3) early bone marrow invasion without bone change at 2 sites; and (4) unknown (3 sites). There were 4 scintigraphy false positives sites (2%); osteoarthritis was the apparent cause. In summary, we found that long-term pamidronate treatment generally did not affect the ability of Tc^{99}MDP bone scintigraphy to identify the presence of bone metastases.

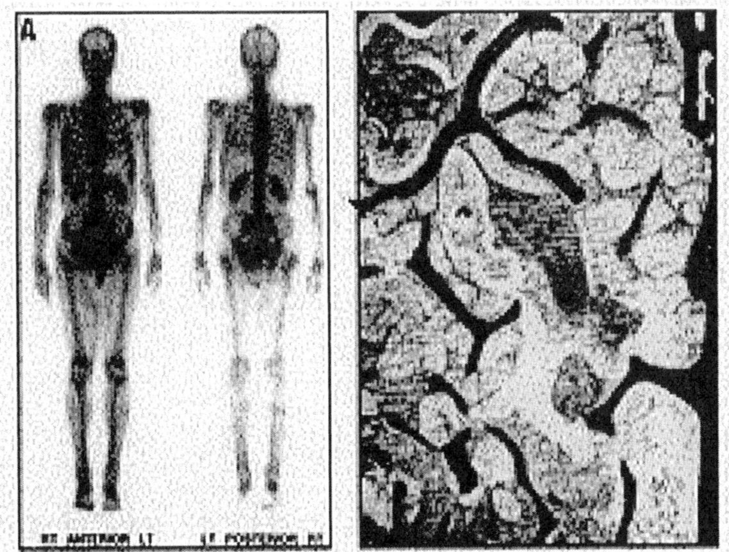

Figure 1. **A**, Negative bone scintigraphy with 12 histologically confirmed bone metastases identified in pelvis, sternum, L1 to L5, T8, T11 and T12. **B**, A representative histological section of a metastasis showing tumor infiltration of the bone marrow without histological evidence of bone reaction (arrows: tumor, Goldner's stain).

Autopsy

The propensity of advanced CaP to metastasize primarily to the bone and lymph nodes has been described since the mid 1800s (Thompson, 1854; Carlier, 1903). The anatomical findings in 8 studies of patients who died of metastatic CaP are summarized in Table 1 (Byar, 1977; de la Monte et al., 1986; Harada et al., 1992; Lamothe et al., 1986; Mintz et al., 1934; Rana et al., 1993; Rubin et al., 2000; Saitoh et al., 1984). These studies reported a predominant localization of CaP bone metastases to the pelvis, with no detailed analysis of skeletal sites. We have recently reported a detailed evaluation of the distribution of CaP metastases in the skeleton (Roudier et al., 2002b). Our Prostate Cancer Donor Rapid Autopsy Program has the goal of obtaining tumor tissue from consented patients within 6 hours of death from advanced CaP. After examining and removing the organs to expose the spine and pelvic bones, large bone core biopsies (5 cm long and 1.2 cm in diameter) from 20 pre-determined sites, including iliac crest, sacrum, vertebrae L1 to L5 and T8 to T12, 7th right anterior rib, proximal epiphysis of humerus, femur, and the sternum, as well as grossly visible rib metastases are obtained. We evaluated 153 bone metastases obtained from 14 patients who died of advanced CaP. All patients had bone metastases at autopsy. The locations of the histologically confirmed non-bone and bone metastases are shown in Table 2. Bone metastasis frequency is shown in Figure 2. Bone metastases had formed in 95% of the pelvic bone biopsies, 92% of the spine biopsies, and 77% of the thoracic cage biopsies. We found a higher frequency of bone metastasis than previously reported. A study done in the early part of the 20th century, when advanced CaP was not treated (Mintz et al., 1934) showed a distribution of CaP metastases similar to ours. Thus, our data suggest that the distribution of CaP metastases has not fundamentally changed in the past century, despite new detection and treatment modalities.

Table -1. Review of the literature where frequency of bone metastases is provided (as % of patients in each series)

	Blummer 1909	Mintz et al., 1934	Vacurg 1977	Saitoh et al., 1984	Harada et al., 1990	Rana et al., 1993	Bubendorf et al., 2000	Rubin et al., 2000	Roudier et al, 2003
	Autopsy	Autopsy	X-ray	Autopsy	Autopsy	B.scan + X-ray	Autopsy	Autopsy	Autopsy
Bone sites	Pts=43	Pts=100	Pts= 103	Pts=1367	Pts=137	Pts= 169	Pts=1589	Pts=14	Pts= 14
Pelvis	83	13	86		26	76			95
Lumbar Spine	81*	20*	71	34*	77*	63	97	64*	92
Thoracic Spine			60			73	66		72
Ribs	69	10	53	11	24	57	18	36	75
Sacrum						47			90
Femur	58	3	48	5	12	28	15**		73
Humerus	35		39		1	18			77
Sternum	37			9	28	14			82
		*all spine					** long bones		

Table 2. Distribution of osseous and non osseous metastases in 13 patients

	Number of patients	Patient # with bone metastases (range of bone metastases)	Patient # with lymph node metastases	Patient # with liver metastases	Patient # with lung metastases
Bone metastases only	2	2 (14, 19)	0	0	0
Minimal involvement in non-bone sites (<10cc)	7	7 (2-19)	6	3	1
Substantial involvement in non-bone sites (≥10cc)	4	4 (1-19)	3	3	1
Non osseous metastases only	0	0	0	0	0

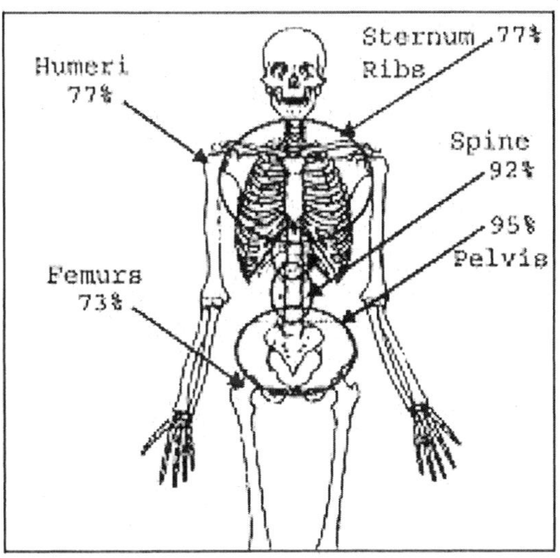

Figure 2. Frequency of bone metastases in 14 rapid autopsy patients.

With regard to non-osseous sites, lymph-node metastases were observed in 80% of patients; these were located along the aorta and in the mediastinum. The largest non-osseous metastases were observed in the liver, reaching 5 cm in diameter, although this size was observed in only 2 of the

14 patients. Only micro-metastases were observed in the lungs. Adrenal, peritoneal, and diaphragm metastases were rare and, when observed, of small size. Finally, in every instance in which the prostate had not been resected as part of the initial treatment, we failed to find tumor in the prostate. This finding suggests that it is more difficult or unusual for tumor cells at the primary site to progress to androgen independence than at the metastatic sites. One might further speculate that the wealth of growth factors in bone and the multitude of cell-cell interactions facilitate survival of bone metastases and/or the development of androgen independence.

PHENOTYPE NATURE OF CAP BONE METASTASES

Histological types

There are no reports in the literature on extensive histological evaluations of CaP bone metastases. The autopsy studies cited in Table 1 provided relatively little data regarding the nature of tumors in the bone. In a small number of patients whose tumors were studied before the era of hormonal treatment, Mintz et al. observed that most metastases retained the morphological features of the primary tumor (Mintz et al., 1934). The effect of hormonal treatment on the histology of bone metastases in patients who have received prolonged androgen blockade therapy has not been studied in depth. De la Monte et al. histologically characterized the tumor cells in patients after androgen ablation with estrogen therapy: these cells had a clear cytoplasm and a prominent degree of atypia (Harada et al., 1992). Reuter reported that androgen deprivation induces a variety of characteristic histological changes; a decreased nuclear:cytoplasmic ratio, cytoplasmic swelling and vacuolization, scattered apoptosis of prostatic epithelial cells, and shrinkage of prostatic glands (Reuter, 1997). In our histological analysis of 153 bone metastases obtained from 14 patients who had been treated with androgen ablation and progressed to androgen independence, none of the bone metastases exhibited the histological features characteristic of androgen deprivation. The cytology of the tumor cells was consistent with that of primary, hormone-sensitive CaP, i.e. cells of intermediate size with regular round or oval nucleus, and prominent nucleolus (Figure 3A). The tumor metastases exhibited five distinct histological patterns (Figure 3A-E). The most frequently observed pattern (10 patients) consisted of tumor cells growing as solid sheets with scattered lumens (Figure 3A). Less frequent patterns were: micro-acinar (one patient, Figure 3B), comedo-carcinoma pattern (one patient, Figure 3C), clear cell carcinoma pattern (one patient, Figure 3D), and a macro-acinar pattern (one patient, Figure 3E). All metastases in a given patient had a similar histological pattern, although the percentage of tumor cells that formed acinar structures varied widely within a patient. Interestingly, our results show that tumor cells in androgen-independent bone metastases exhibited morphology similar to that of androgen-dependent primary tumors.

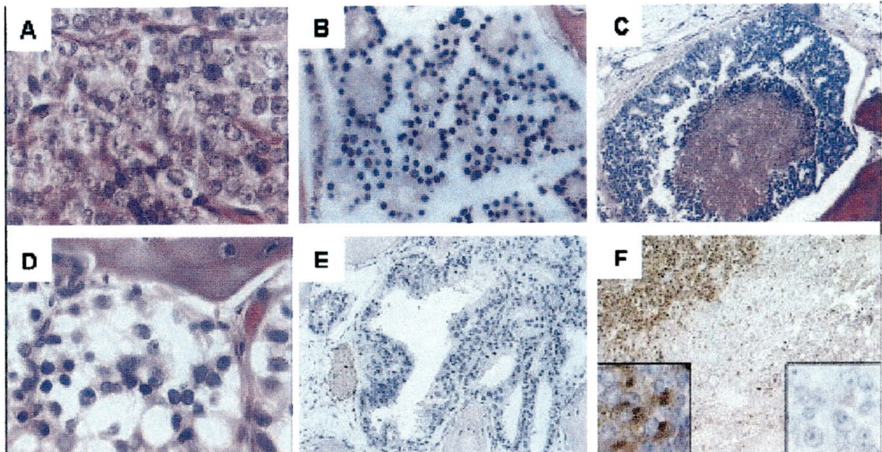

Figure 3. Five different histological patterns (Hand E) observed in androgen-independent bone metastases of 14 patients who died of prostate cancer: **A**, Solid pattern, **B**, Micro-acinar pattern, **C**, Comedocarcinoma pattern, **D**, Clear cell pattern, and **E**, Macro-acinar pattern. **F**, shows the heterogeneity of immunophenotype; two contiguous fields of the same morphological tumor are positive and negative for prostatic specific membrane antigen. Inserts show a magnification of each field.

Immunohistochemical characterization

It has become widely accepted that CaP is a heterogeneous disease. The heterogeneity of CaP is manifested in multiple ways: in the wide range of histological grades of primary tumors, in the variable rate of tumor progression and response to therapy, in the wide range of pre-terminal serum prostate specific antigen (PSA) levels, and, as described above, in the variety of histological patterns in bone metastases. Yet there has been only limited immunophenotyping of CaP bone metastases. Stein et al. reported variable expression of PSA and prostatic acid phosphatase (PAP) in the metastases of 16 autopsied patients (Stein et al., 1984). Cheville et al. reported that 80% of bone metastases of CaP sampled during surgical stabilization of pathological fracture expressed PSA (Cheville et al., 2002). To characterize the immunophenotype of CaP bone metastases in detail, we examined the expression of PSA, human kallikrein 2 (hK2), prostate specific membrane antigen (PSMA), androgen receptor (AR, Her-2/neu, Ki67, and chromogranin A (CGA) in bone metastases acquired in our rapid autopsy program from 14 patients who died of prostate cancer. The results of our study are presented in Figure 4A to G.

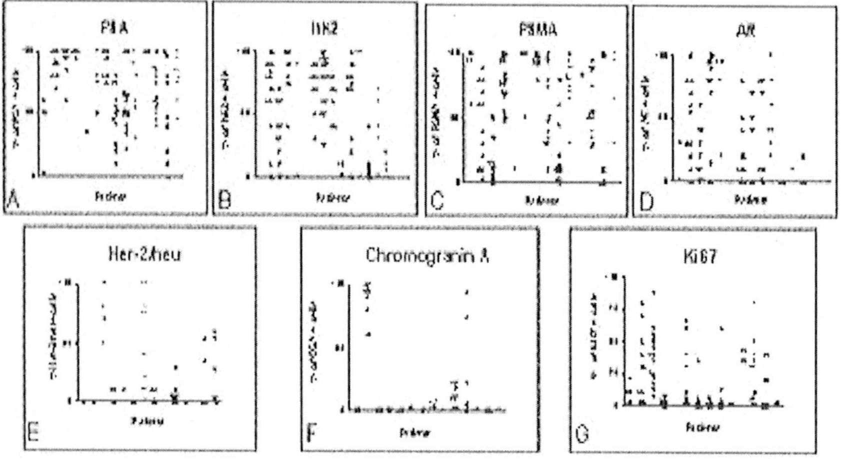

Figure 4. Immunohistochemical analysis of androgen independent prostate cancers in bone metatases of 14 patients. **A**, Prostatic specific antigen, **B**, Human kallikrein 2, **C**, Prostatic specific membrane antigen, **D**, Androgen receptor, **E**, Her-2/neu, only patient #3 met the criteria defined in breast cancer pathology as being positive for Her-2/neu (contiguous strong membranous staining in more than 10% of the tumor cells), all others did not meet these criteria, **F**, Chromogranin A, **G**, Ki67. Note the marked heterogeneity of immunoreactivity in a given patient from one metastasis to another.

PSA and hK2 are serine proteases (human kallikrein 3 and 2, respectively) expressed by prostate epithelial cells (Rittenhouse et al., 1998). PSA expression is down-regulated in poorly differentiated primary prostate carcinomas. In contrast to PSA, hK2 exhibits higher levels of expression in less differentiated adenocarcinomas (Darson et al., 1997; Furuya et al., 2001). In our study, most of the tumor cells in the majority of metastases expressed PSA (average of 75%) (Figure 4A). The range in the percentage of PSA-positive cells in each patient and at each metastatic site was broad: in five patients all tumor sites exhibited greater than 90% PSA immunoreactivity, and in 2 patients, there was a range of 0 to 100% of PSA-immunoreactive cells from one site to another. hK2 exhibited a similar pattern of expression (correlation factor r = 0.85, $P < 0.05$) (Figure 4B).

PSMA is a 100-kDa folate gamma-glutamyl carboxypeptidase of both diagnostic and therapeutic interest. It is an especially attractive therapeutic target because it is up-regulated in androgen-depleted and androgen-independent tumors (Murphy et al., 1998). Radiolabeled anti-PSMA monoclonal antibodies are currently being used in radioimmunoscintigraphy for the detection of metastases (see previous section on scintigraphy). Anti-PSMA monoclonal antibody-toxin conjugates are being evaluated in Phase I and II trials (Chang et al., 1999; Assikis et al., 2002; Shankar et al., 2002). In our study, PSMA was widely and heterogeneously expressed among the bone metastases in a given patient and from one patient to another (Figure 4C). PSMA can be detected in the cytoplasm and/or on the cell membrane, depending upon the specificity of the antibody. In the bone metastases, PSMA staining was frequently observed as a patchy cytoplasmic pattern without membranous localization, although the antibody was immunoreactive with an epitope typically expressed as an external domain in primary CaP.

The growth of CaP is initially dependent on androgen stimulation mediated by the androgen receptor (AR), a member of the steroid hormone receptor family of ligand-dependent nuclear receptors. Although most CaP patients with persistent disease respond initially to androgen ablation therapies, virtually all patients eventually relapse and progress to an androgen-independent state. Many lines of evidence indicate that AR function contributes to tumor-cell survival, even after androgen ablation, and to the growth of androgen-independent prostate cancer. A number of mechanisms are thought to contribute to AR activity in androgen-independent prostate cancer, including AR amplification, AR mutation, altered expression of AR co-activator and co-repressor proteins, and activation of other pathways that can enhance AR function (Balk, 2002). Expression of the AR in androgen-dependent and -independent metastases is a rather controversial area, although the discrepancies are most likely due to differences in reagents, techniques and, based on our data, tissue sampling (vide infra). AR expression has been reported to be decreased in primary tumors in response to androgen ablation (van der Kwast et al., 1996), but has been found to be variable in androgen-independent metastases (Leav et al., 2001). Our results highlight the significant heterogeneity in AR expression among the 153 bone metastases, ranging from 0 to 100% of cells expressing the AR in some patients. AR was highly expressed in 2 patients, heterogeneously expressed in 7 patients and virtually absent in 3 patients (Figure 4D). On average this reveals a decrease in the number of cells that are AR-positive in advanced CaP bone metastases vs. the number of AR-positive cells in primary CaP. Our study also demonstrates that a small number of samples may not be representative of the diversity that exists overall. Since there are now reports that androgen-independent metastases show AR gene amplification (Brown et al., 2002), it will be interesting to correlate gene amplification to protein expression in a comprehensive series of specimens.

Overexpression of Her-2/neu occurs in approximately 25% of mammary carcinomas, where it is associated with poor prognosis and alterations in response to chemotherapy (Slamon et al., 1987; Slamon, 1987). Recently there have been encouraging results from the selection of breast cancer patients who express Her-2/neu for treatment with the Her-2/neu-targeted drug trastuzumab (trade name Herceptin) (Ligibel et al., 2002; Spigel et al., 2002). The frequency of Her-2/neu expression in CaP has varied widely, from frequent (Osman et al., 2001; Signoretti et al., 2000) to infrequent (Jorda et al., 2002; Lara, Jr. et al., 2002) with at least one recent report showing that the frequency of detection is directly correlated with the immunohistochemistry method used (Sanchez et al., 2002). In our set of 14 patients we detected Her-2/neu expression in >20% of cells in 52 of 153 bone metastases specimens, including 15 sites with over-expression, as defined by breast-pathology guidelines (Rhodes et al., 2002) (Figure 4E). However, in this series only one patient (patient #3, Figure 4E) would have been considered Her-2/neu positive by the criteria used to assess breast cancer positivity. Note again the heterogeneity among sites (0-100% Her-2/neu positive cells in a given patient). Our findings have significant ramifications if therapeutic decisions were based on an analysis of inappropriate or insufficiently large sample sets. For example, Morris et al. showed that Her-2/neu was not expressed in three primary tumors but was expressed in the matched androgen-independent metastases (Morris et al., 2002).

Emerging evidence suggests that the evolution and progression of androgen-independent CaP are influenced by growth-modulating factors secreted by neuroendocrine cell constituents of the tumor (Abrahamsson, 1999). Moreover, several investigators have attributed the progression to androgen-independence in some patients to the acquisition by tumor cells of a predominantly neuroendocrine (NE) phenotype. The percentage of NE cells in CaP has been shown to be correlated with (1) the rate of tumor progression (Cohen et al., 1991; Ro et al., 1987) (2) adverse outcome (Weinstein et al., 1996) and (3) surrogate markers of adverse outcome such as tumor grade (Bohrer et al., 1993) and stage (Allen et al., 1995). In addition, NE differentiation in CaP metastases was reported to be more extensive than in the primary tumor; 19% of CaP bone metastases sampled during surgical stabilization of pathological fracture expressed chromogranin A (CGA) (Cheville et al., 2002), one of the most commonly used markers of the NE phenotype. In contrast, in our study, CGA immunoreactivity was found less frequently (Figure 4F). In 11 of 14 patients fewer than 3% of CaP cells expressed CGA, while 8%, 13%, and 88% of CaP cells were CGA-positive in the three remaining patients. The patients with ≥8% CGA positive cells did not have clinical histories that distinguished them from those who had virtually no NE cells in their bone metastases. Therefore our results do not support the hypothesis that a high frequency of NE cells in CaP bone metastases is essential for aggressive, androgen-independent growth.

One of the general characteristics of tumor cells is a higher proliferation rate than seen in normal cells, but in primary prostate cancer the increase is marginal (Berges et al., 1995; Cohen et al., 1991; Sebo et al., 2002). We used immunohistochemical analysis to assess the expression of Ki67, which marks proliferating cells (Figure 4G). Our results revealed that in half of the patients evaluated (7/14) the percentage of Ki67-positive CaP cells was, on average, ten-fold higher in the bone metastases (20% positive cells) than the percentages reported for primary tumors (Cohen et al., 1991; Sebo et al., 2002).

Interestingly, in addition to the wide variability of immunoexpression of the biomarkers described above between patients and also from one bone site to another in the same patient, in several bone metastases we observed distinct but contiguous areas of positivity and negativity with PSA, AR, and PSMA on the same slide (Figure 3F). These observations were highly reproducible, and when sections were immunostained for other biomarkers the pattern was uniform, strongly suggesting that the heterogeneity observed was not due to tissue artifacts. These results might reflect either (1) the seeding and growth of different clones adjacent to one another, or (2) outgrowths from individual clones that have lost expression of a specific biomarker.

In combination with our histology findings, these biomarker expression profiles confirm the extensive heterogeneity that exists from one bone metastasis site to another in a given patient and among patients. The implications of our findings for targeted therapies, such as gene therapy, may be profound. At the very minimum it should heighten the awareness of sampling errors in the study of bone metastases.

The "osteoblastic" response

One of the hallmark features of CaP is perturbation of the normal bone-remodeling process, leading to new bone formation. This process is termed the osteoblastic response, and is in contrast to the perturbation that results in an overall resorption of bone which is referred to as the osteolytic response (Figure 5). Prostate carcinoma is the only cancer that consistently produces osteoblastic rather than osteolytic bone metastases. Early studies concluded that greater than 85% of CaP bone lesions are osteoblastic (Jacobs, 1983; Koutsilieris, 1993). Our analysis of specimens from the rapid autopsies was consistent with these previous studies. Defining the character of CaP bone metastases is a complex process that involves the assessment of multiple parameters. As will be discussed subsequently, it is now recognized that overall osteoblastic lesions often have osteolytic components. Also, within a given patient with CaP bone metastasis, even if the preponderance of bone lesions can be classified as osteoblastic, there may be a subset of lesions with a predominantly osteolytic character. Similarly, even though breast cancer bone metastases are classically osteolytic, two-thirds of bone biopsies from breast cancer have regions of an osteoblastic response (Taube et al., 1994).

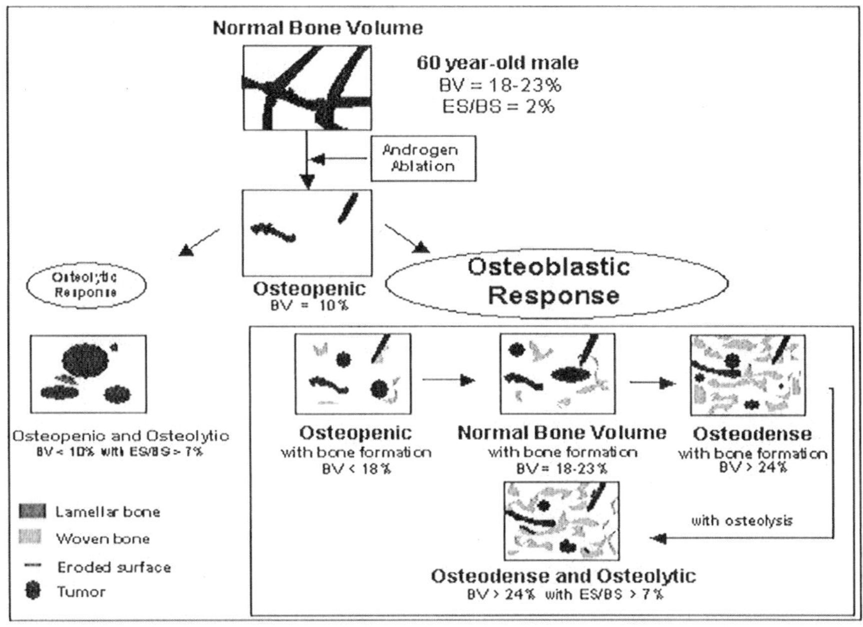

Figure 5. Schematic representation of the different bone remodeling processes associated with prostate cancer bone metastasis

HISTOMORPHOMETRY DATA

A quantitative assessment of the osteoblastic and osteolytic patterns associated with bone remodeling is referred to as bone histomorphometry. In our study we mainly evaluated bone parameters recommended by the American Society of Bone and Mineral Research (Parfitt et al., 1987):

- Bone volume (BV/TV). The proportion (%) of tissue volume (TV) occupied by both mineralized and unmineralized bone.
- Lamellar bone volume (LamBV/TV). The proportion (%) of tissue volume (TV) occupied by lamellar bone observed under polarization.
- Osteoid surface (OS/BS). The proportion (%) of the trabecular bone surface (BS) occupied by unmineralized bone.
- Osteoblast number (Ob/BS). The number of active-appearing plump osteoblasts per millimeter of the trabecular bone surface.
- Osteoid thickness (OTh). The width of osteoid seams measured directly, expressed in microns, and corrected for obliquity.
- Osteoid volume (OV/BV). The unmineralized bone matrix expressed as a percentage of bone volume (BV).

- Eroded surface (ES/BS). The proportion (%) of the bone surface occupied by erosion, assumed to be due to bone resorption. This is defined as a rough crenated surface with a scalloped surface transecting mineralized bone lamellae.
- Osteoclast surface (OcS/BS). The proportion of the fully mineralized bone surface occupied by multinucleated giant cells (osteoclasts) and mononucleated cells with similar morphological characteristics closely applied to the bone and assumed to be osteoclasts.
- Osteoclast number (Oc/BS). The number of multinucleated and mononucleated cells present per millimeter of the trabecular bone surface. Tartrate resistant acid phosphatase (TRAP)-specific staining helps in counting the osteoclasts on the measured surface.

Literature reports on histomorphometric analyses of CaP skeletal metastases is limited to eight studies in which a single iliac bone biopsy from each CaP patient was used to determine the histomorphometric features (Burki et al., 1987; Charhon et al., 1983; Clarke et al., 1991a; Coindre et al., 1985; Heaney, 1994; Percival et al., 1987b; Rico et al., 1990; Taube et al., 1993). Most of these studies focused on the osteomalacia and bone resorption associated with the osteoblastic response. A summary of the results of these eight studies is presented in Table 3. To obtain a better understanding of the processes associated with CaP bone metastases and the diversity among bone metastatic sites we performed initial microscopic assessment of 240 clinical specimens from 12 patients, which yielded 91 samples that exhibited bone marrow infiltrated by CaP cells without evidence of necrosis or osteonecrosis. These specimens were used for the histomorphometric analysis to characterize the various patterns shown in Figure 5. As illustrated, the histomorphometric analysis of CaP bone metastasis is confounded by androgen ablation, which precedes, sometimes by years, evidence of bone metastasis. Androgen ablation significantly reduces the amount of lamellar bone, resulting in decreased BV/TV (Clarke et al., 1993). Thus, prior to bone-remodeling perturbations induced by the CaP cells, the histomorphometric character of the bone is osteopenic. Since the vast majority of CaP bone metastases result in production of new woven bone, the BV/TV will begin to increase when metastasis occurs. If it increases only slightly, to a BV/TV value below that of normal bone which has not been exposed to androgen ablation, then the lesion will still exhibit an osteopenic character. The BV/TV may increase to a level where it is approximately equivalent to that of normal bone, or to a higher level, where it is classified as osteodense. As noted below, sometimes the osteodense patterns show remarkably high BV/TV values, which are even more noteworthy given that the starting point was most likely below that of normal bone. Note in Figure 5 that there is also the occasional CaP bone metastasis that exhibits an overall osteolytic character. In this situation, there is an increase in eroded bone surfaces.

Table 3. Histomorphometric values in osteoblastic metastases

Controls	Bx #	BV/TV %	OV/TV %	OS/BS %	Ob/BS %	Oth μm	ES/BS %	OcS/BS %
Taube *et al.*, 1993	16	19.9 ± 1.6	1.7 ± 0.25	6.7 ± 1.1	0.92 ± 0.2	12.6 ± 1.8	5.3 ± 0.6	0.23 ± 0.1
Charhon *et al.*, 1983	14	46.7 ± 14.4	19.4 ± 16.3	62.9 ± 28.9		26.8 ± 9.9	7.7 ± 5.6	
Urwin *et al.*, 1985	11	52 ± 5			4 ± 1		13 ± 7	
Coindre *et al.*, 1985	10	60.9 ± 16.3	19.1 ± 19.3	59.2 ± 25.1		26.7 ± 19.6	8.5 ± 4.6	
Burki *et al.*, 1987	18	48.5 ± 22	13.5 ± 15.2	50.6 ± 22.4		22.1 ± 15	8.7 ± 4.7	
Percival *et al.*, 1987	11	51.5 ± 3.5	5 ± 1	52.3 ± 4.4	4.0 ± 1.1	14.6 ± 4.7	13.9 ± 2.3	0.8 ± 0.2
Rico *et al.*, 1990	12	48.2 ± 10				31.8 ± 6.2	9.7 ± 1.1	
Clarke *et al*, 1991	21	37 ± 10					22.5 ± 10	
Taube *et al*, 1993	20	36.3 ± 3.7	9.7 ± 2.6	37.6 ± 5.8	5.50 ± 1	18.4 ± 1.6	12.7 ± 1.9	0.94 ± 0.2
Taube *et al.*, 1994 (Breast)	21	45.1 ± 5.6	15.0 ± 4.6	38.8 ± 6.9		17.4 ± 0.9	15.7 ± 2.8	1.23 ± 0.3
Roudier, 2003	12	30.2 ± 19	5.17 ± 5.1	22.5 ± 15.8	1.2 ± 2	9.0 ± 3.6	6.4 ± 6.7	0.6 ± 2.1

Abbreviations: Bx: biopsies, BV/TV: bon volume/tissue volume, OV/TV: osteoid volume/tissue volume, OS/BS: osteoid surface/bone surface, Ob/BS: osteoblast surface/bone surface, Oth: osteoid thickness, ES/BS: eroded surface/bone surface, OcS/BS: osteoclast surface/bone surface.

Different bone patterns

Our data were analyzed using criteria based on historical data from normal bone specimens in older men (Taube et al., 1993). We defined a cut-off value of BV/TV > 24% as indicative of an osteodense pattern, and ES/BS > 7% as indicative of an osteolytic pattern. Of the 91 bone specimens with tumor infiltration, 42 biopsies (46%) were osteodense, 38 biopsies

(42%) were osteopenic, and 11 biopsies (12%) were essentially normal with histological evidence of new bone formation (see Table 4). In those classified as osteodense, the BV/TV ranged from 24% to 73%, whereas the BV/TV range in those classified as osteopenic was 4% to 20%. Both osteodense and osteopenic patterns were associated with a loss of lamellar native bone that was replaced by woven bone. Moreover, in approximately half to two-thirds of the specimens, regardless of the pattern, there was distinctive evidence of an ongoing, concomitant resorptive process. In addition to the three patterns depicted in Figure 5, we observed a fibrotic pattern of the bone marrow that was primarily present in the spine. This was probably a consequence of radiation therapy. Representative examples of these four different histological bone patterns are presented in Figure 6A-D. In our patient population, eight patients exhibited an overall osteoblastic response to the CaP, one was diffusely osteolytic, one patient had predominance of osteolytic metastases, and one patient had extensive infiltration of the bone marrow that was not associated with bone change. Finally, one patient in our study did not have extensive bone metastases; only one of 20 sites was infiltrated by CaP cells. In summary, our results confirmed that there is a wide variability of bone responses to the tumor cells among patients as well as within a given patient. We hypothesize that existence of the various bone metastases patterns may be due to differences in phenotypes of the CaP cells originally infiltrating the bone, differences in the stage of metastatic progression, and to various influences of the normal physiological remodeling process.

Table 4. Histomorphometric values in 80 bone metastases of prostate carcinoma from 12 patients

	Controls Taube, 1993 N=16	Osteodense biopsies N=42	Osteopenic biopsies N=38
Bone volume/ TV%	19.9 ± 1.6	47.3 ± 13.8	12.3 ± 4.2
Osteoid volume/TV%	1.7 ± 0.7	3.1 ± 2.6	7.9 ± 6.2
Woven bone volume/TV%	0	37.8 ± 14.3	6.0 ± 5
Remaining native bone volume/TV%	18.2 ± 1.2	10 ± 6	6.0 ± 3.7

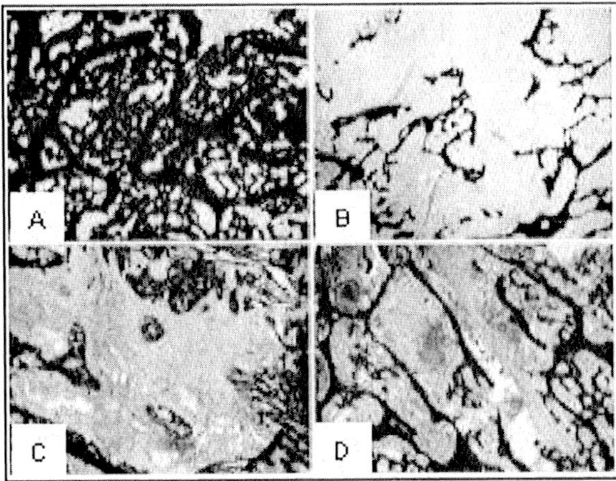

Figure 6. Four histological bone patterns revealed by undecalcified histology (Goldner's stain) in a given patient. **A**, Osteodense, **B**, Osteolytic, **C**, Fibrotic, **D**, Early bone response. Goldner's stain.

Sequence of bone formation

Prostate cancer bone metastases first appear within capillaries in the bone marrow, within the cancellous part of the bone (Suzuki et al., 1994). When the tumor cells invade the marrow space, they develop their own stroma and blood supply. We and others have observed that woven bone and osteoid arise from the tumor stroma within the marrow cavity (Clarke et al., 1991a). The woven bone also grows progressively by apposition on the native bone trabeculae. The progression of woven bone formation in CaP metastasis is shown in Figure 7A-C. Using polarized light that distinguishes lamellar bone from woven bone, we observed woven bone in the majority of osteodense specimens; even where the bone volume was up to 80% of the total tissue volume (Figure 7D). We observed only rare cases in which woven bone was eventually remodeled into lamellar bone. In addition to new bone formation, polarization revealed major destruction of the lamellar bone within osteodense CaP metastases (see Table 4). As previously reported, resorption occurs as part of the response to androgen ablation and also during the overall production of new woven bone (Charhon et al., 1983; Clarke et al., 1991b; Ikeda et al., 1996; Maeda et al., 1997; Percival et al., 1987a; Sebo et al., 2002; Takeuchi et al., 1996).

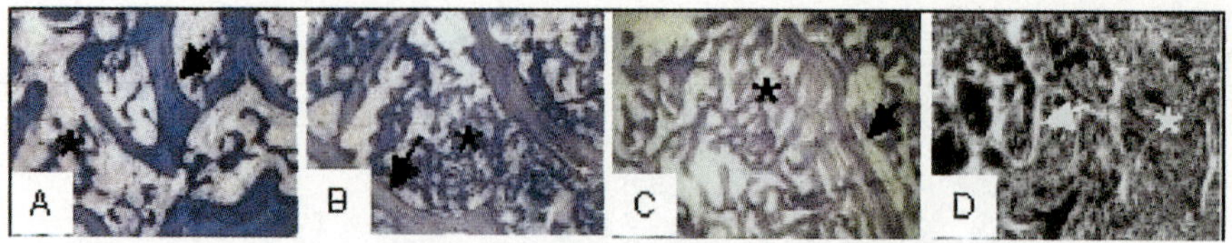

Figure 7. **A-C**, Progression of bone formation progression in an osteoblastic bone metastasis stained with toluidine blue. **D**, The bone induced by the prostate cancer cells is woven (demonstrated by polarized light).

Bone cells observed in the osteoblastic bone response

Our analysis showed that most of the new woven bone is formed in the marrow space and not along the old bone surfaces, and that it is laid down primarily by spindle cells. Spindle cells from the bone marrow stroma appear to lay down woven osteoid (Figure 8A). These cells are then entrapped in the woven bone, at which time they exhibit characteristics of osteocytes (Figure 8B). Alkaline phosphatase activity was detected in these spindle cells as shown in Figure 8C. Therefore, we speculate that these cells may be pre-osteoblast cells. Osteoid secreted by these presumed pre-osteoblasts was mainly observed arising from dense connective tissue stroma surrounding the tumor cords within the marrow cavity. This osteoid matrix was progressively mineralized. We have not observed endochondral bone formation.

Well-differentiated osteoblasts, identifiable as plump cuboidal cells with basophilic cytoplasm lining the osteoid surface, were extremely rare in the "osteoblastic" metastases. When present they were usually observed in repair zones existing around necrotic areas of the tumor and bone. Osteonecrosis and tumor necrosis were quite common, occurring in 118 of the 240 bone metastases and presumably a consequence of chemotherapy or radiation therapy. An example of osteonecrosis, consisting of bone trabeculae with enlarged empty osteocyte lacunae, is presented in Figure 8D. Often tumor cells could still be observed in the dilated bone marrow capillaries. Finally, only small numbers of osteoclasts were present in the metastases, whether or not the patient had been treated with BisPs.

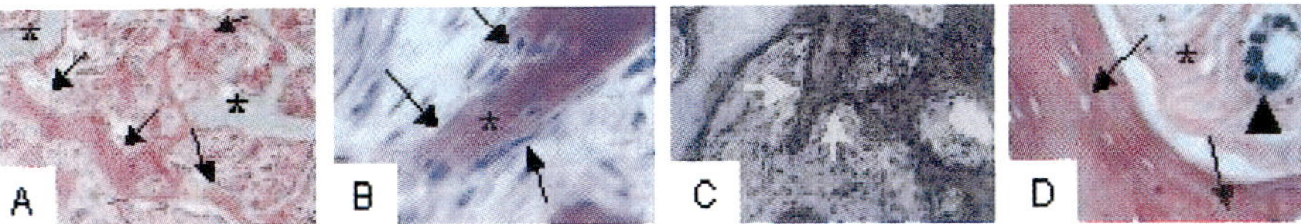

Figure 8. **A**, Osteoid formation in the stroma of the tumor in the bone marrow space (long arrows: osteoid, asterisk: mineralized bone Goldner's stain). **B**, Spindle cells deposting osteoid, Hand E (long arrows: spindle cells, asterisk osteoid) (see also Figure 10). **C**, Spindle cells are alkaline phosphatase positive (NBT/BCIP (long arrows: alkaline phosphatase positive cells) (see also figure 10). D, Effect of radiation therapy on prostate cancer bone metastasis: osteonecrosis (long arrows) and fibrosis (asterisk) of the bone marrow, persistence of tumor in a dilated vessel, HandE.

LUCAP 23.1 OSTEOBLASTIC MODEL OF CAP BONE METASTASIS AND COMPARISON TO CLINICAL SPECIMENS:

Critical to the understanding of how CaP cells interact with the bone microenvironment is the generation of suitable *in vivo* models. A separate chapter of this book is devoted to a review of existing models of bone disease. Here we briefly summarize the characteristics of our osteoblastic model of CaP bone metastasis, which is generated by direct injection of PSA-producing LuCaP 23.1 CaP xenograft cells into the tibiae of SCID mice (Corey et al., 2002a). Since this model does not involve spontaneous metastasis to bone from a distant site, it cannot be used to study trafficking, but it is a good model for investigating the bone/tumor cellular responses. In order to characterize the bone response to LuCaP 23.1, animals were sacrificed based on the radiographic appearances of the tibiae at early, intermediate, and late stages of the osteoblastic response (Figure 9A). The progressive histological host response is illustrated in Figure 9B. At the early stage, bone formation was observed in the vicinity of solid sheets of tumor cells. Shortly thereafter at mid-stage, numerous small, irregular bone trabeculae were scattered throughout the tumor stroma. Eroded surfaces were observed on these bone trabeculae and on cortical bones. Paralleling our observations of the bone metastases in patients, the new bone trabeculae arise from the stroma of the tumor and new bone are laid down by spindle cells that are alkaline phosphatase-positive (Figure 10A-C). At the late stage, extensive amounts of new bone with small cavities filled with tumor cells have replaced the medullary cavity. Most of the tumor burden was now present under the periosteum and outside the bone. From the central bone core, spicules of bone induced by periosteal osteoblasts were observed radiating toward the skin surface. There was a strong correlation (r = 0.87, *P* < 0.05) when all of the bone histomorphometry data from the osteodense bone metastases from patients were compared to those of LuCaP 23.1 intra-tibial tumors. Other similarities between the bone response and histological features, e.g., spindle cells forming bone and woven bone arising from the stroma of the tumor, suggest that common mechanisms of cellular interactions exist in this model and in man. Accordingly, the model has proven fruitful in the study of new treatment modalities for CaP bone metastasis (Corey et al., 2002b) and may provide much needed insight regarding the cellular interactions occurring within the bone microenvironment that allow prolific tumor growth and induction of an overall osteoblastic response.

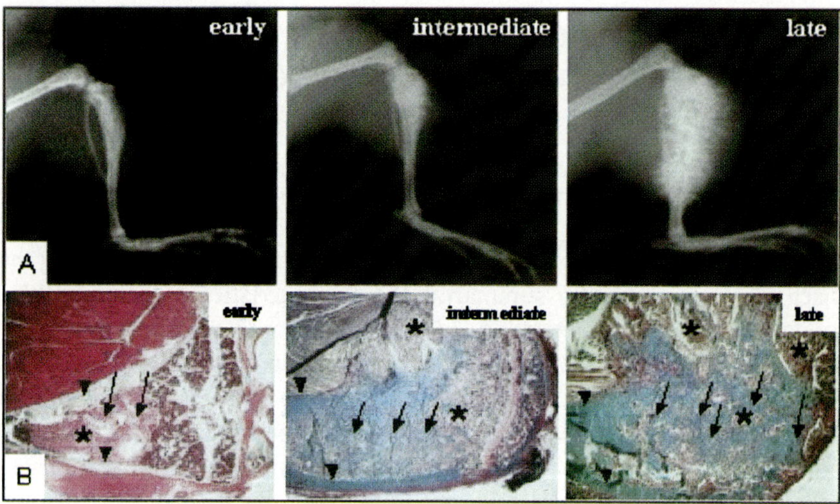

Figure 9. **A**, Early, intermediate and late stage development of the LuCaP 23.1 intratibial tumor by X-ray. **B**, Early, intermediate and late stage development of LuCaP 23.1 intratibial tumor using undecalcified specimens and Goldner's stain (arrowheads: cortical bones, long arrows: new bone formation, asterisks: tumor). Note the increase of bone volume in the medullary cavity.

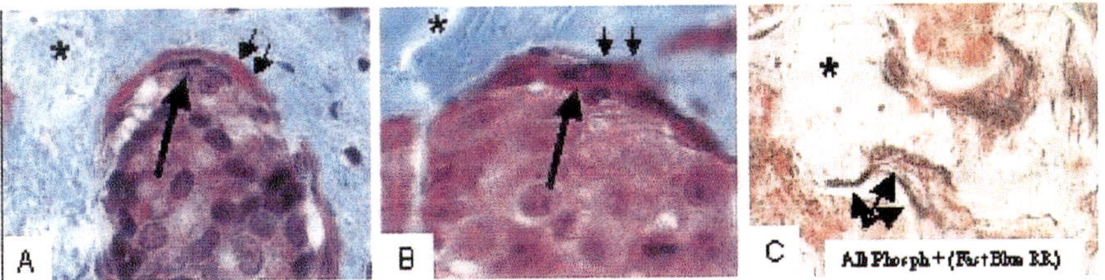

Figure 10. **A**, Spindle cells depositing osteoid in a human bone metastasis (long arrow: spindle cell, double arrow: osteoid, asterisk: mineralized bone), **B**, Spindle cells depositing osteoid in LuCaP 23.1 (long arrow: spindle cells, double arrows: osteoid, asterisk: mineralized bone). C, in LuCaP23.1 the spindle cells are alkaline phosphatase positive (long arrows: positive spindle cells, asterisk: mineralized bone (Fast Blue RR).

CONCLUSIONS

This chapter reveals the tremendous heterogeneity of CaP bone metastases among patients and within the same patient. This heterogeneity was exhibited by each of the parameters evaluated: histological features, histomorphometric criteria, and immunophenotype. This heterogeneity represents one of the major difficulties in defining the mechanisms that give rise to the characteristic osteoblastic response. Others in this book provide useful information regarding the multitude of factors derived from the tumor, stroma, and cells within the normal bone environment that are or may be critically involved in the growth of tumor cells in the bone marrow and perturbation of normal bone remodeling, but many questions remain unanswered. Availability of clinical specimens and appropriate in vitro and in vivo models is one of the absolute requirements to begin to address these questions. We have demonstrated in this chapter the value of a rapid autopsy program dedicated to the acquisition of multiple bone metastases from each patient and the potential of an intra-tibial xenograft model that exhibits many attributes of CaP bone metastases in man. Likewise, others are making their clinical resources and models available for study. Through the process of sharing and collaboration will arise the best opportunities to reveal new mechanistic insights, and the stimulus to conceive of and test new therapeutic strategies.

ACKNOWLEDGMENTS:

The authors gratefully acknowledge the help and support of several individuals without which this work would not have been possible: William Ellis, M.D., Paul Lange, M.D., Janna

Harada, M., Iida, M., Yamaguchi, M. and Shida, K. (1992) Analysis of bone metastasis of prostatic adenocarcinoma in 137 autopsy cases. Prostate Cancer and Bone Metastasis. Edited by J.P.Karr and H Yamanaka, Plenum Press, New York, 173-182.

Heaney, R.P. (1994) The bone-remodeling transient: implications for the interpretation of clinical studies of bone mass change. *Journal of Bone and Mineral Research*, **9**, 1515-1523.

Ikeda, I., Miura, T. and Kondo, I. (1996) Pyridinium cross-links as urinary markers of bone metastases in patients with prostate cancer. British Journal of Cancer, **77**, 102-106.

Jacobs, S.C. (1983) Spread of prostatic cancer to bone. *Urology*, **21**, 337-344.

Jacobson, A.F., Stomper, P.C., Cronin, E.B. and Kaplan, W.D. (1990) Bone scans with one or two new abnormalities in cancer patients with no known metastases: reliability of interpretation of initial correlative radiographs. *Radiology*, **174**, 503-507.

Jemal, A., Thomas, A., Murray, T. and Thun, M. (2002) Cancer statistics, 2002. *CA-A Cancer Journal for Clinicians*, **52**, 23-47.

Jorda, M., Morales, A., Ghorab, Z., Fernandez, G., Nadji, M. and Block, N. (2002) Her2 expression in prostatic cancer: a comparison with mammary carcinoma. *Journal of Urology*, **168**, 1412-1414.

Koutsilieris, M. (1993) Osteoblastic metastasis in advanced prostate cancer. *Anticancer Research*, **13**, 443-449.

Krasnow, A.Z., Collier, B.D., Isitman, A.T., Hellman, R.S. and Ewey, D. (1988) False-negative bone imaging due to etidronate disodium therapy. *Clinical Nuclear Medicine*, **13**, 264-267.

Lamothe, F., Kovi, J., Heshmat, M.Y. and Green, E.J. (1986) Dissemination of prostatic carcinoma: an autopsy study. *Journal of the National Medical Association*, **78**, 1083-1086.

Lara, P.N., Jr., Meyers, F.J., Gray, C.R., Edwards, R.G., Gumerlock, P.H., Kauderer, C., Tichauer, G., Twardowski, P., Doroshow, J.H. and Gandara, D.R. (2002) HER-2/neu is overexpressed infrequently in patients with prostate carcinoma. Results from the California Cancer Consortium Screening Trial. *Cancer*, **94**, 2584-2589.

Leav, I., Lau, K.M., Adams, J.Y., McNeal, J.E., Taplin, M.E., Wang, J., Singh, H. and Ho, S.M. (2001) Comparative studies of the estrogen receptors beta and alpha and the androgen receptor in normal human prostate glands, dysplasia, and in primary and metastatic carcinoma. *American Journal of Pathology*, **159**, 79-92.

Ligibel, J.A. and Winer, E.P. (2002) Trastuzumab/chemotherapy combinations in metastatic breast cancer. *Seminars in Oncology*, **29**, 38-43.

Macro, M., Bouvard, G., Le Gangneux, E., Colin, T. and Loyau, G. (1995) Intravenous aminohydroxypropylidene bisphosphonate does not modify 99mTc-hydroxymethylene bisphosphonate bone scintigraphy. A prospective study. *Revue du rhumatisme* (English ed), **62**, 99-104.

Maeda, H., Koizumi, M., Yoshimura, K., Yamauchi, T., Kawai, T. and Ogata, E. (1997) Correlation between bone metabolic markers and bone scan in prostatic cancer. *Journal of Urology*, **157**, 539-543.

Masarachia, P., Weinreb, M., Balena, R. and Rodan, G.A. (1996) Comparison of the distribution of 3H-alendronate and 3H-etidronate in rat and mouse bones. *Bone*, **19**, 281-290.

McCarthy, E.F. (1997) Histopathologic correlates of a positive bone scan. *Seminars in Nuclear Medicine*, **27**, 309-320.

Mintz, R. and Smith, G.G. (1934) Autopsy findings in 100 cases of prostatic cancer. *New England Journal of Medicine*, **211**, 481-487.

Morris, M.J., Reuter, V.E., Kelly, W.K., Slovin, S.F., Kenneson, K., Verbel, D., Osman, I. and Scher, H.I. (2002) HER-2 profiling and targeting in prostate carcinoma. *Cancer*, **94**, 980-986.

Murphy, G.P., Elgamal, A.A., Su, S.L., Bostwick, D.G. and Holmes, E.H. (1998) Current evaluation of the tissue localization and diagnostic utility of prostate specific membrane antigen. *Cancer*, **83**, 2259-2269.

Osman, I., Scher, H.I., Drobnjak, M., Verbel, D., Morris, M., Agus, D., Ross, J.S. and Cordon-Cardo, C. (2001) HER-2/neu (p185neu) protein expression in the natural or treated history of prostate cancer. *Clinical Cancer Research*, **7**, 2643-2647.

Oyama, N., Akino, H., Kanamaru, H., Suzuki, Y., Muramoto, S., Yonekura, Y., Sadato, N., Yamamoto, K. and Okada, K. (2002) 11C-acetate PET imaging of prostate cancer. *Journal of Nuclear Medicine*, **43**, 181-186.

Parfitt, A.M., Drezner, M.K., Glorieux, F.H., Kanis, J.A., Malluche, H., Meunier, P.J., Ott, S.M. and Recker, R.R. (1987) Bone histomorphometry: standardization of nomenclature, symbols, and units. Report of the ASBMR Histomorphometry Nomenclature Committee. *Journal of Bone and Mineral Research*, **2**, 595-610.

Paulson, D.F. (1980) Assessment of anatomic extent and biologic hazard of prostatic adenocarcinoma. *Urology*, **15**, 537-541.

Pecherstorfer, M., Schilling, T., Janisch, S., Woloszczuk, W., Baumgartner, G., Ziegler, R. and Ogris, E. (1993) Effect of clodronate treatment on bone scintigraphy in metastatic breast cancer. *Journal of Nuclear Medicine*, **34**, 1039-1044.

Percival, R.C., Urwin, G.H., Harris, S., Yates, A.J., Williams, J.L., Beneton, M. and Kanis, J.A. (1987a) Biochemical and histological evidence that carcinoma of the prostate is associated with increased bone resorption. *European Journal of Surgical Oncology*, **13**, 41-49.

Rana, A., Chisholm, G.D., Khan, M., Sekharjit, S.S., Merrick, M.V. and Elton, R.A. (1993) Patterns of bone metastasis and their prognostic significance in patients with carcinoma of the prostate. *British Journal of Urology*, **72**, 933-936.

Reuter, V.E. (1997) Pathological changes in benign and malignant prostatic tissue following androgen deprivation therapy. *Urology*, **49**, 16-22.

Rhodes, A., Jasani, B., Anderson, E., Dodson, A.R. and Balaton, A.J. (2002) Evaluation of HER-2/neu immunohistochemical assay sensitivity and scoring on formalin-fixed and paraffin-processed cell lines and breast tumors: a comparative study involving results from laboratories in 21 countries. *American Journal of Clinical Pathology*, **118**, 408-417.

Rico, H., Uson, A., Hernandez, E.R., Prados, P., Paramo, P. and Cabranes, J.A. (1990) Hyperparathyroidism in metastases of prostatic carcinoma: a biochemical, hormonal and histomorphometric study. *European Urology*, **17**, 35-39.

Rittenhouse, H.G., Finlay, J.A., Mikolajczyk, S.D. and Partin, A.W. (1998) Human Kallikrein 2 (hK2) and prostate specific antigen (PSA): Two clossely related, but distinct, kallikreins in the prostate. *Critical Reviews in Clinical Laboratory Sciences*, **35**, 275-368.

Ro, J.Y., Tetu, B., Ayala, A.G. and Ordonez, N.G. (1987) Small cell carcinoma of the prostate. II. Immunohistochemical and electron microscopic studies of 18 cases. *Cancer*, **59**, 977-982.

Roudier,M.P., Vesselle,H., True,L.D., Higano,C.S., Vessella,R. (2003) Concordance between bone histology and Technetium[99] methylene diophosphonate bone scintigraphy in advanced prostate cancer patients with special reference to Pamidronate treatment. *Clinical and Experimental Metastasis*, in press.

Roudier, M.P., True, L.D., Higano, C.S., Vesselle, H., Ellis W.J., Lange, P.H. and Vessella, R.L. (2002) Phenotypic heterogeneity of androgen-independent prostate cancer bone metastases. *Human Pathology*, (submitted).

Rubin, M.A., Putzi, M., Mucci, N., Smith, D.C., Wojno, K., Korenchuk, S. and Pienta, K.J. (2000) Rapid ("warm") autopsy study for procurement of metastatic prostate cancer. *Clinical Cancer Research*, **6**, 1038-1045.

Ryan, P.J., Gibson, T. and Fogelman, I. (1992) Bone scintigraphy following intravenous pamidronate for Paget's disease of bone. *Journal of Nuclear Medicine*, **33**, 1589-1593.

Saad, F., Gleason, D.M., Murray, R., Tchekmedyian, S., Venner, P., Lacombe, L., Chin, J.L., Vinholes, J.J., Goas, J.A. and Chen, B. (2002) A randomized, placebo-controlled trial of zoledronic acid in patients with hormone-refractory metastatic prostate carcinoma. *Journal of the National Cancer Institute*, **94**, 1458-1468.

Saitoh, H., Hida, M., Shimbo, T., Nakamura, K., Yamagata, J. and Satoh, T. (1984) Metastatic patterns of prostatic cancer. Correlation between sites and number of organs involved. *Cancer*, **54**, 3078-3084.

Sanchez, K.M., Sweeney, C.J., Mass, R., Koch, M.O., Eckert, G.J., Geary, W.A., Baldridge, L.A., Zhang, S., Eble, J.N. and Cheng, L. (2002) Evaluation of HER-2/neu expression in prostatic adenocarcinoma: a requested for a standardized, organ specific methodology. *Cancer*, **95**, 1650-1655.

Sandler, E.D., Parisi, M.T. and Hattner, R.S. (1991) Duration of etidronate effect demonstrated by serial bone scintigraphy. *Journal of Nuclear Medicine*, **32**, 1782-1784.

Sebo, T.J., Cheville, J.C., Riehle, D.L., Lohse, C.M., Pankratz, V.S., Myers, R.P., Blute, M.L. and Zincke, H. (2002) Perineural invasion and MIB-1 positivity in addition to Gleason score are significant preoperative predictors of progression after radical retropubic prostatectomy for prostate cancer. *American Journal of Surgical Pathology*, **26**, 431-439.

Shankar, G., Kelley, H., Samadzadeh, L., Lodge, A., Boynton, A., Papandreou, C., Logothetis, C., Belldegrun, A. and Elgamal, A. (2002) Induction of tumor antigen-specific immune responses in hormone-refractory priostate cancer patients treated with DCVax-Ptostate in a Phase I/II clinical trial. *Proceedings of the American Association for Cancer Research*, **43**, 144, #716.

Signoretti, S., Montironi, R., Manola, J., Altimari, A., Tam, C., Bubley, G., Balk, S., Thomas, G., Kaplan, I., Hlatky, L., Hahnfeldt, P., Kantoff, P. and Loda, M. (2000) Her-2-neu expression and progression toward androgen independence in human prostate cancer. *Journal of the National Cancer Institute*, **92**, 1918-1925.

Slamon, D.J. (1987) Proto-oncogenes and human cancers. *New England Journal of Medicine*, **317**, 955-957.

Slamon, D.J., Clark, G.M., Wong, S.G., Levin, W.J., Ullrich, A. and McGuire, W.L. (1987) Human breast cancer: correlation of relapse and survival with amplification of the HER-2/neu oncogene. *Science*, **235**, 177-182.

Spigel, D.R. and Burstein, H.J. (2002) HER2 overexpressing metastatic breast cancer. *Current Treatment Options in Oncology*, **3**, 163-174.

Stein, B.S., Vangore, S. and Petersen, R.O. (1984) Immunoperoxidase localization of prostatic antigens. Comparison of primary and metastatic sites. *Urology*, **24**, 146-152.

Suzuki, T., Shimizu, T., Kurokawa, K., Jimbo, H., Sato, J. and Yamanaka, H. (1994) Pattern of prostate cancer metastasis to the vertebral column. *Prostate*, **25**, 141-146.

Takeuchi, S.I., Arai, K., Saitoh, H., Yoshida, K.I. and Miura, M. (1996) Urinary pyridinoline and deoxypyridinoline as potential markers of bone metastasis in patients with prostate cancer. *Journal of Urology*, **156**, 1691-1695.

Taube, T., Beneton, M.N., Williams, J.L., McCloskey, E.V. and Kanis, J.A. (1993) Distinction between focally accelerated bone formation and osteomalacia in carcinoma of prostate metastasised to bone. *British Journal of Urology*, **72**, 98-103.

Taube, T., Elomaa, I., Blomqvist, C., Beneton, M.N. and Kanis, J.A. (1994) Histomorphometric evidence for osteoclast-mediated bone resorption in metastatic breast cancer. *Bone*, **15**, 161-166.

Thompson, H. (1854) Comments. *Transactions of the Pathology Society of London*, **5**, 204.

Van der Kwast, T.H. and Tetu, B. (1996) Androgen receptors in untreated and treated prostatic intraepithelial neoplasia. *European Urology*, **30**, 265-268.

Watt, I. and Hill, P. (1981) Effects of acute administration of ethane hydroxydiphosphonate (EHDP) on skeletal scintigraphy with technetium-99m methylene diphosphonic acid (Tc-MDP) in the rat. *British Journal of Radiology*, **54**, 592-596.

Weinstein, M.H., Partin, A.W., Veltri, R.W. and Epstein, J.I. (1996) Neuroendocrine differentiation in prostate cancer: enhanced prediction of progression after radical prostatectomy. *Human Pathology*, **27**, 683-687.

Whitmore, Jr.W.F. (1990) Natural history of low-stage prostatic cancer and the impact of early detection. *Urologic Clinics of North America*, **17**, 689-697.

Yao, D., Trabulsi, E.J., Kostakoglu, L., Vallabhajosula, S., Joyce, M.A., Nanus, D.M., Milowsky, M., Liu, H. and Goldsmith, S.J. (2002) The utility of monoclonal antibodies in the imaging of prostate cancer. *Seminars in Urologic Oncology*, **20**, 211-218.

Index